EXERCISE PRESCRIPTION AND THE BACK

EXERCISE PRESCRIPTION AND THE BACK

WENDELL LIEMOHN, PH.D.

Department of Exercise Science
University of Tennessee
Knoxville, Tennessee

McGRAW-HILL
Medical Publishing Division

New York St. Louis San Francisco Auckland Bogota
Caracas Lisbon Madrid Mexico City Milan Montreal
New Delhi San Juan Singapore Sydney Tokyo Toronto

McGraw-Hill

*A Division of The **McGraw·Hill** Companies*

EXERCISE PRESCRIPTION AND THE BACK

1 2 3 4 5 6 7 8 9 0 DOC DOC 0 9 8 7 6 5 4 3 2 1 0

ISBN 0-8385-2325-0

This book was set in New Baskerville at V&M Graphics, Inc.
The editors were Stephen Zollo and Nicky Panton.
The production supervisor was Richard Ruzycka.
The cover designer was Aimee Nordin.
The index was prepared by Coughlin Indexing Services, Inc.

R.R. Donnelley and Sons Company was printer and binder.

This book is printed on acid-free paper.

Library of Congress Cataloging-in-Publication Data

Liemohn, Wendell.
    Exercise prescription and the back / Wendell Liemohn.
        p.   ;   cm.
    Includes bibliographical references and index.
    ISBN 0-8385-2325-0
        1. Backache—Exercise therapy. 2. Backache—Prevention. I. Title.
        [DNLM: 1. Low Back Pain—rehabilitation. 2. Exercise Therapy—methods. WE 755
    L719e2001]
    RD771.B217 L54 2001
    617.5′64062—dc21   00–055029

I would like to dedicate

this book to my dear wife Meredith,

who often did things solo in order

that I could commit the time necessary

to complete this project.

CONTENTS

CONTRIBUTORS

BRUCE E. BECKER, M.D.
Medical Director
St. Luke's Rehabilitation Institute
Spokane, Washington
Chapters 9, 10

JULIE BOWDEN, P.T.
Career Staff Unlimited
Nolensville, Tennessee
Chapter 4

JULIE M. FRITZ, P.T., A.T.C., Ph.D.
Assistant Professor
Department of Physical Therapy
University of Pittsburgh
Pittsburgh, Pennsylvania
Chapter 8

LAURA HORVATH GAGNON, P.T.
Ph.D. Student
Department of Exercise Science
(and Physical Therapist, Tennessee Sports
Medicine Group)
University of Tennessee
Knoxville, Tennessee
Chapters 6, 12

JAMES E. GRAVES, Ph.D., FACSM
Professor of Exercise Science
Associate Dean for Graduate Studies & Research
School of Education
Syracuse University
Syracuse, New York
Chapter 11

GREGORY E. HICKS, P.T., A.T.C.
Department of Physical Therapy
University of Pittsburgh
Pittsburgh, Pennsylvania
Chapter 8

WENDELL LIEMOHN, Ph.D., FACSM
Department of Exercise Science
University of Tennessee
Knoxville, Tennessee
Chapters 1, 2, 4, 5, 6, 12

JOHN M. MAYER, D.C., Ph.D.
Director of Research
U.S. Spine and Sport
San Diego, California
Chapter 11

MARISA A. MILLER, A.T.C., Ph.D.
Program Director, Assistant Professor
Entry-Level Graduate Athletic Training Program
The University of Tennessee, Chattanooga
Chattanooga, Tennessee
Chapter 5

JEANNE NELSON, P.T., M.S.
Department of Physical Therapy
University of Tennessee Medical Center
Adjunct Instructor, Exercise Science
University of Tennessee
Knoxville, Tennessee
Chapter 7

GINA PARISER, P.T., Ph.D.
Department of Physical Therapy
Louisiana State University Medical School
New Orleans, Louisiana
Chapters 2, 4

JEFFREY L. YOUNG, M.D., M.A., FACSM
Department of Physical Medicine and
Rehabilitation
Hospital for Special Surgery
New York, New York
Chapter 3

JOSEPH P. ZUHOSKY, M.D.
Attending Physiatrist
Miller Orthopedic Clinic
Clinical Instructor
Department of Physical Medicine & Rehabilitation
Carolinas Medical Center
Charlotte, North Carolina
Chapter 3

PREFACE

In addition to being a major problem in medicine, low back pain (LBP) presents as a major problem in sport, for dependent upon the sport, LBP is often seen across strata of skill levels, whether they be seen in a weekend athlete or in a highly toned professional athlete. LBP is a condition that does not appear to be related to gender from the perspective of susceptibility, thus although the incidence of LBP in sports such as tennis and swimming may be comparable between genders, gymnastics may present more low back injuries for females (with age accounting for some of this disparity), and American football would of course present more back injuries for males.

This book could be used as an adjunct text in courses in physical therapy, athletic training, and exercise science. Because of its research basis, it could also be used as a reference by the aforementioned as well as a reference for physicians. The contributing authors include five physical therapists (two are also ATC's and three are Ph.D.'s and two are working on their Ph.D.), three M.D.'s (all physiatrists), and four Ph.D.'s (one is an ATC and one is a D.C.).

Part I of the book is entitled *Musculoskeletal Form and Function of the Back*. It includes a chapter on the anatomy and biomechanics of the trunk that endeavors to provide the reader with a basic foundation, based on a synthesis of the most recent research, for the ensuing chapters. Because flexibility can be an important element in both exercise therapy and in prevention, the second chapter in this section is devoted to it. In addition to addressing factors that specifically relate to the functioning of the spine, this chapter also reviews generic aspects of flexibility including range of motion improvement programs.

Part II of the book is entitled *Epidemiology and Diagnosis*. The first chapter in this section (Ch. 3) is written by two M.D.'s; they present the reader with techniques of assessing the individual who presents with low back pain. Chapter 4 addresses the role of aerobic condition and the spine. It is followed by a chapter that examines different sports and the types of stresses incumbent in each that can lead to low back pain.

Part III of the book is entitled *Exercise Prescription*. The first chapter of this section (Ch. 6) reviews exercise protocols starting with the one proposed by Williams in the 1930's; this is followed by a discussion of the respective programs popularized by McKenzie and the San Francisco Spine Institute (i.e., lumbar stabilization). In the next chapter, the Feldenkrais and Alexander techniques are discussed. Chapter 8 presents exercise protocols for those low back conditions. Both Chapters 9 and 10 are on aquatic therapy; the first gets into history and hydrodynamics and the next gets into aquatic exercise per se. Chapter 11 presents the latest research on back strength development. The concluding chapter presents research on the efficacy of clinically controlled trials of exercise regimens.

ACKNOWLEDGMENTS

I would like to thank Gene Asprey, my M.S. and Ph.D. advisor at the University of Iowa, who initially kindled my interest in the low back many years ago. With tongue in cheek, I express my thanks for having had the opportunity to have an acute disc problem, for this experience enabled me to better appreciate the nuances of LBP for it helped teach me what I could do to combat it.

I would like to thank Tinah Utsman for her photography and my former students who posed as subjects. Although cited in the figure captions, I also am most appreciative of the pictures that were courtesy of the Lady Vol Media Relations Office, the Vol Sports Information Office, and Football Time in Tennessee. I am particularly indebted to Flora Shrode, Associate Professor and Science Coordinator, University of Tennessee Libraries, who volunteered and proofread the majority of the chapters and offered extremely helpful advice.

I would also like to pay particular thanks to my editors at McGraw-Hill. Steve Zollo, Medical Editor, who has been wonderful to work with and who has been exceptionally supportive and encouraging in this endeavor ever since McGraw-Hill acquired the contract that I had signed with another publisher. Nicky Panton, Editing Supervisor, who took in stride many late changes that without a doubt presented challenges exceeding the ordinary. Lastly from McGraw-Hill, I would like to thank Charissa Baker, Illustration Manager; she not only carefully monitored the figures to be included but she also persisted in showing me how her artist could markedly improve many of the figures that I had planned to use.

EXERCISE PRESCRIPTION AND THE BACK

PART I

MUSCULOSKELETAL FORM
AND FUNCTION OF THE BACK

CHAPTER 1

ANATOMY AND BIOMECHANICS OF THE TRUNK

Wendell Liemohn

INTRODUCTION

The purpose of this chapter is to present a review of those aspects of anatomy and biomechanics that are pertinent to the functioning of the spine and low back pain (LBP). This synthesis will include a review of anatomy, a discussion of vertebrae and disc biomechanics, an examination of trunk flexion exercises, and a description of pertinent synergies of the muscular and connective tissues of the trunk. The latter will be followed by a brief discussion on some research on lifting, and how it relates to trunk stabilization (also called trunk bracing). The San Francisco Spine Institute (1) was one of the first entities to espouse trunk stabilization as a technique to be used in rehabilitation. Learning to stabilize the trunk when it is in a neutral and pain-free position is a major element in therapeutic exercise in most back rehabilitation programs.

THE SPINE

The segmental mobile spinal column, coupled with its fascia and muscular counterparts, has been called a biomechanical masterpiece (2). Its uniqueness is attributed in part to its being able to balance lordotic curves in the cervical and lumbar regions, with kyphotic curves in the thoracic and sacral regions. This results in a double "S" curvature that enables the spine to absorb vertical forces in spring-like fashion (Fig. 1-1).

The spine is an important contributor to many movements; however, its role in these movements is often overlooked. After seeing negligible differences in spine movement in a man engaged in bipedal locomotion compared with that of a man without legs walking on his ischial tuberosities, Gracovetsky contended that the spine and its surrounding tissues are in essence the primary "engine" of locomotion in the human species (3,4). Many examples depicting an "engine role" for the spine in sports exist; for example, shot putters and hammer and discus throwers in particular display how a winding and unwinding rotation-type movement

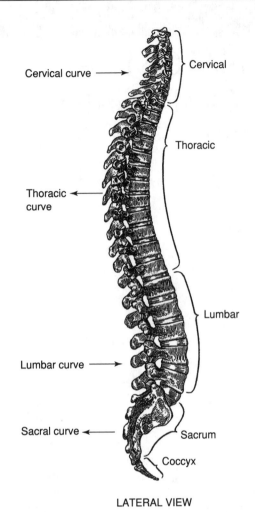

LATERAL VIEW

Fig. 1-1 Lateral view of the spinal column. (From Pansky, B. *Review of Gross Anatomy.* © 1996. Reprinted with permission from the McGraw-Hill Companies, Inc.)

of the spine contributes to success in their athletic activities (Fig. 1-2).

Architecture of the Spine

The architecture of the spine that will be included in this section includes spine curvatures, the vertebral and intervertebral disc components and their articulations, and the ligaments of the spine.

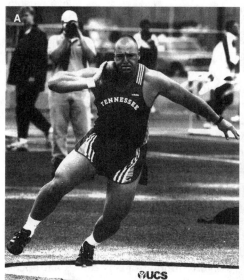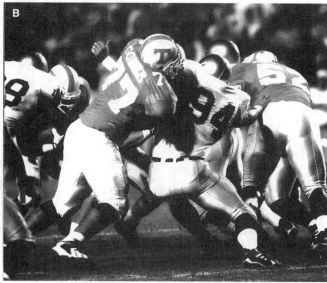

Fig.1-2 **(A)** In a properly executed shotput the spine can serve as an "engine" as it moves body parts (*Courtesy of the Vol Sports Information Office*). **(B)** The spine of number 94 is obligated to resist torsional and lateral flexion and translation force (*Courtesy of Football Time in Tennessee*).

Curvatures of the Spine

The natural curvatures of the spine as viewed from the side include a concavity in the cervical and lumbar regions and a convexity in the thoracic and sacral regions. These curves are viewed as normal, although they are described as lordotic and kyphotic, respectively (see Fig. 1-1). If these curves are excessive, they are often called hyperlordosis in the lumbar area (or a swayback) and a dorsal kyphosis or round upper back in the thoracic area.

When viewed from the back, the spine is in an almost straight vertical line; an appreciable lateral deviation would be called *scoliosis*. Lordotic, kyphotic, and scoliotic deviations are functional if they can be removed voluntarily by modifying posture; they are structural if postural adjustments do not immediately affect the deviation.

Lordosis   The lumbar lordosis is dictated primarily by two factors: the shapes of both the lumbosacral intervertebral disc and the fifth lumbar vertebra (Fig. 1-3). The disc between L5 and S1 and the L5 vertebra are thicker anteriorly than posteriorly, about 6 to 7 mm and 3 mm, respectively (5). Although this positioning might suggest a degree of precariousness because of an apparent shear stress (e.g., L5 slipping over S1), this factor is counterbalanced by the reinforced structure of the superior and inferior articular processes of L5 and a strong reinforcing ligamentous structure.

However, if injury occurs to the supporting structures, slippage of L5 over S1 or of L4 over L5 can occur and result in the condition spondylolisthesis. Fujiwara et al. (6) studied the morphology of the iliolumbar ligament and found that its length and direction can be a predisposing factor to the development of disc degeneration between L5 and S1 and subsequent spondylolisthesis. Nagaosa et al. (7) and Berlemann et al. (8) independently found facet orientation to be a pathoanatomic risk predisposing one to the development of degenerative spondylolisthesis.

A lumbar lordotic curve helps the discs in cushioning compressive forces and shocks. Although it

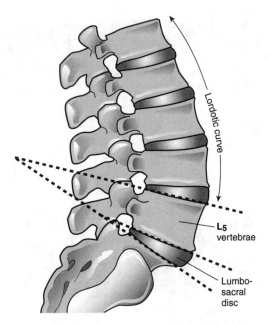

Fig. 1-3 Shape of the lumbar lordosis. The lordotic curve is due to the wedge-shapes of the lumbosacral disc and the L5 vertebra.

has been a common belief that excessive lordosis is a risk factor for LBP, a relationship between the shape of the lumbar lordosis and low back symptomatology is not evident (9). Intrinsic features set the lumbar curve; extrinsic factors such as overweight, use of high heels, or shortened muscles can modify it. Although strength-training programs have not been effective in reducing the lordotic curve (10), tightness in the hip flexors (e.g., psoas) could serve to increase the curve, whereas tightness in the hamstrings could reduce it. Aging is another factor that affects the curve because the lumbar lordosis often decreases with age (5).

Kyphosis   In activities of daily living, spinal extension movements and postures are used less often than spinal flexion ones. Continued flexion postures

(e.g., slouching) could cause an increased dorsal kyphotic curve in the thoracic area. This faulty posture is characterized by muscle imbalances including (a) stretched and weakened thoracic erector spinae and scapulae retractors (rhomboids and trapezius) and (b) tight anterior shoulder girdle muscles (pectoralis minor and serratus anterior). A greater than average thoracic kyphosis is also frequently associated with a compensatory increase in the cervical and lumbar lordoses; however, these postures have not been proven to predispose one to LBP (11).

Scoliosis   Although most spines when viewed from the posterior would not be perfectly straight, a marked deviation or a lateral curvature of the spine is called *scoliosis*. Although many causes have been identified for scoliosis, the cause is usually unknown (12). It is not surprising that leg length discrepancy, leading to pelvic obliquity, is associated with both scoliosis and LBP. Nevertheless, little hard evidence of scoliosis causing LBP exists in the general population (13). Junghanns (2) noted that hammer and discus throwers had a high percentage of scoliosis and subsequent LBP. Because of this finding, he contended that an extreme number of throws per year leads to (a) asymmetric trunk strength development and scoliosis and (b) annular tears in the intervertebral discs due to torsional stresses.

Vertebrae

The seven cervical vertebrae display a lordotic curve and rest on the 12 thoracic vertebrae. The thoracic vertebrae display a kyphotic curve and provide anchorage for the ribs, which contributes to circumferential stability (see Fig. 1-1). The last thoracic vertebra rests on the first lumbar vertebra; the lumbar vertebra and its four counterparts are stacked lordotically on top of the sacrum.

Panjabi et al. (14) detailed the differences of the thoracic and lumbar vertebrae by doing a three-dimensional surface anatomy study. They found that L4 and L5 seemed transitional toward the sacral region, whereas L1 and L2 seemed transitional toward the thoracic region.

The primary curves (i.e., those present at birth) are the thoracic and sacral curves. Cervical and lumbar curves are referred to as secondary curves; they are not present at birth and develop during the process of maturation. The five fused segments of the sacrum transmit weight laterally through the sacroiliac joints to the pelvis; caudally, the fifth segment provides attachment for the vestigial coccyx. As depicted in Figure 1-1, the vertebrae become progressively larger from the cervical to the lumbar spine as their load-bearing functions increase.

The vertebrae are cancellous (trabecular) bone with a thin cortical shell. They adjust to stress as defined by Wolff's law; thus the positioning and density of the vertical and transverse trabeculae within the cortical shell of each vertebra change with the stresses placed on the spine (15,16). The extremes of how much bone mineral density are present are exemplified by vertebrae's (a) inability to support body weight and collapsing in osteoporosis of the spine (2) and (b) being able to support 28,000 N (>6000 lb) in world-class weight lifters (16).

A vertebra is often subdivided into three functional components, namely the body, intermediary pedicle, and posterior elements (Fig. 1-4). Two vertebrae and their intervening disc are called a *motion segment* (or a functional structural unit); a motion segment of the lumbar spine is presented in Fig. 1-5. A motion segment is the smallest func-

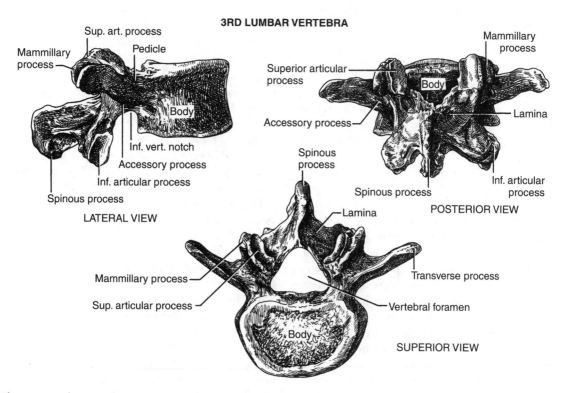

3RD LUMBAR VERTEBRA

Sup. art. process
Pedicle
Mammillary process
Body
Inf. vert. notch
Accessory process
Inf. articular process
Spinous process
LATERAL VIEW

Mammillary process
Superior articular process
Body
Accessory process
Lamina
Spinous process
Inf. articular process
POSTERIOR VIEW

Spinous process
Lamina
Mammillary process
Sup. articular process
Transverse process
Vertebral foramen
Body
SUPERIOR VIEW

Fig. 1-4 Lumbar vertebrae. (From Pansky, B. *Review of Gross Anatomy.* © 1996. Reprinted with permission from the McGraw-Hill Companies, Inc.)

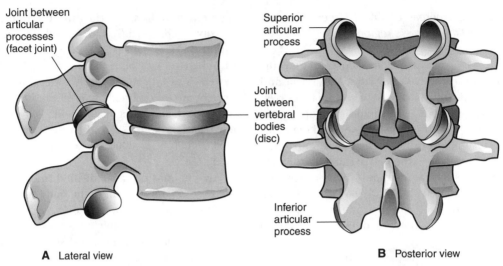

Fig. 1-5 Lateral **(A)** and posterior **(B)** views of a motion segment. The segment includes the junction of the intervertebral disc with its two adjacent vertebrae. In the posterior view, the joints between the superior and inferior articular processes can be seen; these joints are referred to as zygoapophyseal or facet joints.

tional unit of the spine; the joints that comprise it include the anterior joints between the vertebral bodies and the disc and the posterior joints between the paired facets (superior and inferior articular processes).

Intervertebral Discs

Intervertebral discs act as spacers and shock absorbers in addition to absorbing rotational stresses (Fig. 1-6). Although most low back problems in young athletes originate in the posterior elements (e.g., in the pars interarticularis as seen in spondylolysis and spondylolisthesis or facet joint injury), in adults the disc is the site of most of the problems. The disc consists of the annulus fibrosis, nucleus pulposus, and the vertebral endplates.

Annulus Fibrosis   The annulus fibrosis contains 10 or more collagen reinforced concentric rings oriented in alternating angles of alignment; thus,

if rotational stresses are placed on the spine, the fibers of the disc are so oriented that some fibers can always resist this strain (see Fig. 1-6). If strained excessively, for example, with repetitive microtrauma, the outer fibers of the annulus have nociceptors and therefore pain is perceived. The annulus is about 60 to 70% water and the concentration of collagen is about two to three times that of the proteoglycan.

Nucleus Pulposus   The nucleus pulposus is a dense, randomly arranged network of collagen fibers and proteoglycan gel; it is without nociceptors. The nucleus pulposus is approximately 70 to 90% water, with the concentration of proteoglycans about three to four times that of collagen (5). Both the proteoglycan cells and their water imbibing properties are known to decrease with age and injury. Because the nucleus pulposus and the annulus fibrosis are similar in makeup, their lines of demarcation are not as definitive as those displayed in Figure 1-6. In vivo, the layers of the annulus fibrosis become less distinct as they approach and merge with the nucleus. In diseased discs, the differentiation between the nucleus and annulus is even less distinct.

Vertebral Endplate A third component of discs but not depicted in Figure 1-6 is the vertebral endplate. The vertebral endplate separates each disc from the adjacent vertebra. When compressive forces are placed on the spine, the nucleus pulposus of the affected discs exerts pressure in all directions against their more rigid periphery (Fig. 1-7). A disc under a load would exert radial pressure against the annulus fibrosus; cephalically and

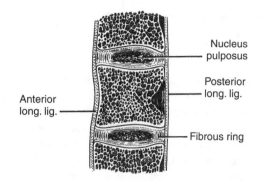

SAGITTAL SECTION — LUMBAR REGION

Fig. 1-7 Weight transmission in an intervertebral disc. Compression raises the pressure in the nucleus pulposus circumferentially; the tension in the annulus redirects some of this pressure in the direction of the vertebral endplates. (From Pansky, B. *Review of Gross Anatomy.* © 1996. Reprinted with permission from the McGraw-Hill Companies, Inc.)

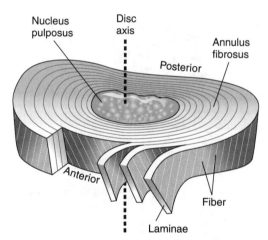

Fig. 1-6 Intervertebral disc. The outer portion, the annulus fibrosis, is composed of laminated collagen fibers oriented to resist rotational/torsional stress from either direction. Although not seen in this figure, the vertebral endplates complete the enclosure of the nucleus and anchor the disc to the ring apophysis. (Adapted with permission from Borenstein, D.G. and Wiesel, S.W. *Low Back Pain—Medical Diagnosis & Comprehensive Management.* 1989, Philadelphia: W.B. Saunders.)

caudally, pressure would be placed against the vertebral endplates. Although the annuli fibrosi distend to help dissipate the stress, if the annulus is healthy and the compression force is too great, something has to give, and it is usually the vertebral endplate (17). Thus, the vertebral endplate is often the weak link of the spine. Once a disc is injured or degenerates beyond its physiologic capacity, it becomes less viscoelastic than a healthy disc. A diseased disc would not provide as much shock absorption as a healthy one.

A diminishment in disc height is an example of creep, a viscoelastic property of connective tissue. In this scenario, creep is temporary because disc height returns to its prestanding value within an hour or two after the recumbent position is assumed (18). In the morning, the back is generally stiffer because of the long period of rehydration of the discs; not coincidentally, disc injuries are also most common in the mornings (5). Interestingly, after long periods of weightlessness, as seen by astronauts during space travel, fluid gain to the disc can result in a 3% increase in body height (18).

Functional Adaptations of Discs   Because the disc is avascular, its nutrition requires continual hydration and rehydration of its contents; this is best accomplished when the disc undergoes periods of small loading (e.g., horizontal positions as in sleeping) followed by periods of dehydration that occur because of loading, as in movement activity. Because discs account for nearly a quarter of the height of the vertebral column, such a fluid loss can result in an individual being 1 to 2% shorter at the end of the day (13). Disc nutrition is dependent on diffusion from the vertebral endplates and the annuli fibrosi; the process that results in this transmission of nutrients is called *imbibition.* Muscular contraction enhances the process of imbibition; conversely, bed rest would be deleterious to the nutrition and functioning of discs. In experimental animals, it has been shown conclusively that moderate exercise enhances disc nutrition (19). Good disc nutrition enhances disc resiliency and shock absorption capability because the nucleus translates vertically applied pressure circumferentially against the annulus (see Fig. 1-7). As the collagenous tissue of the annulus stretches, the force transmitted to each subsequent vertebra up the kinetic chain is reduced. Although the disc resists most burdens, its frailties may become manifest when it is subjected to compromising stress. If the disc degenerates or ruptures or if its nucleus is removed, disc height is permanently lost; the facet joints would then be obligated to assume a greater portion of the load. The motion segment may then become hypermobile and clinically less stable because the spinal ligaments would be on slack (20,21). Similarly, Haughton et al. (21) found that radial tears of the intervertebral disc reduced its stiffness and thus increased its motion under applied torque. This would be analogous to a radial tire of a car that has lost a significant amount of air pressure, thus rendering the vehicle less stable when cornering.

Under these circumstances, the capsular ligaments of the facet joint may become chronically and excessively stretched and strained; this would make the motion segment more vulnerable to further injury (Fig. 1-8). Goel et al. (22) were among the first researchers to provide quantitative data that showed that increased movement across a spinal motion segment is the first sign of degenerative change. Abnormally large amounts of intervertebral motion can cause compression or stretching of the pain receptors in spinal ligaments, joint capsules, and annular fibers (23). A reduction in disc height also reduces the diameter of the intervertebral foramen; this condition is called *stenosis* (see Fig. 1-8). In addition to pain, the next occurrence in this degenerative cascade is a stiffening of the motion segment and a decrease in motion magnitude (21).

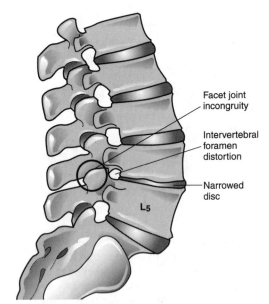

Facet joint incongruity

Intervertebral foramen distortion

Narrowed disc

L5

Fig. 1-8 A reduction in disc height also reduces the size of the intervertebral foramen; the latter condition is referred to as stenosis. Disc height reduction also stretches the capsular ligaments of the facet joints. (From Pansky, B. *Review of Gross Anatomy.* ©1996. Reprinted with permission from the McGraw-Hill Companies, Inc.)

Facet (Zygapophyseal) Joints

The junction of the superior and inferior articular processes is called a *zygapophyseal* or *facet joint* (Fig. 1-9). Facet joints are synovial joints and, therefore, articular cartilage lines the joint surfaces. From Figure 1-9 it can readily be seen that the facet joint surfaces of the lumbar vertebrae are vertical in the sagittal plane; this joint structure permits little rotation. Because the facet joints also provide an additional antishear component, they are a major factor in controlling movement between vertebrae and improving the stability of the spine.

Facet joints are gliding joints and therefore belong to the classification of diarthrodial joints. Thus, fhyaline cartilage lines each facet joint articular surface, and a joint capsule is present. These joint surfaces and the adjacent tissue are highly

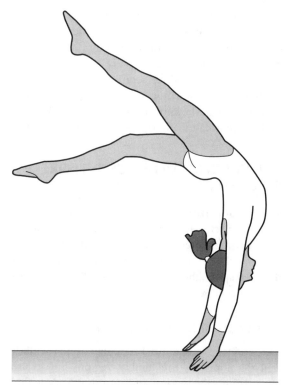

Fig. 1-10 Extension movements can load the facet joints; continual and/or extreme such movements can compromise facet joint function.

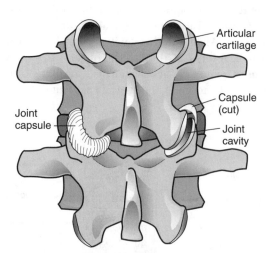

Fig. 1-9 Facet joints. This is a posterior view of L4–L5 facet joints. The capsule of the joint is intact on the left. On the right, the capsule has been removed to show the articular cartilage and the joint cavity. In hyperextension of the vertebral column, the inferior articular processes bottom out on the lamina of the vertebra beneath it. Continued movement of this sort can have a deleterious effect on the joint capsule of the facet joint.

innervated and are subject to inflammatory changes should the joint become injured. Acute strain of the capsular ligaments and damage to the articular cartilage can result when it is forced into extreme ranges of motion or when it is subject to motions of high velocity (e.g., ballistic activity).

When hyperlordotic postures are assumed, facet joints are obligated to assume a greater share of the load than in a less lordotic posture (Fig. 1-10). If disc height is reduced because of degeneration or dehydration, the facet joint would similarly be obligated to assume a greater portion of the load. The joint capsule in such an afflicted articulation would be subject to chronic and excessive stretch. This would make the motion segment even more vulnerable to further injury. A chronically stretched facet joint capsule may remain inflamed and painful for extended periods. Thus, an intersegmental motion problem at one level (e.g., articulation between L4 and L5) could place additional stress at contiguous motion segments (e.g., L3–L4, L5–S1) (24,25). Further mobility problems would then be probable; moreover, the stage might be set for the inflammatory process of arthritis (11).

MUSCULOLIGAMENTOUS SUPPORT STRUCTURES

The support structures of the spine include ligaments, muscles, tendons/aponeuroses, and fascia. A functional integration between these support tissues exists in a healthy spine. In an injured or diseased spine, these tissues are keys to the rehabilitation process.

Ligaments of the Spine (Fig. 1-11)

The anterior longitudinal ligament is particularly well developed in the lumbar region, but it also extends into the sacrum and into the thoracic and cervical regions. It is suited to resist vertical separation and, with the annulus fibrosus, helps stabilize the lordotic curve. The thin and narrow posterior longitudinal ligament extends the entire length of the spine within the vertebral canal, attaching to the annuli fibrosi and the posterior margins of the vertebral bodies (5). This ligament resists separation of the posterior margins of the vertebral bodies. Because the posterior longitudinal ligament is abundantly innervated and highly irritable to pressure from a damaged disc and from the outer fibers of the annulus fibrosis, it can warn of a herniating and rupturing disc when placed under stress. The ligamentum flavum lies immediately behind the vertebral canal; its high percentage of elastin differentiates it from the other vertebral ligaments. An advantage of this elastic nature over that of the more typical collagenous ligament is that it not only enables the ligamentum flavum to resist laminae separation, but, unlike a collagenous ligament, it is not as apt to buckle and compromise nerve roots when the laminae are approximated (e.g., become closer together as in hyperextension). The interspinous ligament is so positioned to limit forward bending moments and to oppose separation of the spinous processes. Adding to this stability would be the capsular ligaments of the facet joints and the supraspinous ligament. These ligaments contribute to the stability of the spine and they are sometimes called the *midline ligaments*.

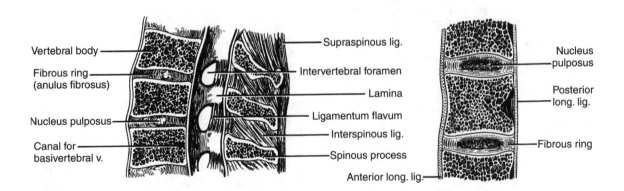

MEDIAN SECTION — LUMBAR REGION   SAGITTAL SECTION — LUMBAR REGION

Fig. 1-11 Ligaments of the spine. Five of the ligaments that contribute to the stability of the motion segments of the spine are identified. The two capsular ligaments (i.e., zygapophyseal or facet) also make a contribution. (From Pansky, B. *Review of Gross Anatomy.* © 1996. Reprinted with permission from the McGraw-Hill Companies, Inc.)

The iliolumbar ligament and the corresponding size of the transverse processes of L5 also enhance spine stability (Fig. 1-12). Iliolumbar ligaments connect the transverse process of the fifth lumbar vertebra to the ilium; they present a very strong antishear force against forward displacement of L5 over the sacrum. The size of the transverse processes is believed to be due to the enormous forces transmitted by the iliolumbar ligament (5). This would be another example of an application of Wolff's law.

Muscles and Related Connective Tissue

Because weakened trunk musculature has been an important risk indicator for low back problems (26–30), most therapeutic exercise programs include activities that develop these muscles. This is most logical; other than by an invasive technique, the muscular component provides the only mechanism by which we can effectively influence the structure and function of the spine. Before discussing the nuances related to the muscular component, some comments should be made on the trunk flexion movement because of misconceptions that have existed with respect to this function.

Considerations in Prescribing Trunk Flexion Exercises

In the past two decades an evolutionary change in the prescription of abdominal strengthening activities has occurred. Although evidence supporting change in abdominal strength training protocols from

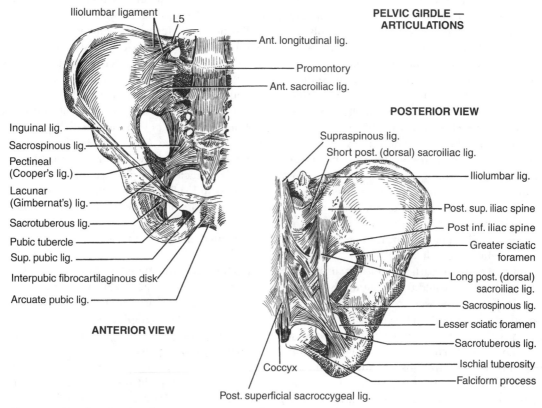

Fig. 1-12 Sacral and pelvic ligaments. (From Pansky, B. *Review of Gross Anatomy.* © 1996. Reprinted with permission from the McGraw-Hill Companies, Inc.)

sit-ups to other types of abdominal exercises such as crunches has been present for sometime (31,32), it has not always been followed or understood because the conventional sit-up is still in use (33).

Over the years, research on trunk flexion exercises has typically been presented from either mechanical or physiologic perspectives. Most recently, some very prodigious research has been conducted that bridges the mechanical and physiologic perspectives. Relevant research from each of these perspectives (i.e., mechanical, physiologic, and combined mechanical/physiologic) will be discussed in the next sections.

Examination of Mechanical Considerations Normal spine movement capabilities in all planes are depicted in Figure 1-13. Figure 1-13B displays motion in the sagittal plane; lumbosacral flexion is in essence limited to the removal of the lordotic curve. Any subsequent flexion in the sagittal plane occurs at the iliofemoral joint, as displayed in Figure 1-13A. This should make it clear that, if the trunk is raised from the recumbent position, as when performing a sit-up, the abdominal muscles are used dynamically only in the very first phase of the movement (e.g., elevating the scapulae from the exercise surface). This view should be kept in mind whenever abdominal strengthening exercises are considered. As the shoulders are raised from the floor, there typically is a concurrent posterior rotation of the pelvis as end range of motion (ROM) in the lumbosacral area is reached. Because the abdominal muscles do not cross the iliofemoral joint, they obviously cannot produce flexion at this joint. The hip flexor musculature, in particular the iliacus, psoas, and rectus femoris, would then assume the dominant role *if* the trunk were to be raised farther. Although the abdominal muscles would still be working if the movement were continued and a full sit-up were performed, their contraction would only be isometric throughout the remainder of the ROM (34). Although it would be unlikely to be seen in athletic populations, individuals with weak abdominal muscles often perform full sit-up–type exercises entirely with their

hip flexors (34). The role of the hip flexors in this type of sit-up becomes even more dominant if the feet are held (35).

Examination of Physiologic Considerations Nachemson (36), using pressure transducers placed within the nucleus pulposus of the intervertebral disc between L3 and L4, studied the effects of body postures on intradiscal pressures. When he examined trunk flexion exercises, he noted that intradisc pressures were higher in the bent-leg sit-up than the straight-leg sit-up that it replaced in different fitness testing protocols (Fig. 1-14). More important, however, Nachemson's research showed that sit-up exercises can produce intradisc pressures comparable to those seen in light lifting tasks and in other postures contraindicated for many individuals with LBP. This would suggest that straight-leg or bent-leg sit-ups that formerly were recommended as therapeutic exercise for the low back could theoretically exacerbate a LBP condition. The more recent and more definitive research conducted by Axler and McGill (37) and by Juker et al. (38) has verified Nachemson's contention that psoas activity increases spinal compressive forces. In both training and in particular rehabilitation programs, the major objective is to challenge the abdominal musculature and minimize the compressive loading on the spine. As Juker et al. (38) noted, using electrodes implanted within the psoas, when this muscle contracts it can place substantial shear and compressive loading forces on the lumbar spine. Further discussion on the advantages and disadvantages of different abdominal strengthening exercises is presented elsewhere (32,34).

Interaction of Mechanical/Physiologic Considerations In a very thorough study on abdominal strengthening exercises, Axler and McGill (37) looked at electromyographic (EMG) data and indirect measures of joint forces as subjects did a variety of abdominal strengthening exercises. Their objective was to determine the challenge-to-cost index for each exercise; they did this by dividing the maximum EMG value for a given exercise by the corresponding maximum disc compression value that the exercise would cause.

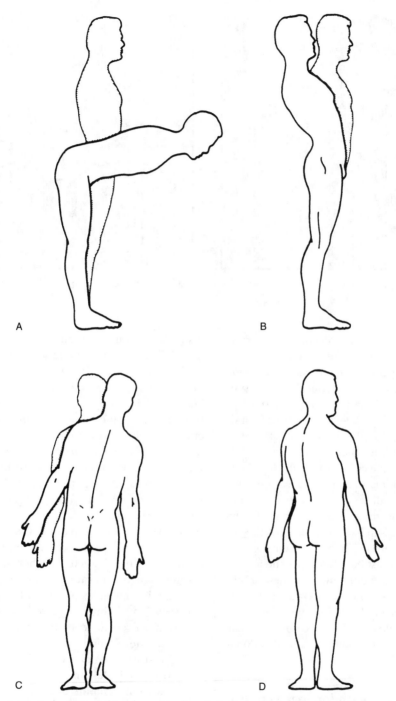

Fig. 1-13 A depiction of trunk range of motion occurring in all planes. (Adapted with permission from White, A.A., and Panjabi, M.M. *Clinical Biomechanics of the Spine*, 2nd ed. 1990, Philadelphia: J.B. Lippincott p. 63.)

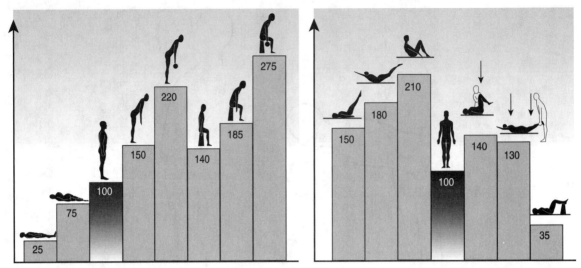

Fig. 1-14 Intradiscal pressure is a function of posture and of any external load. (Adapted with permission from Nachemson, A.L. *Spine* 1976, 1: p. 59.)

The highest peak flexion moment was observed in the bent-leg sit-up, with the straight-leg sit-up being a close second; the compression forces for each exercise were essentially identical, further supporting the contention that the psoas is most active in the performance of the bent-leg sit-up. Axler and McGill found that, for the development of the upper and lower rectus abdominis, the hanging straight-leg raise and the curl-ups with the feet fixed had the highest (optimal) challenge-to-compressive cost indices. For the development of the external oblique, the hanging straight-leg raise and the dynamic cross-knee curl-up had the best challenge-to-compressive cost indices. Their research suggests that several factors must be weighed in the assignment of abdominal strengthening exercises for athletes with and without low back symptomatology. Subsequently, Juker et al. (38) studied the safety of different flexion exercises by using intramuscular electrodes within the psoas and the lateral abdominals (Table 1-1).

Other Nuances of the Abdominal Muscles

The abdominal muscles are presented in Figure 1-15. A strong flexion component is provided by the rec-

tus abdominis in the sagittal plane. Although the internal and external obliques also contribute to flexion, the rectus abdominis is typically dominant in crunch- or curl-type exercises (39). To attain a better understanding of this point, if it is not clear, the reader is encouraged to perform 5 to 10 crunches while palpating the lateral abdominal muscles. Next, try a variation of this exercise in which the abdominal muscles are hollowed (i.e., the umbilicus is brought as close as possible to the spine as the exercise is done). Again, palpate the lateral abdominal muscles as the exercise is done. In this version of the crunch, more dependence on the internal and external oblique muscles should have been noted. Another way to increase involvement of the lateral abdominal muscles is through isometric exercise. Although isometric exercises have been considered passé in exercise programs in recent years, they can be most effective in the development of the trunk musculature (36). Most abdominal muscles come into play in isometric trunk flexion activities. Moreover, it is very easy to incorporate isometric activity into the performance of a crunch or a diagonal curl. For example, an exerciser could do diagonal curls but hold the "up" position for 5 to 15 s (or more) for each repetition. As the individual becomes stronger, either the number of repetitions or the lengths of isometric contractions could be increased. These and other methods that can be used to develop the lateral abdominal musculature are delineated in Figure 1-16.

On the ipsilateral side, the internal and external oblique muscles are positioned approximately 90 degrees to each other. Their teamwork is evident if an internal oblique on one side is considered a continuation of the external oblique on the contralateral side. Note also how their connecting aponeuroses envelop the rectus abdominis. Working together, the paired contralateral external and internal oblique muscles can provide a strong turning moment because of their distance from the axis of rotation (i.e., the spine). It is for

this mechanical reason that this pair of muscles is deemed more important in trunk rotation movements than the multifidus (5). The transversus abdominis contributes to a "corseting effect" of the trunk with the internal and external oblique muscles; its role has become more appreciated in recent years and it will be discussed. The oblique muscles of the same side also work with the ipsilateral erector spinae (in particular the iliocostalis and quadratus lumborum) to provide lateral flexion (Figs. 1-17 and 1-18). The abdominal muscles are also important for routine activities of daily living such as walking and rising to a stand from a seated position. If their structure is studied, it can clearly be seen that their multidirectional stratified layers form a strong protective girdle around the viscera.

Table 1-1   Challenge to the Psoas, Rectus Abdominus, and Obliques During Various Flexion Exercises.*
Mean % MVC (SD)

	MUSCLE								
	PSOAS†			RECTUS ABDOMINIS		ABDOMINAL WALL‡			
RANK	P1	P2		RA		EO	IO	TA	
1	5 (±3)	4 (±4)	Cross curl up	74 (±25)	Isom. hand-to-knee	44 (±16)	42 (±24)	44 (±33)	Dyn. side support
2	7 (±8)	10 ±14)	Curl-up	62 (±22)	Curl-up	68 (±14)	30 (±28)	28 (±19)	Isom. hand-to-knee
3	21 (±17)	12 (±8)	Isom. side support	58 (±24)	Cross curl-up	43 (±13)	36 (±29)	39 (±24)	Isom. side support
4	15 (±2)	24 (±7)	Straight leg sit-up	55 (±16)	Bent knee sit-up	51 (±14)	22 (±14)	20 (±13)	Press heels sit-up
5	24 (±19)	12 (±5)	Push up from feet	51 (±20)	Press heels sit-up	23 (±20)	24 (±14)	20 (±11)	Cross curl-ups
6	24 (±15)	13 (±8)	Bent knee leg raise	48 (±18)	Straight leg sit-up	44 (±9)	15 (±15)	11 (±9)	Straight leg sit-up
7	26 (±18)	13 (±5)	Dyn. side support	41 (±20)	Dyn. side support	43 (±12)	16 (±14)	10 (±7)	Bent knee sit-up
8	17 (±10)	28 (±7)	Bent knee sit-up	37 (±24)	Straight leg raise	19 (±14)	14 (±10)	12 (±9)	Curl-up
9	35 (±20)	33 (±8)	Straight leg raise	32 (±20)	Bent knee leg raise	26 (±9)	9 (±8)	6 (±4)	Straight leg raise
10	28 (±23)	34 (±18)	Press heels sit-up	29 (±10)	Pushup from feet	29 (±12)	10 (±14)	9 (±9)	Push up from feet
11	56 (±28)	58 (±18)	Isom. hand-to-knee (right hand left knee)	21 (±13)	Isom. side support	22 (±7)	8 (±9)	7 (±6)	Bent knee leg raise

SOURCE: Reproduced with permission from Juker, D., McGill, S., Kropf, P., and Steffen, T. Quantitative intramuscular myoelectric activity of lumbar portions of psoas and the abdominal wall during a wide variety of tasks. *Med Sci Sports Exerc*, 30(2):301–310.

*This table presents the challenge that flexion exercises bring to the psoas and the abdominal muscles in terms of percentages of maximum voluntary contraction as determined by intramuscular electrodes. Psoas first rank corresponds to lowest activity level; for the abdominal muscles, first rank corresponds to highest activity levels.

†Psoas first rank corresponds to lowest activity level.

‡Abdominals first rank corresponds to the highest activity level.
 EO, external oblique; IO, internal oblique; TA, transverse abdominis.

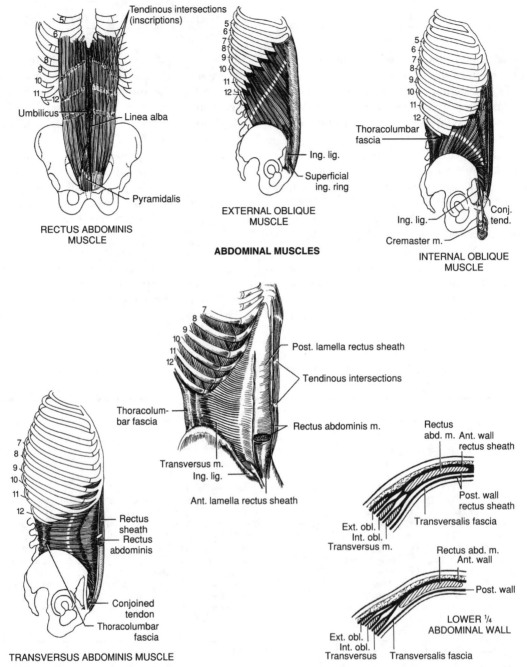

Fig. 1-15 The abdominal muscles are uniquely engineered. The aponeurosis of the external and internal obliques, along with that of the transversus abdominis, envelop and provide a sheath for the rectus abdominis. This is most evident in the last figure of the sequence. Thus, if the three pairs of lateral abdominal muscles contract, they can place tension on the connective tissue sheath that envelops the rectus abdominis. This prominent function will be again mentioned when stabilization exercises are discussed. Although not emphasized in these figures, an internal oblique muscle on one side can be viewed as a continuation of the external oblique on the contralateral side; they also work together, with assistance from the transversus abdominis, in trunk rotation. (From Pansky, B. *Review of Gross Anatomy.* © 1996. Reprinted with permission from the McGraw-Hill Companies, Inc.)

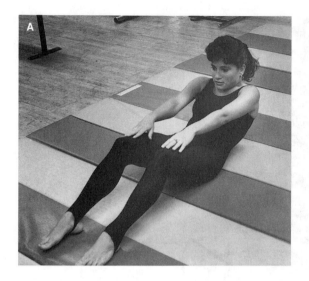

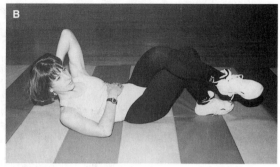

Fig. 1-16 **(A)** The abdominal curl or crunch. Note that the shoulders do not have to be elevated far to attain maximal lumbar flexion. **(B)** The diagonal (or oblique) curl. This exercise is particularly effective for the oblique muscles. (For variety an isometric hold of 5 to 10 s can be incorporated in either exercise.)

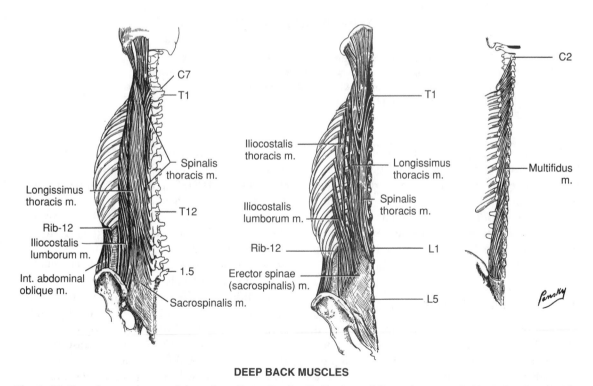

DEEP BACK MUSCLES

Fig. 1-17 Dorsal musculature of the spine. (From Pansky, B. *Review of Gross Anatomy.* © 1996. Reprinted with permission from the McGraw-Hill Companies, Inc.)

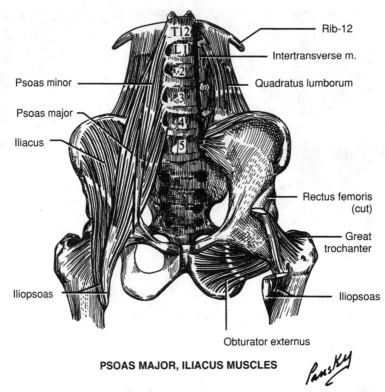

Fig. 1-18 The psoas major and the quadratus lumborum are particularly important to low back function. (From Pansky, B. *Review of Gross Anatomy.* © 1996. Reprinted with permission from the McGraw-Hill Companies, Inc.)

The uniquely engineered structure of the abdominal muscle group with its stratified layers of muscle and aponeuroses can form a strong protective girdle anteriorly and laterally. Figure 1-15 also shows how the aponeurosis of the lateral abdominal muscles sheathes the rectus abdominis; thus, these muscles can have an anterior bracing and corseting effect on the rectus abdominis.

Dorsal Fascia and Musculature

It should be noted that part of this muscular girdle provided by the lateral abdominal muscles adjoins with the thoracolumbar fascia posteriorly at a junction that Bogduk (40) called the lateral raphe. As can also be seen in Figure 1-19, the deep and super-ficial layers of the fascia of the lateral abdominal muscles in essence envelop the erector spinae muscle; Williard (41) referred to this connective tissue arrangement as a ligamentous stocking. This arrangement permits portions of the transversus abdominis and, to a lesser extent, the internal obliques to exert lateral tension on this "connective tissue" envelope of the erector spinae. The implications for this will be discussed in the next section.

Traditionally, the extensor musculature of the spine has been viewed as just bridging the lumbar area as a bowstring from its common origin to its diverse insertions (42,43). In contrast, Bogduk (5,40) noted that the erector spinae and multi-fidus are in reality a laminated series of short muscle fibers, each with a unique orientation. He furthermore contended that fibers to a given verte-bra could contract independently. Bogduk (5) hypothesized that the force vectors of the lumbar erector spinae were too small to enable one to lift heavy objects from the ground. After performing microdissection, he contended that neither the iliocostalis lumborum nor the longissimus thoracis has the necessary force vector to be an effective extensor of the spine, and that the former (Fig. 1-20) and the latter (Fig. 1-21) are much better suited for lateral flexion and stabilization than for extension. Although he believed that the multi-fidus has a good force vector for extension, its mass limits it to nothing more than nominal exten-sion movements (Fig. 1-22).

Although not discussed here, even the smallest muscles of the spine can have important roles in maintaining spine health. For example, McGill (30) believed that the rotatores and intertransversarii act *as position transducers at each lumbar joint because they are endowed with a large number of muscle spindles.*

Because lifting heavy objects from the ground can put excessive stress on structures of the spine, the biomechanics of lifting have been an area of research interest. Although some research con-ducted in Bogduk's laboratories is less relevant to the mechanics of lifting than originally perceived, it would appear to have extreme relevance to trunk splinting or bracing, a popular form of exercise therapy for the spine (1). Therefore, research perti-nent to this area will be reviewed.

Mechanical Considerations Inherent in Lifting

Possibly many taboos about lifting objects from the ground were based on early biomechanical models.

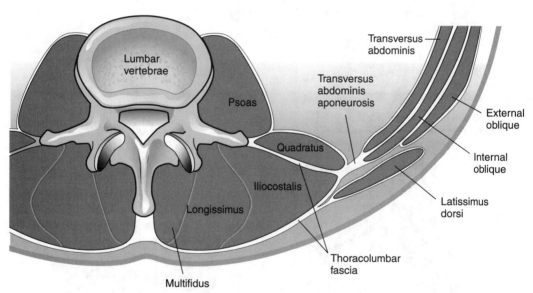

Fig. 1-19 A cross section of the lateral and dorsal trunk musculature. Note how the fibers of the transversus abdominis and the internal oblique attach to the thoracolumbar fascia; Bogduk calls this site the lateral raphe. The transversus abdominis has an extensive attachment on this fascia; thus, it can exert lateral tension on the erector spinae, which can contribute to trunk stabilization. (Adapted from Pansky, B. *Review of Gross Anatomy.* © 1996. Reprinted with permission from the McGraw-Hill Companies, Inc.)

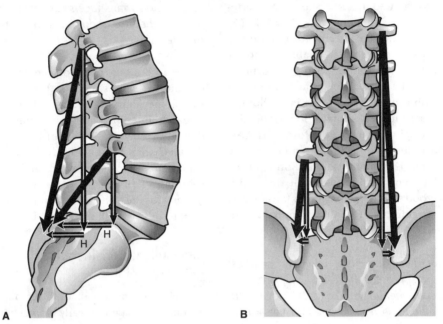

A   **B**

Fig. 1-20 The force vectors of the lumbar iliocostalis. **(A)** lateral view; **(B)** posterior view. (Adapted from Bogduk, N. *Clinical Anatomy of the Lumbar Spine and Sacrum.* 1998, London: Churchill Livingstone.)

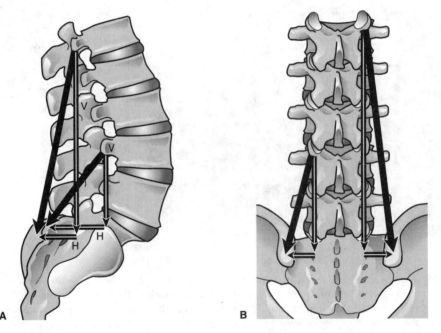

A   **B**

Fig. 1-21 The force vectors of the longissimus. **(A)** lateral view; **(B)** posterior view. (Adapted from Bogduk, N. *Clinical Anatomy of the Lumbar Spine and Sacrum.* 1998, London: Churchill Livingstone.)

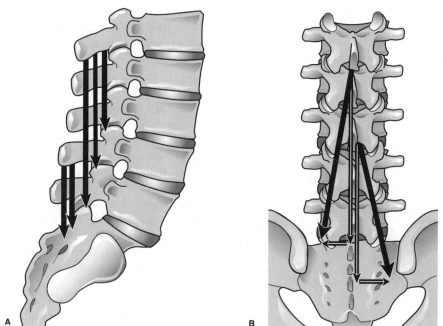

Fig. 1-22 The force vectors of the multifidus. **(A)** lateral view; **(B)** posterior view. (Adapted from Bogduk, N. *Clinical Anatomy of the Lumbar Spine and Sacrum.* 1998, London: Churchill Livingstone.)

Strait et al. (44) calculated that if a 180-lb man performed a dead lift from a position of 60 degrees of forward bending (i.e., without lifting anything other than his upper body), his erector spinae musculature would have to contract with a force of more than 450 lb (approximately 2000 N) for him to maintain equilibrium (Fig. 1-23). They estimated that the erector spinae acted at an average angle of only 12 degrees with the spine; thus, force vectors for sagittal extension rotation were small. The same researchers contended that, if this individual were holding a 50-lb (23-kg) weight in his hands, the same muscles would have to increase their contractile force by 70%. According to the calculations of Strait et al., this could place a compression force of more than 850 lb (approximately 3800 N) on the fifth lumbar vertebra. If their model were correct, because of their poor force vectors the erector spinae would produce extremely large compression components on the vertebrae and intervertebral discs when individuals lifted heavy weights or performed some athletic activities.

The preceding discussion underscores the fact that the musculature of the spine does not always have optimal leverage for spinal extension, particularly when heavy loads are lifted; this is also supported by more recent research (29,40). Although there is a consensus that the object lifted should be held as close as possible to the lifter's body to reduce the object's turning moment, several additional factors have influenced thoughts on the topic of lifting. Research relating to these issues will now be reviewed; they include the roles of the flexion–relaxation response, intraabdominal pressure, and the active and passive extensors of the spine, including the thoracolumbar fascia.

Flexion–Relaxation Response

Floyd and Silver (45) found, by using both surface and needle electrodes, that, from the starting position of standing, the erector spinae initially contracted eccentrically as a forward bending posture was assumed; however, the erector spinae became

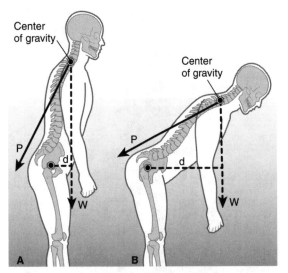

Fig. 1-23 Comparative moments of gravitational pull on the trunk in two positions of flexion.

quiescent as the movement continued into full flexion (Fig. 1-24). They proposed that this was a type of reflex inhibiting mechanism that thrusts the support of the trunk to the ligaments of the spine. In the return to the upright position, they found that the erector spinae became active in extension at a position approximating that in which relaxation in flexion occurred; this finding emphasized the fact that hip extension, for which the erector spinae play no role, can play a dominant role in trunk extension, at least when moderate loads are lifted.

Floyd and Silver's flexion–relaxation response finding is supported by research of others (46–48). However, its actual duration and onset differ with increased loads (49,50) and pelvic posture (51,52), and it is different in the chronic idiopathic LBP patient (53). Bogduk (5) called this phenomenon the *critical point* and defined it as a point at which there is "locking" of the facet joints and increased

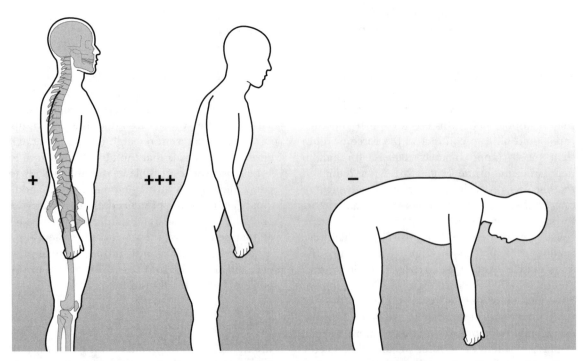

Fig. 1-24 This figure depicts the flexion–relaxation response that occurs in forward bending. Between 60 and 90 degrees of bending the muscles relax, and the mid-line ligaments are obligated to support the head and trunk.

tension in the posterior ligaments. Furthermore, he contended that it does not occur in all individuals. Under heavy loading conditions, this relaxation may not occur as the back musculature takes an active role (51). Recent research on the flexion–relaxation response will be discussed in a subsequent section.

Intraabdominal Pressure

Bartelink (54) noted that, in cadaver specimens, discs yielded with an average compression force of 710 lb (approximately 3150 N). He theorized that intraabdominal pressure (IAP) counterbalanced much of the compression force. His EMG research suggested that the transversus abdominis, followed by the internal and external obliques, contributed most to the IAP in lifting maneuvers. Bartelink concluded that IAP could help balance forward bending moments and lessen the load on the spine by "several hundred pounds." Morris et al. (55) expanded on Bartelink's work by examining intrathoracic pressure, IAP, and muscle action potential; they calculated that the compressive force on lumbosacral discs could be reduced by approximately 30% by the IAP factor in a heavy lifting task.

A couple of points should be raised with respect to this research on IAP. One significant factor to consider is the bone mineral density of vertebral bodies. Granhed et al. (16) found that, in world-class weight lifters, a vertebra may withstand up to 38 kN of compressive force. Although not all athletes would be expected to have this much bone density, most would be much higher than that seen in Bartelink's cadaveric specimens. Moreover, although IAP is important in lifting (48,56,57), it has also been noted that it (a) correlated well with static but not with dynamic loading conditions (58), (b) had a negligible relationship, if any, with abdominal muscle strength (59), (c) did not decrease muscle contraction forces or spine compression forces (60,61), and (d) may have to be higher than systolic pressure to ease lifting heavy objects (3). Even though subsequent research did not support Bartelink's original contention that IAP markedly reduced the pressure

on the spine in lifting tasks, its role is believed to be important. More recently, Cholewicki et al. (62) found that the IAP mechanism can increase spine stability in tasks such as lifting and jumping that demand a trunk extensor moment and that this mechanism may do this without necessitating further erector spinae coactivation.

Thoracolumbar Fascia

In their endeavor to explain how heavy lifts could be performed, Bogduk and Macintosh (63) also performed a detailed dissection of the structure of the thoracolumbar (lumbodorsal) fascia. They pointed out that the superficial lamina, chiefly the aponeurosis of the latissimus dorsi (Fig. 1-25), fuses with the deep lamina fibers at the border of the erector spinae (Fig. 1-26). They contended that this junction (i.e., the lateral raphe) permits the transversus abdominis (and to a lesser extent the internal oblique) to pull laterally on this connective tissue sheath and provide a modest antiflexion moment (Figs. 1-19 and 1-27) (63,64). The important point is that the transversus abdominis and, to a lesser extent, the internal oblique are contiguous with the thoracolumbar fascia. Because the thoracolumbar fascia encapsulates the erector spinae and multifidus, these two lateral abdominal muscles are positioned to enhance trunk stabilization; theoretically, they can accomplish this by tightening the thoracolumbar fascia that envelops the erector spinae.

Bogduk's dissections led to the research by Gracovetsky and Farfan (65) in which they used an optimization technique to study a champion weight lifter performing the dead lift (i.e., ground lift). The dead lift was chosen because it produces the maximum moments that the spine is apt to encounter in voluntary activity (Fig. 1-28). These investigators contended that the major components to this mathematical model of lifting are passive, namely the posterior ligamentous system (PLS) is driven by the powerful hip extensors (i.e., gluteus maximus aided by the hamstrings) (Fig. 1-29). The PLS consists of the mid-line ligaments (supraspinous, interspinous, capsular, ligamentum flavum, posterior longitudinal) and the thoracolumbar

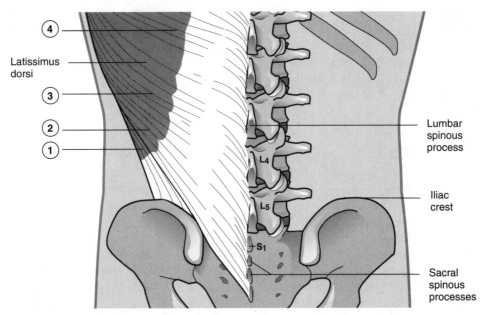

Fig. 1-25 The superficial lamina of the posterior layer of the lumbodorsal fascia. The latissimus dorsi are differentiated into four segments, namely fibers (1) attaching to the ilium, (2) reaching L5 and sacral spinous processes, (3) reaching L3 and L4 spinous processes, and (4) that cover the erector spinae. (Adapted from Bogduk, N. *Clinical Anatomy of the Lumbar Spine and Sacrum.* 1998, London: Churchill Livingstone.)

fascia, with the aponeurotic portions of the latissimus dorsi as a prime element. Gracovetsky and Farfan contended that the PLS, when taut, was analogous to a steel cable driven by the hip extensors.

This group of researchers (64–66) further contended that the passive component could be supplemented nominally by an active antiflexion component, namely the contraction of the transversus abdominis and part of the internal oblique through their lateral raphe origin. In other words, they believed that as the transversus abdominis (and to a lesser extent the internal oblique) contracted they could exert an antiflexion component. However, subsequent research by McGill and Norman (67) showed that the contribution of this active component to trunk extension was very small (i.e., less than 4% contribution to extensor torque). Nevertheless, the tension that the transversus abdominis and internal oblique exert on the thoracolumbar fascia through the lateral raphe is important in trunk stabilization and thus may help control shearing forces (68).

Further Research on Lifting

Research from McGill's laboratory subsequently inferred that the Gracovetsky model did not adequately explain how extremely heavy weights could be lifted. They contended that the passive extensor moment could not permit lifting heavy weights because it would place excessive tensile forces on the mid-line structures lying close to the center of movement; they also believed that maintaining the lumbar lordosis was critical to obtain maximum leverage from the extensor musculature of the spine (60,67,69,70).

Dolan et al. (52) assumed a stance somewhere between those taken by Gracovetsky and McGill, for they showed that the passive extensor moment could make a viable contribution to lifting. Dolan et al. partitioned the passive extensor moment into deep and more superficial structures. The deep structures included the interspinous ligaments and facet joint capsules, all very close to the center of movement. The more superficial structures were the lumbodorsal (i.e., thoracolumbar) fascia, the supraspinous ligament, and the noncontractile tissue of the erector spinae muscles. They found that the deep structures contributed less than 25% of the total passive extensor moment and that the largest majority was provided by the superficial structures. Because the superficial structures can provide a high passive extensor moment without placing high tensile forces on the deep structures (e.g., excessive compressive penalties on the discs), this research supports the role of these passive structures in lifting. Dolan et al. also gave credence to the role of the hip extensors in increasing the passive extensor moment, the importance of IAP, and that the flexion–relaxation response can only occur in the absence of lumbar lordosis.

Bogduk (5) recently reported that the hydraulic amplifier effect originally proposed by Gracovetsky (3) could enhance the back muscles up to 30% in lifting tasks. Bogduk also stated that the passive tension provided by the dorsal muscles of the spine could be the major component of the PLS in lifting

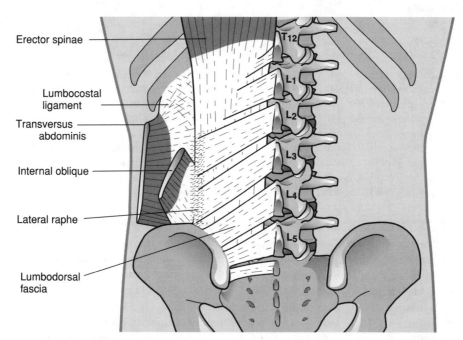

Fig. 1-26 The deep lamina of the posterior layers of the thoracolumbar (lumbodorsal) fascia is represented as bands of fibers; fibers from L4 and L5 attach to the iliac crest, fibers from L2 and L3 end in the lateral raphe, and fibers from T12 and L1 become membranous over the erector spinae. The internal oblique attaches to the lateral raphe fibers opposite from L3; the transversus abdominis arises from the middle layer of the lumbodorsal fascia anterior and above the internal oblique and forms the lumbocostal ligament. (Adapted from Bogduk, N. *Clinical Anatomy of the Lumbar Spine and Sacrum.* 1998, London: Churchill Livingstone.)

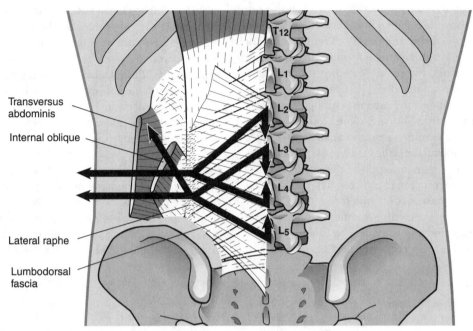

Fig. 1-27 Mechanics of the lumbodorsal fascia. The transversus abdominis (TA) and, to a lesser extent, the internal oblique are in a position to exert lateral tension against the lateral raphe (LR). This tension is then transmitted upward through the deep lamina and downward through the superficial layer; because of the obliquity of these lines of force, a downward vector is generated by the deep lamina and an upward vector by the superficial lamina. The resulting vectors tend to approximate or oppose the separation of the spinous processes between L2 and L4 and between L3 and L5. (Adapted from Bogduk, N. *Clinical Anatomy of the Lumbar Spine and Sacrum.* 1998, London: Churchill Livingstone.)

tasks when the erector spinae are quiescent due to the flexion–relaxation response. Gracovetsky and Farfan (65) had contended that the PLS was composed of passive tissue only (e.g., ligaments and fascia); however, McGill and Norman (67) showed that this was not feasible. If the fascia of the dorsal muscles of the spine were included as part of the PLS, it would appear that the disagreements between the stands taken by Gracovetsky and McGill (and the latter's cohorts) are weakened. Bogduk suggested that there was an additional and very plausible but important responsibility for the lateral abdominal muscles in lifting tasks, namely to keep the weight in the mid-line in the sagittal plane and thus help avert twisting moments.

When Toussaint et al. (50) conducted recent research on the flexion–relaxation response, they assumed that their EMG normalization procedure would enable them to find the erector spinae active at full flexion in the lumbar area. Although they did not find EMG activity in the lumbar area in any of their subjects, they did find EMG activity in the thoracic erector spinae. Their findings agreed with Bogduk's deduction that the thoracic fibers of the erector spinae are attached to the lumbar and sacral spinous processes through an erector spinae aponeurosis (40); they also agree with the contention of McGill and Norman (71) that the thoracic fibers can produce lumbar extension torque independent of the lumbar fibers. To contract independently, Toussaint et al. concluded that an "intricate coordinating mechanism" apportions the load to the active thoracic part of the erector spinae and the passive lumbar structures (i.e., thoracolumbar fascia, erector spinae aponeuroses). These recent findings tend to minimize the discordant arguments of Gracovetsky and McGill with respect to the role of thoracolumbar fascia in the performance of ground lifts.

More recently, others (41,72) have also examined the posterior layer of the thoracolumbar fascia. The research discussed previously emphasized the significance of the superficial fibers of the latissimus dorsi to the thoracolumbar fascia (5,40,63,64); however, this research ignored the role that the gluteus maximus played in the mechanics of the thoracolumbar fascia. The point that Vleeming et al. emphasized is that the gluteus maximus and the contralateral latissimus dorsi tense the

posterior layer of the thoracolumbar fascia (41,72). Furthermore, they contended that this force is perpendicular to the sacroiliac joints and that this coupling is an important aspect of trunk rotation and load transfer (Fig. 1-30). These researchers also believed that, as the erector spinae muscle contracts under a load, it will increase the tension on the deep lamina and dilate the posterior layer of the thoracolumbar fascia. This, too, would contribute to splinting or bracing the trunk.

The previously discussed research by Toussaint et al. (50) showed that the lumbar fibers of the erector spinae are affected by the flexion–relaxation response but the thoracic fibers are not. When this is considered with the preceding discussion, the polarization that existed on the role of the passive extensor moment may be diminished. This may be the reason Fortin (29) surmised that, from a practical sense, a degree of lordosis could be maintained (e.g., McGill's

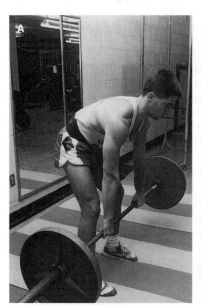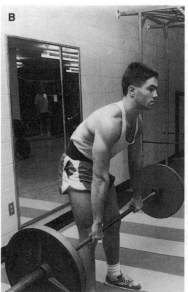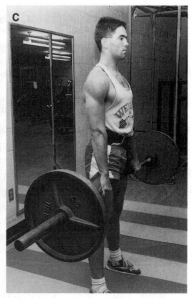

Fig. 1-28 Three stages of the dead lift as proposed in the Gracovetsky model. The prime muscular force that enables movement from the starting position **(A)** to the second position **(B)** is supplied by the gluteus maximus; because there is no lordosis, the posterior ligamentous system (PLS) remains taut as the upper torso is raised. Position **(C)**, in which a lordotic curve is seen, is brought about by contraction of the erector spinae (in particular the multifidus).

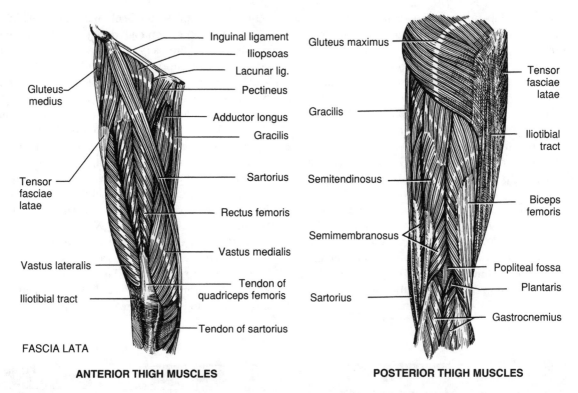

Fig. 1-29 Anterior and posterior views of the lower extremity musculature. (From Pansky, B. *Review of Gross Anatomy.* © 1996. Reprinted with permission from the McGraw-Hill Companies, Inc.)

contention) and that one could still use the passive extensor moment in lifting heavy loads (e.g., Gracovetsky's contention). Because osteophyte formation and facet hypertrophy are related to aging (36), it is possible that the passive (i.e., ligamentous) system would become more important as one ages. Although Parnianpour et al. (51) did not specifically address the issue of age, they emphasized that the anthropometry of the lifter affects lifting style. Thus, with the decrease in lean body mass associated with aging, the role of the passive extensor moment may be of increased importance.

Trunk Bracing

The stabilizing role that the abdominal muscles play in trunk bracing is most important in the rehabilitation process. Anyone who has cracked one or more ribs has appreciated their role even in mundane tasks such as getting into or out of an automobile. An injury such as this provides a foreboding challenge to this seemingly simple task because the abdominal muscles are important stabilizers in transitional movements such as rising from a seated position. As the individual with the cracked ribs attempts the movement, the nociceptors in the injured area are quick to recommend its cessation. This bracing role played by the trunk muscles is the basis for a popular low back therapeutic exercise regimen dependent on trunk stabilization (1). The basis for trunk stabilization will be briefly introduced here; in Chap. 6 there will be more discussion on it and specific exercises in its use will be presented in Chap. 8.

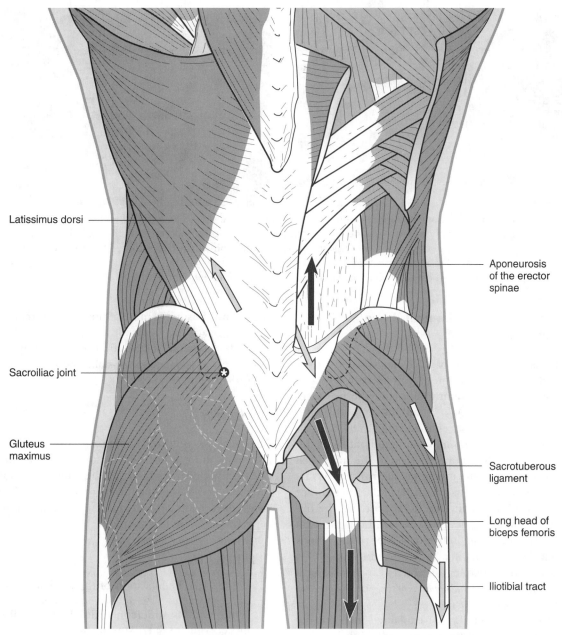

Fig. 1-30 This schematic shows the functional linking between structures such as the **(A)** latissimus dorsi, thoracolumbar fascia, gluteus maximus, and iliotibial tract, and **(B)** midline ligament/erector spinae, sacrotuberous ligament, and long head of biceps. (Adapted from Vleeming A., Snijders, C.F., Stoeckart, R., et al. The role of the sacroiliac joints in coupling between spine, pelvis, legs, and arms. In Vleeming et al. (eds). *Movement, stability, and low back pain-the essential role of the pelvis.* 1997, London: Churchill Livingstone, p. 63.)

Latissimus dorsi

Sacroiliac joint

Gluteus maximus

Aponeurosis of the erector spinae

Sacrotuberous ligament

Long head of biceps femoris

Iliotibial tract

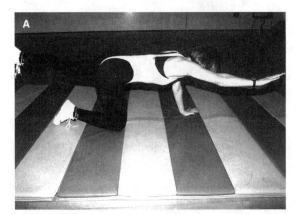 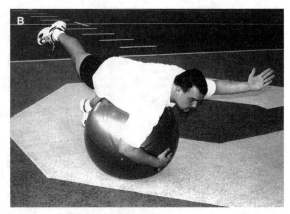

Fig. 1-31 Example of the bracing/stabilization exercises. This activity should be initiated with the controlled extension of only one arm or one leg; emphasis should be placed on keeping the trunk in neutral position, with the shoulders and hips level. **(A)** After the individual has mastered this movement, the contralateral limbs can be raised slowly. **(B)** Use of a therapy ball provides greater challenge because of the increased emphasis on core stabilization and proprioception.

Neutral Spine/Abdominal Brace/ Trunk Stabilization

At least initially, most back problems could be isolated to a motion segment; this includes two vertebrae, their intervening disc, and the two facet joints (see Fig. 1-5). If a motion segment is diseased or injured, nociceptive endings in the annular fibers of the disc, posterior longitudinal ligament, or in the facets continually remind the individual that certain movements are not appropriate at that time. However, if persons so affected learn to brace their trunk in a pain-free ROM position, the diseased motion segment will not send out the pain signals and these individuals can resume their usual activity. This led to a procedure based on martial arts principles called *stabilization training*; it is sometimes called *abdominal bracing* or the *neutral spine technique* (1).

Richardson et al. (68) explained in detail the importance of the transversus abdominis in maintaining hoop tension for the abdominal area. They described its role in increasing IAP and in tensing the thoracolumbar fascia; both are critical to bracing the trunk, which is necessary in stabilization training. Although stabilization training may be used with individuals presenting with spondylolysis

and spondylolisthesis, most of the research reporting its efficacy has been with disc patients (73). Examples of spinal stabilization exercises appear in Figure 1-31; further spinal-stabilization activities are presented in Chap. 8.

SUMMARY

The purpose of this chapter was to present a review of those aspects of anatomy and biomechanics that are pertinent to the functioning of the spine and to therapeutic exercise for LBP. The succeeding chapters will build upon many precepts presented in this chapter.

REFERENCES

1. White, A.H. Stabilization of the lumbar spine, in *Conservative Care of Low Back Pain*, A.H. White and R. Anderson, editors. 1991, Baltimore: Williams & Wilkins. p. 106–111.
2. Junghanns, H. *Clinical Implications of Normal Biomechanical Stresses on Spinal Function*. 1990, Rockville, MD: Aspen. p. 480.
3. Gracovetsky, S. *The Spinal Engine*. 1988, New York: Springer-Verlag. p. 505.
4. Gracovetsky, S. Linking the spinal engine with the legs: a theory of human gait, in *Stability &*

Low Back Pain, A. Vleeming, et al., editors. 1997, Churchill Livingstone: New York.

5. Bogduk, N. *Clinical Anatomy of the Lumbar Spine and Sacrum*, 3rd ed. 1998, London: Churchill Livingstone. p. 261.

6. Fujiwara, A., Tamai, K., Kurihashi, A., et al. Relationship between morphology of ilio lumbar ligament and lower lumbar disc degeneration. *J Spinal Disord* 1999, 12(4): p. 348–352.

7. Nagaosa, Y., Kikuchi, S., Hasue, M., et al. Patho-anatomic mechanism of degenerative spondylolisthesis. *Spine* 1998, 23(13): p. 1447–1451.

8. Berlemann, U., Jeszenszky, D.J., Buhler, D.W., et al. The role of lumbar lordosis, vertebral endplate inclination, disc height, and facet orientation in degenerative spondylolisthesis. *J Spinal Disord* 1999, 12(1): p. 68–73.

9. Hansson, T., Bigos, S., Beecher, P., et al. The lumbar lordosis in acute and chronic low-back pain. *Spine* 1986, 11: p. 154.

10. Pope, M.H., Bevins, T., Wilder, D.G., et al. The relationship between anthropometric, postural, muscular, and mobility characteristics of males ages 18–55. *Spine* 1985, 10: p. 644–648.

11. Pope, M.H. Risk indicators in low back pain. *Ann Med* 1989, 21: p. 387.

12. Borenstein, D.G. and S.W. Wiesel. *Low Back Pain-Medical Diagnosis and Comprehensive Management*, 3rd ed. 1989, Philadelphia: W.B. Saunders. p. 563.

13. Twomey, L.T. and J.R. Taylor. Lumbar posture, movement and mechanisms, in *Physical Therapy of the Low Back*, L.T. Twomey and J. Taylor, editors. 1987, New York: Churchill Livingstone. p. 51–84.

14. Panjabi, M.M., Goel, V. Oxland, T., et al. Human lumbar vertebrae-quantitative 3-dimensional anatomy. *Spine* 1992, 17(3): p. 299–306.

15. Nordin, M. and V.H. Frankel. Biomechanics of bone, in *Biomechanics of the Musculoskeletal System*, M. Nordin and V. Frankel, editors. 1989, Philadelphia: Lea and Febiger. p. 3–29.

16. Granhed, H., Jonson, R., Hansson, T., et al. The loads on the lumbar spine during extreme weight lifting. *Spine* 1987, 12(2): p. 146–149.

17. Natarajan, R.N., Ke, J.H., Andersson, G.B.J. A model to study the disc degeneration process. *Spine* 1994, 19(3): p. 259–265.

18. van Dieen, J.H. and H.M. Toussaint. Spinal shrinkage as a parameter of functional load. *Spine* 1993, 18(11): p. 1504–1514.

19. Holm, S., and A. Nachemson. Variations in the nutrition of the canine intervertebral disc induced by motion. *Spine* 1983, 8: p. 866–873.

20. Kirkaldy-Willis, W.H. Three phases of the spectrum of degenerative disease, in *Managing Low Back Pain*, W.H. Kirkaldy-Willis and C.V. Burton, editors. 1992, New York: Churchill-Livingstone. p. 105–119.

21. Haughton, V.M., Lim, T.H., An, H. Intervertebral disk appearance correlated with stiffness of lumbar spinal motion segments. *Am J Neuroradiol* 1999, 20(6): p. 1161–1165.

22. Goel, V.K., Kong, W., Han, J.S., et al. A combined finite element and optimization investigation of lumbar spine mechanics with and without muscles. *Spine* 1993, 18: p. 1531.

23. Panjabi, M.M. The stabilizing system of the spine, Part I. Function, dysfunction, adaptation, and enhancement. *J Spinal Disord* 1992, 5(4): p. 383–389.

24. Yong-Hing, K. and W.H. Kirkaldy-Willis. The pathophysiology of degenerative disease of the lumbar spine. *Orthop Clin North Am* 1983, 14(3): p. 491–504.

25. Kim, Y.E., Goel, V.K., Weinstein, J.N., et al. Effect of disk degeneration at one level on the adjacent level in axial mode. *Spine* 1991, 16(3): p. 331–335.

26. Basmajian, J.V. and C.J. DeLuca. *Muscles Alive-Their Functions Revealed by Electromyography*. 1985, Baltimore: Williams & Wilkins.

27. Biering-Sorensen, F. Physical measurements as risk indicators for low-back trouble over a one-year period. *Spine* 1984, 9(2): p. 106–19.

28. Cady, L.D., Bischoff, D.P., O'Connell, E.R., et al. Strength and fitness and subsequent back injuries in firefighters. *J Occup Med* 1979, 21(4): p. 269–72.

29. Fortin, J.D. Weight lifting, in *The Spine in Sports*, R.G. Watkins, et al., editors. 1996, St. Louis: Mosby. p. 484–498.

30. McGill, S.M. Low back exercises: evidence for improving exercise regimens. *Phys Ther* 1998, 78(7): p. 754–765.

31. LaBan, M.M., Raptov, A.D., Johnson, E.W. Electromyographic study of function of iliopsoas muscle. *Arch Phys Med Rehabil* 1965, 45: p. 676–679.

32. Liemohn, W.P., Snodgrass, L.B., Sharpe, G.L. Unresolved controversies in back management. *J Orthop Sports Phys Ther* 1988, 9(7): p. 239–244.

33. Department of the Army. *Physical Fitness Training*. 1999, Washington, D.C.

34. Kendall, F.P., McCreary, E.K., Provance, P.G. *Muscles: Testing and Function*. 1993, Baltimore: Williams & Wilkins.

35. Mutoh, Y. Low back pain in butterfliers, in *Swimming Medicine IV*, B. Eriksson and B. Furberg, editors. 1978, Baltimore: University Park Press.

36. Nachemson, A.L. The lumbar spine-an orthopaedic challenge. *Spine* 1976, 1: p. 59–71.

37. Axler, C.T. and S.M. McGill. Low back loads over a variety of abdominal exercises: searching for the safest abdominal challenge. *Med Sci Sports Exerc* 1997, 29(6): p. 804–811.

38. Juker, D., McGill, S., Kropf, P., et al. Quantitative intramuscular myoelectric activity of lumbar portions of psoas and the abdominal wall during a wide variety of tasks. *Med Sci Sports Exerc* 1998, 30(2): p. 301–310.

39. Sparling, P.B., Millard-Stafford, M., Snow, T.K. Development of a cadence curl-up test for college students. *Res Q Exerc Sport*, 1997, 68(4): p. 309–316.

40. Bogduk, N. A reappraisal of the anatomy of the human lumbar erector spinae. *J Anat* 1980, 131(3): p. 525–540.

41. Williard, F.H. The muscular, ligamentous and neural structure of the low back and its relation to back pain, in *Movement, Stability & Low Back Pain*, A. Vleeming, et al., editors. 1997, New York: Churchill Livingstone. p. 3–35.

42. Gray, H. *Anatomy, Descriptive and Surgical*. Revised American edition, from the 15th English edition. 1978, New York: Bounty Books. p. 1257.

43. Lockhart, R.D., Hamilton, G.F., Fyfe, F.W. *Anatomy of the Human Body*. 1959, Philadelphia: J.B. Lippincott. p. 705.

44. Strait, L.A., Inman, V.T., Ralston, H.J. Sample illustrations of physical principles selected from physiology and medicine. *Am J Phys* 1947, 15: p. 375.

45. Floyd, W.F. and P.H.S. Silver. The function of the erectores spinae muscles in certain movements and postures in man. *J Physiol* 1955, 129: p. 184.

46. Dolan, P. and M.A. Adams. The relationship between EMG activity and extensor moment generation in the erector spinae muscles during bending and lifting activities. *J Biomech* 1993, 26(4/5): p. 513–522.

47. Kippers, V. and A.W. Parker. Posture related to myoelectric silence of erectores spinae during trunk flexion. *Spine* 1984, 9(7): p. 740–745.

48. Tveit, P., Daggfeldt, K., Hetland, S., et al. Erector spinae lever arm length variations with changes in spinal curvature. *Spine* 1994, 19: p. 199.

49. Hemborg, B., Moritz, U., Hamberg, J., et al. Intra-abdominal pressure and trunk muscle activity during lifting-III. Effect of abdominal muscle training in chronic low-back patients. *Scand J Rehabil Med* 1985, 17: p. 15–24.

50. Toussaint, H.M., de Winter A.F., de Hass, Y., et al. Flexion relaxation during lifting: implications for torque production by muscle activity and tissue strain at the lumbo-sacral joint. *J Biomech* 1994, 28(2): p. 199–210.

51. Parnianpour, M., Bejjani, F.J., Pavlidis, L. Worker training: the fallacy of a single, correct lifting technique. *Ergonomics* 1987, 30: p. 331–334.

52. Dolan, P., Mannion, A.F., Adams, M.A. Passive tissues help the back muscles to generate extensor moments during lifting. *J Biomech* 1994, 27(8): p. 1077–1085.

53. Ahern, D.K., Hannon, D.J., Goreczny, A.J. Correlation of chronic low-back pain behavior and muscle function examination of the flexion–relaxation response. *Spine* 1990, 15: p. 92.

54. Bartelink, D.L. The role of abdominal pressure in relieving the pressure on the lumbar intervertebral discs. *J Bone Joint Surg* 1957, 39B: p. 718.

55. Morris, J.M., Lucas, D.B., Bresler, B. The role of trunk muscles in stability of the spine. *J Bone Joint Surg* 1961, 43A: p. 327.

56. Harman, E.A., Frykman, P.N., Clagett, E.R. Intra-abdominal and intra-thoracic pressures during lifting and jumping. *Med Sci Sports Exerc* 1988, 20(2): p. 195–201.

57. Kapandji, I.A. *The Physiology of Joints, Vol III. The Trunk and the Vertebral Column*. 1982, New York: Churchill Livingstone.

58. Leskinen, T.P.J., Stalhammer, H.R., Kuorinka, I.A.A., et al. Hip torque, lumbosacral compression, and intraabdominal pressure in lifting and lowering tasks, in *Biomechanics IX-B International*

Series on Biomechanics, R.P. Winter, et al., editors 1983, Champaign, IL: Human Kinetics. p. 55.

59. Hemborg, B. and U. Moritz. Intra-abdominal pressure and trunk muscle activity during lifting-II. Chronic low-back patients. *Scand J Rehabil Med* 1985, 17: p. 5–13.

60. McGill, S.M. and R.W. Norman. 1986 Volvo Award in Biomechanics-partitioning of the L4–L5 dynamic moment into disc, ligamentous, and muscular components during lifting. 1986, 11: p. 666.

61. Nachemson, A.L., Andersson B.J., Schultz, A.B. Valsalva maneuver biomechanics: effects on lumbar trunk loads of elevated intraabdominal pressures. *Spine* 1986, 11: p. 476.

62. Cholewicki, J., Juluru, K., McGill, S.M. Intra-abdominal pressure mechanism for stabilizing the lumbar spine. *J Biomech* 1999, 32(1): p. 13–17.

63. Bogduk, N. and J.E. Macintosh. The applied anatomy of the thoracolumbar fascia. *Spine* 1984, 9: p. 164–170.

64. Macintosh, J.E., Bogduk, N., Gracovetsky, S. The biomechanics of the thoracolumbar fascia. *Clin Biomech* 1987, 2: p. 79–83.

65. Gracovetsky, S. and H. Farfan. The optimum spine. *Spine* 1986, 11(6): p. 543–571.

66. Gracovetsky, S. The abdominal mechanism. *Spine* 1985, 10(4): p. 317–324.

67. McGill, S.M. and R.W. Norman. Potential of lumbodorsal fascia forces to generate back extension moments during squat lifts. *J Biomed Eng* 1988, 10(July): p. 312.

68. Richardson, C., Jull, G., Hodges, P., et al. *Therapeutic Exercise for Spinal Stabilization in Low Back Pain-Scientific Basis and Clinical Approach.* 1999, London: Churchill Livingstone. p. 191.

69. Cholewicki, J., McGill, S.M., Norman, R.W. Lumbar spine loads during the lifting of extremely heavy weights. *Med Sci Sports Exerc* 1991, 23(10): p. 1179–1186.

70. Potvin, J.R., McGill, S.M., Norman, R.W. Trunk muscle and lumbar ligament contributions to dynamic lifts with varying degrees of trunk flexion. *Spine* 1991, 16: p. 1099.

71. McGill, S.M. and R.W. Norman. Effects of an anatomically detailed erector spinae model on L4/L5 disc compression and shear. *J Biomech* 1987, 20: p. 591–600.

72. Vleeming, A., Pool-Goudzwaard, A.L. Stoeckhart, R., et al. The posterior layer of the thoracolumbar fascia: its function in load transfer from spine to legs. *Spine* 1995, 20(7): p. 753–758.

73. Saal, J.A. and J.S. Saal. Nonoperative treatment of herniated lumbar intervertebral disc with radiculopathy-an outcome study. *Spine* 1989, 14(4): p. 431–437.

CHAPTER 2

FLEXIBILITY, RANGE OF MOTION, AND LOW BACK FUNCTION

Wendell Liemohn

Gina Pariser

INTRODUCTION

Flexibility relates to the capacity to move a joint throughout its range of motion (ROM). Range of motion deficiencies in the spine and its supporting structures are viewed as prognostic indicators of low back pain (1–3). Maintenance of good ROM at the iliofemoral joint and in the spinal articulations is paramount to having a healthy back. Moreover, in individuals with chronic low back pain, exercise regimens to improve trunk and hip joint ROM are viewed as therapeutic.

Range of motion, rather than the term *flexibility*, is often a better descriptor when discussing this concept because it implies that movement can be measured in more than one direction. For example, the individual in Figure 2-1 shows an exceptional degree of hyperextensibility; however, to call hyperextensibility flexibility can be confusing. Although the terms *flexibility* and *ROM* are often used interchangeably and in essence can have the same meaning, in this text the acronym *ROM* will be used more often than the term *flexibility*. The major topics to be covered in this chapter include kinematics of the spine, kinematics of the ilio-femoral joint, assessing ROM as it relates to low back function, and improving ROM.

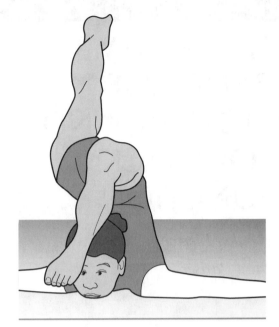

Fig. 2-1 *Flexibility* is the appropriate word to use to describe this athlete's hyperextensibility. Using the word *flexibility* to describe an extension movement can be confusing; for this reason *range of motion* is often used instead.

KINEMATICS

Kinetics is the study of forces and motions. Kinematics is that aspect of mechanics pertaining only to the study of motion without considering forces such as those imposed by muscle contraction, gravity, or collision forces that occur in contact sports.

Kinematics of the Spine

The possible motions of a vertebra are rotation and translation. Rotation implies that movement occurs about some fixed point or axis; it is measured in degrees and is exemplified by flexion and extension in the sagittal plane, lateral flexion (or bending) in the frontal plane, and rotation in the transverse (horizontal) plane. The movement translation occurs when all particles of the body (e.g., a vertebra) have the same direction of motion (e.g., up or down, forward or backward). Intervertebral translation within a healthy motion segment is very slight and is measured in millimeters. In the condition of spondylolisthesis, translation of L5 over S1 may exceed 2 cm in severe cases. In athletics, spondylolisthesis is the result of exceptional forces placed on the lumbosacral junction.

Under normal conditions the instantaneous center for flexion-extension and lateral flexion in a lumbar spine motion segment is within the disc (4). If injury or damage to an intervertebral disc occurs, the instant center or axis of rotation may migrate, and then the structure may become less stable as compensatory adjustments occur (5).

The limits and representative values of lumbosacral ROM are presented in Table 2-1. Lumbosacral ROM (LROM) diminishes in a caudalcephalic direction with respect to movement in the sagittal plane. In lateral bending in the frontal plane, ROM diminishes in a cephalocaudal direction. Similarly, the least amount of rotation in the transverse plane is seen in the last motion segment (i.e., L5–S1); facet joint orientation restricts rotational movements among all lumbar vertebrae but particularly between L5 and S1 (Fig. 2-2). Figure 1-13 in Chap. 1 presents trunk ROM information pictorially in all planes. Figure 1-13B warrants particular attention; it depicts ROM extremes from lumbosacral hyperextension to lumbosacral flexion. Lumbar flexion is, in essence, a removal of the lordotic curve. Under normal conditions, no further flexion than the removal of the lordotic curve occurs. Figure 2-3 shows the flexion limitations in the sagittal plane. Although the supraspinous and interspinous ligaments and the ligamentum flava restrict flexion in the sagittal plane, the facet joint ligaments are primarily responsible for the limitation (6). Bony impaction of the inferior articular processes on the lamina of the vertebra below is the chief factor that limits hyperextension movements in the sagittal plane (6) (see Fig. 1-13B, Chap. 1). These movement constraints are important considerations in the analysis and prescription of trunk ROM activities.

Kinematics of the Iliofemoral Joint

Iliofemoral ROM is less ambiguous than lumbar ROM. In the sagittal plane, 10 degrees of extension and 125 degrees of flexion are the norms (7). In the frontal plane, 45-degree abduction and 10-degree adduction are expected; in the transverse plane, 45 degrees is the norm for both lateral and medial rotation (7). Besides the joint capsule, hip joint extension is limited by the iliacus and psoas muscles. When extension occurs at the knee joint, hip joint flexion is limited by the two joint hamstring muscle groups.

Table 2-1   Representative Values of Ranges of Rotation in the Lumbar Spine

INTERSPACE	COMBINED FLEXION/EXTENSION (±X-AXIS ROTATION)		ONE SIDE LATERAL BENDING (Z-AXIS ROTATION)		ONE SIDE AXIAL ROTATION (Y-AXIS ROTATION)	
	LIMITS OF RANGES (DEGREES)	REPRESENTATIVE ANGLE (DEGREES)	LIMITS OF RANGES (DEGREES)	REPRESENTATIVE ANGLE (DEGREES)	LIMITS OF RANGES (DEGREES)	REPRESENTATIVE ANGLE (DEGREES)
L1–L2	5–16	12	3–8	6	1–3	2
L2–L3	8–18	14	3–10	6	1–3	2
L3–L4	6–17	15	4–12	8	1–3	2
L4–L5	9–21	16	3–9	6	1–3	2
L5–S1	10–24	17	2–6	3	0–2	1

(Adapted from White, A.A., and Panjabi, M.M., *Clinical Biomechanics of the Spine*, 2nd edition. Philadelphia: J.B. Lippincott, 1990, p. 107.)

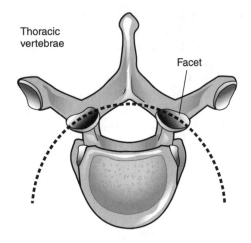

Thoracic vertebrae

Facet

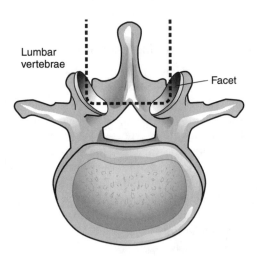

Lumbar vertebrae

Facet

Fig. 2-2 Note the difference in facet orientation between the thoracic and lumbar vertebrae. In the lumbar vertebrae, this orientation minimizes rotation movements.

Because the pelvis is the foundation for the spine, tightness in the flexors or extensors of the iliofemoral joint will affect spinal integrity. These muscles crossing the hip joint can be viewed as "guy wires" that control pelvic positioning; if any of the guy wires are too tight, the affected individual will have difficulty controlling pelvic position with the trunk musculature (Fig. 2-4). For example, tightness in the psoas, iliacus, or rectus femoris muscles can cause hyperlordosis. Conversely, tightness in

the hamstrings can obliterate the lumbar curve and cause a flat back. Tightness in either the hip flexors or hip extensors will severely limit the effectiveness of the abdominal musculature (even if these muscles are strong) in protecting the spine and helping it react to the forces to which it is subjected.

For example, tight hamstrings may preclude postural compensation at the iliofemoral joint as an individual accidentally steps in a hole. In such a scenario, the spine may be obligated to give with the unexpected stress because of hamstring tightness. Even if the healthy spine can usually absorb stresses such as this, these incidents can eventually take their toll.

An important point to remember is that pelvic control with the trunk musculature is fundamental

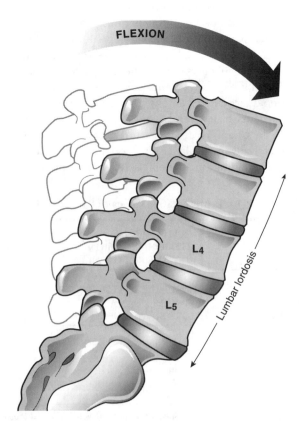

FLEXION

L4

L5

Lumbar lordosis

Fig. 2-3 Lumbosacral flexion is in essence an unfolding and straightening of the lumbar lordosis.

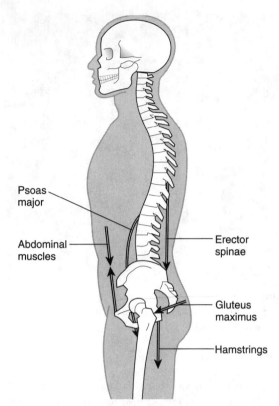

Psoas major

Abdominal muscles

Erector spinae

Gluteus maximus

Hamstrings

Fig. 2-4 The major muscles that cross the hip joint can be viewed as guy wires that control the posture of the pelvis. Because the pelvis is the foundation for the spine, the spine can be vulnerable to injury if these muscles are too tight.

to having good spinal function and a healthy back; vulnerability to low back pain will increase if pelvic positioning cannot be controlled by the abdominal and back musculature. Because tightness in the hamstrings is more prevalent than tightness in the hip flexors, these muscles are usually the culprits, particularly in males. Hip flexor tightness is not seen as often as hip extensor tightness and it may be more often seen in females than in males.

Range of motion in joints distal to the hip joint is also important to the absorption of forces to which the spine may be subjected. For example, decreased ROM in the ankle will affect the biomechanics of foot strike and take off. Tightness in the Achilles tendon may preclude heel strike and, hence, there is less distance available to absorb the

force in stepping; similarly, tightness in the anterior compartment muscles may preclude force absorption in the forepart of the foot. If a runner made much noise with each foot strike rather than cushioning the feet from the most distal to the proximal joints of the lower extremities, running, which is usually viewed as an activity that can enhance function of the spine, could be detrimental because of the jarring the spine is obligated to absorb if cushioning does not occur in distal joints.

Special Factors Affecting Kinematics

Many different factors can influence the kinematics of the spine and the iliofemoral joint. Disease or injury to the spine would obviously be expected to affect joint kinematics. Less obvious are the effects of age and sex. These factors will now be discussed.

Effects of Age and Disease on LROM   Figure 1-13A and B show iliofemoral and spine ROM in flexion in the sagittal plane. Kendall et al. (7) proposed that, during the pubertal growth spurt, hamstring muscle tightness and disproportionate limb length gains adversely affect flexibility. However, in a recent study done with more than 600 adolescent students, the results suggested that growth during this period of their lives could not lead to a decrease in flexibility (8). Nevertheless, research suggests that a progressive decline in spinal mobility occurs with aging (3,9–11). Twomey and Taylor (12) reported diminishment in spinal LROM with age, particularly in extension movements; however, this has not always been noted (11). For individuals who are not active, it is not known how much of this ROM diminution is due to aging per se or to the activity reduction that occurs with aging. One reason offered for the decline of extension ROM is the contention that extension movements are used less than flexion movements as a person ages (10).

The research on decrements in ROM in individuals with low back pain presents mixed findings. Mellin (3) found a greater diminishment in flexion movements in this population. In agreement with that finding, McGregor et al. (13), using computerized potentiometric techniques, found that

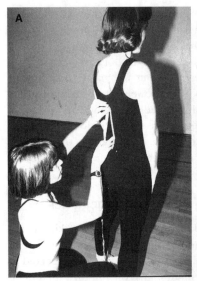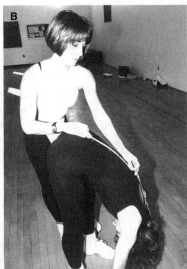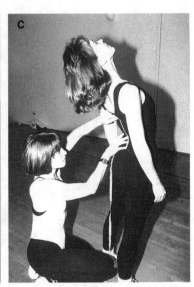

Fig. 2-5 In the modified-modified Schober method, **(A)** a mark is made at the mid-line between the two posterior superior iliac spines; a second mark is then made 15 cm superior to this point. The distance between the two markers is measured in maximum flexion **(B)** and extension **(C)**.

subjects with low back pain had much lower flexion LROM than asymptomatic subjects; however, they did not see significant differences in extension, lateral flexion, or rotation LROM. In contrast, Youdas et al. (14), in a study of males with low back pain, found decrements in extension and rotation LROM to be greater than those seen in flexion LROM. When both age and low back pain were variables, Ensink et al. (15) did not find a correlation between age and LROM.

The loss of LROM associated with physiologic aging is caused by an increased stiffening of the intervertebral discs due to histologic changes; the idea that LROM is reduced by the thinning of discs with age is no longer believed to be the case (6). Although no research was found to support the idea that ROM improved after reaching adulthood purely as a process of aging, McGregor et al. (13) found that age alone could not explain the variability that they saw in spine LROM. The findings of Buchalter et al. (16) were in agreement; thus, the only conclusions that can be drawn are that lifestyle plays a definite role in LROM diminishment with

age and LROM variability increases with age (17). Other disease processes also would affect LROM; for example, the presence of osteophytes is related to age and would restrict movement (18).

Effects of Sex on LROM   There is no unanimity with respect to the exact effect that sex has on LROM. MacRae and Wright (19) and McGregor et al. (13) found greater LROM in flexion in men than in women. White and Panjabi (5) reported that, in the sagittal plane, male mobility exceeded female mobility; however, in the frontal plane, the converse was true. Ensink et al. (15) however, did not find a correlation between sex and LROM in back patients.

ASSESSING LUMBOSACRAL AND ILIOFEMORAL ROM

Flexibility, or ROM, is joint specific; determining the ROM of a few joints does not provide an indicator of the flexibility in other joints even if the same joint movement is measured in the opposite limb. The tests used to measure flexibility (i.e., as they relate to the low back) range from the simple to the more complex; a sampling of the more commonly used clinical measurements, including their advantages and shortcomings, will now be discussed.

Lumbosacral ROM

The tests that purport specifically to measure LROM distinctly from hip joint ROM are described in this section. They include both skin distraction and inclinometer techniques.

Skin Distraction Techniques   The original Schober test as described by Ensink et al. (15) and subsequent modifications of this original test (19,20) are frequently cited in the literature as skin distraction techniques. These tests rely on taking measurements between two reference points as the subject (a) first stands with normal upright posture and (b) then assumes the fingertips-to-floor position. As the subject bends forward, the distance between the two reference points increases (i.e., distraction of the skin). The distance between the two points in standing is then subtracted from the distance between the two points in the bent-over position.

In the original Schober test, the subject's lumbosacral junction is the reference point (15). After marking this point, the examiner makes a second mark 10 cm above the L-S junction while the individual is assuming a relaxed standing posture. After the subject assumes a finger-tips-to-floor posture, the distance between the two marks is measured. An increased distance of at least 5 cm (i.e., 15 cm between marks) is considered a normal value. One problem specific to this technique is being able to find the lumbosacral junction (21).

MacRae and Wright (19) modified the original Schober test by placing reference points 5 cm below and 10 cm above a midline mark in the line connecting the "dimples of Venus" that approximates the lumbosacral junction. They contended that the reference point was easier to find than the lumbosacral junction. An increased distance of at least 5 cm is considered a normal value. Although the dimples of Venus are easier to find than the

L-S junction, approximately one-fourth of the general population may not have this landmark (21).

Williams et al. (20) modified the Schober technique further. The inferior reference point (i.e., 0-cm mark) was the spinal intersection of a horizontal line drawn between the usually easily identifiable posterior superior iliac spines (PSIS) (Fig. 2-5). (It should be noted, however, that the PSIS are at the level of the second sacral vertebrae.) The superior landmark is then marked at a distance of 15 cm above this reference point. In addition to the measurement of flexion ROM, the same researchers determined that extension ROM can be measured with this technique. When the hyperextension posture is assumed, the reference points approximate (i.e., are less than 15 cm apart). Williams et al. (20) computed both interrater (Pearson product moment) and intrarater (intraclass correlation) coefficients for this technique; most of their correlations were quite good. In our initial use of this technique with three cohorts, intraclass correlation coefficients for repeated measurements by the same tester were 0.92 to 0.98 for flexion and 0.92 to 0.94 for extension (22).

Critique of Skin Distraction Techniques. Although Mayer and Gatchel (23) did not critique the modified Schober technique just described, they contended that (a) the anatomic reference points for the two earlier versions of the Schober tests were too difficult to find, (b) the Schober techniques do not consider extreme variances in height, and (c) only flexion ROM could be measured. Although the technique by Williams et al. (20) averts the first and third shortcomings listed by Mayer and Gatchel (23), extremes in body size are still not factored into this technique. For example, the 15-cm distance would cover different motion segments on a 150-cm individual than it would on a 170-cm individual. Nevertheless, if patients are being compared with themselves as they participate in rehabilitation, the drawbacks are less severe. Of the three Schober techniques described, our testers were most comfortable using the PSIS as the starting reference point as advocated by Williams et al. (20) rather than the lumbosacral junction or the dimples of

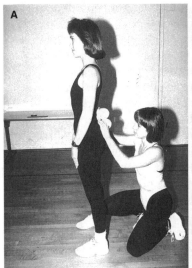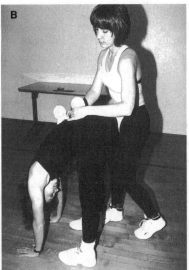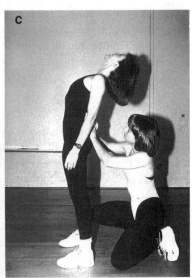

Fig. 2-6 Inclinometer (M.I.E. Medical Research, Leeds, UK). Once the instrument is placed on the body part to be moved, the rotating dial of the inclinometer is set to zero. After the passive or active movement is accomplished, the number of degrees moved can readily be seen. Depicted is the determination of lumbar mobility with the Keeley et al. (24) inclinometer test. Inclinometers are positioned over the T12-L1 interspace and the sacrum (**A**); marking these positions with a felt pen is recommended. The subject tested assumes a maximum forward leaning position (**B**); after both inclinometers are read, the subject returns to the starting position. The hands are then placed on the hips, and, with the knees locked, the subject then assumes a maximum hyperextension position and the inclinometers are read (**C**). The range of motion for each inclinometer is then totaled.

Venus as advocated in the other Schober protocols described.

Inclinometer Tests   The goniometer can be used effectively in measuring limb ROM; however, it is less effective in measuring spinal ROM. A fluid inclinometer (there is also an electronic inclinometer) presents an option to the traditional goniometric techniques (Fig. 2-6). Mayer et al. (21) developed an inclinometer protocol that can delineate sagittal lumbar mobility from that occurring at the hip joint. Moreover, besides reporting excellent reliability, these investigators found that their single inclinometer technique compared very favorably when contrasted with x-ray analyses. Subsequently, individuals from this group developed a double inclinometer protocol that also permitted evaluating ROM in extension (24).

Critique of Inclinometer Tests.   Although Keeley et al. (24) reported reliability scores in the low 0.90s for their administration of the double inclinometer test, those reported by Williams et al. (20) for the same test were very low for two of their testers. In our research with the double inclinometer technique, our intraclass correlation coefficients (ICCs) have ranged from 0.95 to 0.98 (for flexion) and from 0.87 to 0.96 (for extension) (22). However, the high coefficients were obtained at the expense of using two testers (i.e., one per inclinometer) to make the measurements. However, similarly high ICCs were obtained in subsequent research in our laboratory by a single investigator (25). In a more extensive study, Saur et al. (26) validated the inclinometer technique against radiologic techniques; although total lumbar ROM ($r = 0.94$) and flexion ROM ($r = 0.88$) coefficients were high between the two techniques, extension ROM correlation was much lower ($r = 0.42$), suggesting that the latter needs refinement. (However, the subsequent discussion explores whether the validity of the extension test might be improved if the measurement is taken from the prone position rather than from the standing position; this eliminates the subject's fear of falling.)

In comparison to the goniometer, the inclinometer may be easier to use for at least some limb ROM measurements; moreover, the potential of the inclinometer for measuring transverse plane spine ROM (e.g., cervical or lumbar rotation) is much better than that of the goniometer. Our test-retest reliability coefficients for measuring performance on the passive straight-leg raise were 0.98. Keeley et al. (24) also reported a technique for measuring spinal rotation with the inclinometer; however, the reliability

coefficients they reported were too low for research purposes. Nevertheless, there may be clinical implications for using an inclinometer to measure spinal rotation ROM when monitoring a patient's progress provided that the flexibility measurements are made by the same individual.

Combination Skin Distraction and Inclinometer Technique   The Back Range of Motion (BROM) Instrument (Performance Attainment Associates, Roseville, MN) has recently been developed; it includes two measurement devices. One combines skin distraction measurement with inclinometer measurement for measuring flexion and extension ROM. The second unit can be used to measure both lateral flexion and rotation ROM. However, because the instrument was developed so recently, the research conducted with it is limited (Fig. 2-7).

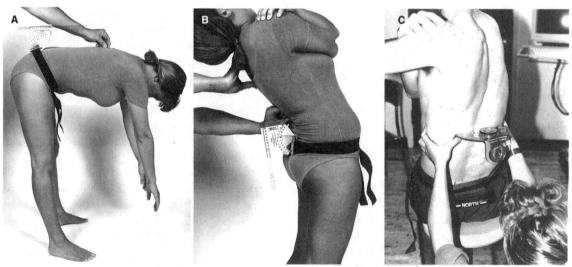

Fig. 2-7 The Back Range of Motion Instrument. With the patient standing, the body of the flexion-extension unit is placed on the sacrum and the arm unit is placed at the T12-L1 interspace. After reading the pelvic tilt, have the patient assume a fingertips-to-toes position while maintaining the arm unit on the T12-L1 interspace; take readings at maximum forward flexion **(A)**. After the patient returns to the standing position, a hyperextended posture is assumed and the readings are taken **(B)**. The lateral flexion-rotation unit is placed on T12, and the lateral flexion is noted on the inclinometer (not depicted). When rotation measurements are taken **(C)**, the horizontal dial is in essence a compass, and a magnet obviates any pelvic movement that might occur. (In our research with this instrument, subjects sat on a stool with a fixed seat.) (Courtesy of *Performance Attainment Associates,* Roseville, MN.)

BROMS Flexion-Extension Unit (see Fig. 2-7A, B). The unit used in measuring flexion and extension movement combines inclinometer and skin distraction techniques. A stand-alone inclinometer is held on S1 and can be used to measure sacral tilt (i.e., iliofemoral ROM) after the patient assumes the fingertips-to-floor position. The other hand manipulates the sliding arm. It is used to measure the distance to the T12-L1 interspace as the subject stands upright, bends forward, and then bends backward. One tester can easily take the measurements with the BROM without assistance.

In our use of the BROM flexion-extension unit for patients and asymptomatic individuals, ICCs were in the 0.80s for degrees (i.e., inclinometer reading) and 0.90s for skin distraction (i.e., centimeter reading) (22). Breum et al. (27) combined the latter degree and centimeter readings and found coefficients for intrarater and interrater to be quite satisfactory for flexion ROM [Intratester correlation coefficients (ICCs) = 0.91 and 0.77, respectively]; however, extension ROM coefficients were much lower for the two variables (ICCs = 0.57 and 0.36, respectively). Madson et al. (28), also with asymptomatic subjects, followed a similar procedure in combining the degree and centimeter measurements. However, they found very low ICCs for both lumbar flexion and lumbar extension (ICCs = 0.67 and 0.78, respectively).

RELIABILITY CONSIDERATIONS IN ROM MEASUREMENT: *It should be noted that in estimating reliability across several trials, intraclass correlation coefficients are more stringent than Pearson coefficients (29–31). The Pearson coefficient is a bivariate statistic that is appropriate in the correlation of two different variables; however, reliability is viewed as a univariate statistic in that the comparison is between performances on the same variable (30). Moreover, the computation of a Pearson coefficient is limited to use with two variables; hence, tests with multiple trials must be averaged together to produce only two scores (30,31). The interclass correlation was limited further in that trial-to-trial variation within tests cannot be detected (31).*

However, if the intraclass correlation is used, one can analyze changes in means and standard deviations from trial to trial; moreover, intraclass correlation can be used to correlate several trials of univariate measures in determining reliability (31).

BROMS Lateral Flexion/Rotation Unit (see Fig. 2-7C). The frame of this unit houses an inclinometer in the frontal plane and a compass in the transverse plane; when either measurement is taken, the frame is positioned at the T12-L1 interspace. Lateral flexion is measured as the subject bends left or right, and the inclinometer shows the movement in degrees. The rotational measurement uses a compass to determine movement in the transverse plane. To measure the latter, it is necessary to provide a stable magnetic field to partial out the effect that hip movement can contribute to the rotation score; this is achieved with two encased magnets attached to a velcro belt secured to the subject's waist between T12 and S1.

In our research with the BROM rotation instrument in a one-tester repeated measures design with 50 male and 50 female asymptomatic individuals as subjects, very high intraclass reliability coefficients were found (ICCs = 0.98) (32). Although trunk rotation can be measured from the standing position, we found that better control can be achieved by having the subject sit on a stationary stool. Madson et al. (28) found quite satisfactory ICCs when they measured lumbar rotation (ICCs = 0.88 and 0.93 for left and right, respectively) and lumbar lateral flexion (ICCs = 0.91 and 0.95 for left and right lateral flexion, respectively). However, Breum et al. (27) found poor intra- and interexaminer reliability (ICCs = 0.57 and 0.36, respectively) when they used the same instrument for their asymptomatic subjects.

Flexible Curve (Fig. 2-8) A draftsman's flexible curve may be used to measure lumbosacral mobility in the sagittal plane. This instrument can be used to measure anterior and posterior pelvic tilt, or lumbar flexion and extension. Youdas et al. (33) used this instrument to determine sagittal mobility.

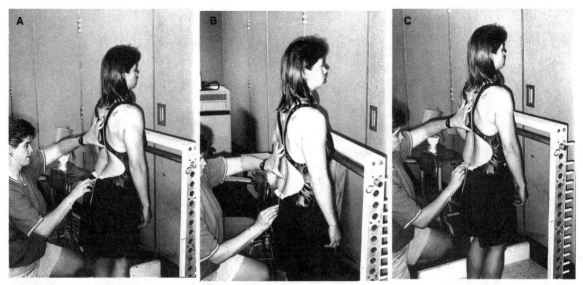

Fig. 2-8 Using a flexible curve to measure **(A)** Anterior pelvic tilt; **(B)** Neutral spine, and **(C)** Posterior pelvic tilt.

Their intratester reliability coefficients (ICCs) were 0.82 to 0.98 with the tangent method and 0.84 to 0.98 with the trigonometric method. They concluded that the tangent method is preferable to the trigonometric method for these movements because it is less time consuming. Miller et al. (25) found that a draftsman flexible rule permitted contrasting neutral spine posture with relaxed standing posture.

Alternate Techniques for Measuring Forward and Backward Bending   In our ROM research, most of the subjects in the data pool have been asymptomatic university students. These individuals did not show any particular uneasiness in assuming postures requiring forward and backward bending. However, the uneasiness that symptomatic or older subjects may experience in assuming maximum flexion or hyperextension movements can preclude getting good measurements on these individuals. If this is the case, the testing protocol delineated by Mellin et al. (34) or by Sullivan et al. (10) would be an option for subjects uncomfortable in end ROM in either standing extension or standing flexion (Fig. 2-9). Moreover, their recommendations on subject positioning could be used with all of the sagittal plane ROM techniques described in this section.

HYPEREXTENSION MOVEMENT CONSIDERATIONS: *Because hyperextension of the spine is an issue often ignored or misinterpreted, a few general comments are desirable. Spinal hyperextension is a natural movement, and it is in the best interest of the biomechanics of one's spine to maintain this mobility. However, it is acknowledged that ballistic-hyperextension movements of the spine are inappropriate; as bad, if not worse, would be ballistic rotation movements. Nevertheless, slow and controlled passive hyperextension movements are generally most appropriate for inclusion in exercise programs for those with disc symptomatology (9,35); however, active extension (as when using the Roman chair) beyond one's normal lordosis is seldom recommended (36). For individuals with posterior element symptomatology such as facet damage or spondylolisthesis, hyperextension movements would doubtfully be appropriate because extension beyond neutral could aggravate the prob-*

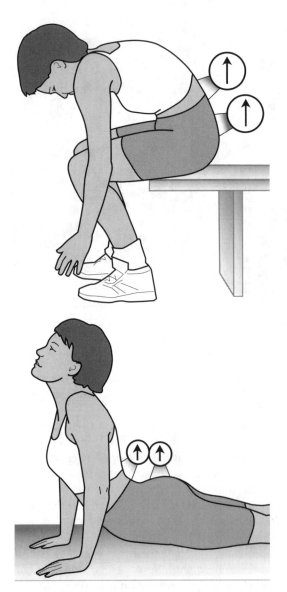

Fig. 2-9 Inclinometer measurements and most other sagittal plane range of motion measurements can be made from stable positions for those patients who have difficulty with balance.

lem and make it worse. It is important that movements such as hyperextension exercises be carefully taught because some individuals do not have a very *good kinesthetic awareness of their body parts when they do some exercises.*

In addition to the clinical back extension ROM tests previously discussed, there are simpler back extension ROM field tests; one is shown in Figure 2-10A. In this test the individual being evaluated places the hands under the shoulders as if doing a push-up. In doing the movement the pelvis must maintain contact with the floor as the individual elevates the chest with arm action. This is a passive test of spinal extension because only the arm and shoulder girdle muscles are used; the muscles of the spine should be quiescent. For readers familiar with the McKenzie back exercise protocol, the movement is comparable; however, in the latter the movements are repeated (9). Because weakness in the low back muscles is not often seen (7), an active strength test from the prone position is sometimes used (Fig. 2-10B).

Iliofemoral ROM

As stated previously, the biomechanics of the spine will be adversely affected if too much tightness in any of the muscle groups crossing the iliofemoral joint exists. The psoas muscles are typically called one-joint hip flexors, although they cross the spinal articulations from L1 to S1. Because each psoas is paired with an iliacus and their tendons of insertion run together, the collective name *iliopsoas* is frequently used, although the function of the psoas is more complex because of its attachment to mobile vertebrae.

Hip Joint Flexion ROM (Thomas Test)   The Thomas test can be used to measure tightness in the one-joint and two-joint hip flexors; the two-joint test is shown in Figure 2-11. It is important that individuals using this test are familiar with its nuances. For example, if the contralateral leg is brought too close to the chest, the posterior rotation of the pelvis incumbent in this movement may raise the ipsilateral leg. This would be an example of a false positive (i.e., a suggestion of hip flexor tightness but in reality the tightness was due to inappropriate posturing of the patient).

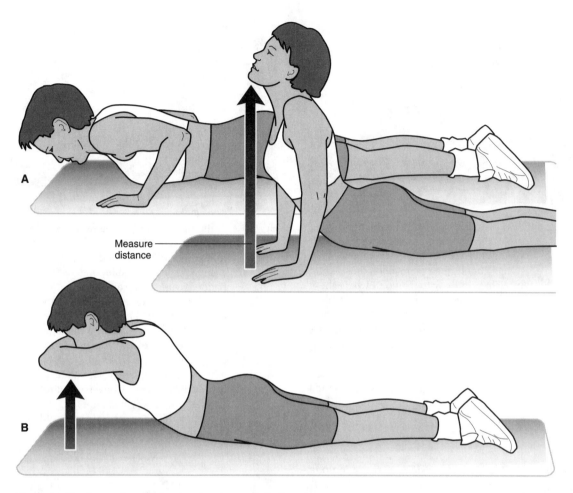

Measure distance

Fig. 2-10 Passive and active back extension range of motion.

Hip Joint Extension ROM   The straight-leg raise (SLR) has been used for a number of years. More recently, the active-knee extension test has gained in popularity. Each will be discussed in the next sections.

Straight-Leg Raise Test.   A passive straight-leg raise test is often used to measure tightness in the hamstrings. In the version of the SLR advocated by Kendall et al. (7), the starting position is one in which the individual being tested first posteriorly rotates the pelvis until the low back is snug against an *uncushioned* table or surface. The examiner

then raises one leg until tightness precludes further movement while concurrently placing a hand on the knee of the other leg to ensure that the pelvis does not rotate posteriorly and bias the results (Fig. 2-12). Although Kendall et al. stated that 80 to 85 degrees of hip flexion is normal, we believe that this may be a conservative goal for an athletic population. A drawback to this test is that all testers may not raise the leg for a given subject the same amount because of different perceptions of resistance to stretch (37). We found that, with the knee joint splinted, the active SLR presents an option to the passive SLR (38).

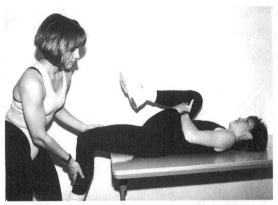

Fig. 2-11 Two-joint Thomas test. After the tester assists the patient to a supine position that permits the knee of the leg being tested to hang freely, the contralateral thigh is brought back only to the point where the low back is in firm contact with the table. Positive signs of shortness would be if the posterior thigh raised from the table surface (tight iliopsoas) or the knee straightened appreciably (tight rectus femoris). A false positive may be seen if the thigh of the contralateral leg is brought too close to the trunk and the pelvis rotates too much posteriorly.

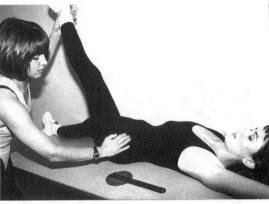

Fig. 2-12 In the passive straight-leg raise test advocated by Kendall et al. (7), the pelvis is rotated posteriorly until the low back is snug against the table (preferably unpadded); one leg is raised while ensuring that the other one remains stationary. It is essential that the patient assume the correct posture; for example, if the leg opposite to the one tested is flexed at the knee joint, a posterior rotation of the pelvis will allow a greater range of motion (approximately 10 degrees). Conversely, if rotated anteriorly (i.e., low back not in contact with the table), the movement would be restricted.

An important key in administering any of the hamstring length tests is the position of the pelvis. For example, if the hook lying starting position is assumed, the posterior rotation of the pelvis incumbent in this posture will permit the leg to be raised a few degrees farther (e.g., about 10 degrees) before tightness precludes movement. Subtleties such as this should be understood; consistency in these is essential.

Active Knee Extension Test (Fig. 2-13). The active knee extension (AKE) test has gained in popularity in recent years (37,39,40). In the starting position, both hip and knee joints are at 90 degrees, so it is also called the 90-90 test. The AKE is preferred by many testers because passive soft tissue stiffness, contractile response to stretch, and limb mass are not as apt to contaminate results as they are in the

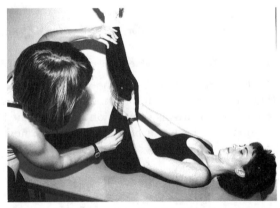

Fig. 2-13 Active knee extension (90-90 test). For the scoring scheme most typically used, complete extension has a score of 0, movement of the leg 80 degrees has a score of 10, and so forth.

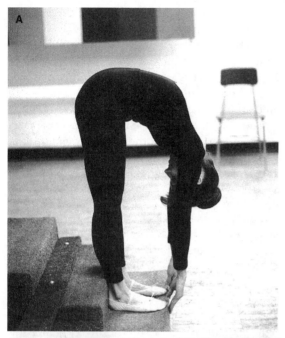

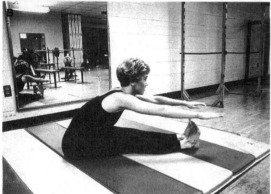

Fig. 2-14 The fingertips-to-floor (**A**) and the sit-and-reach (**B**) tests essentially measure hamstring length, but there is less pelvic movement in the sit-and-reach test.

passive SLR test (37,40). Unlike the passive SLR, with the AKE the tester does not have to estimate whether he or she is truly taking the limb to end–ROM because it is an active test and the subject is responsible for showing ROM. In the protocol described by Worrell et al. (40), individuals using this test for research purposes brace the subject's thigh of the

tested leg at 90 degrees of hip flexion, with the knee joint also at 90 degrees; the subject then extends the leg until the thigh "breaks" from this brace. Either an inclinometer or a goniometer can be used to take the measurement.

Combination Tests (Fingertips-to-Toes and Sit-and-Reach) For purposes of differentiation, tests purporting to measure both hamstring length and lumbosacral mobility are referred to as *combination tests* in this text. These include the fingertips-to-floor (FTF) and the sit-and-reach (SR); each is depicted in Fig. 2-14.

Safety Considerations. Besides questions on the validity of the FTF and the SR tests, the movement inherent in both has been questioned with respect to endangerment of the spine. For example, if either activity is done repeatedly and if the exerciser has tight hamstrings, the subject's limited excursion at the iliofemoral joint can transfer the stress to the structures of the spine (41,42). Adams and Hutton (43) showed that, when a forward bending movement of this sort occurs without muscular control (e.g., doing the fingertips to toes rapidly), the supraspinous, interspinous, and capsular ligaments are subject to sprain.

Cailliet (41) argued that, aside from the danger, as an exercise the SR will not appreciably improve hamstring length; he recommended his "protective

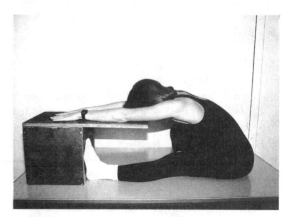

Fig. 2-15 Cailliet's protective hamstring stretch.

hamstring stretch" as a substitute (Fig. 2-15). Cailliet contended that doing such a unilateral SR stretch prevents excessive flexion and stress in the lumbosacral area. We tested Cailliet's hypothesis by using an Ady-Hall Lumbar Monitor to record LROM as 40 asymptomatic young adults (20 male and 20 female) performed Cailliet's protective hamstring stretch and the conventional SR (44). Lumbosacral flexion was greater when the subjects performed the conventional SR as opposed to Cailliet's protective hamstring stretch, although these differences were not statistically significant. Our subjects who showed a preference were more comfortable performing Cailliet's test than the SR with both legs extended. Intuitively it would appear that the posterior rotation of the pelvis incumbent in Cailliet's protective hamstring stretch should diminish the moment of inertia of the torso in forward bending; this may suggest that intradiscal pressures would be lower in the performance of Cailliet's protective hamstring stretch (one leg extended) than in the conventional SR (both legs extended concurrently).

Although the one-leg extended version of the SR would take approximately twice as long to administer as the two-leg extended version, it would permit checking for symmetry. Although asymmetry with respect to hamstring length has not been cited as increasing the likelihood of having low back problems, asymmetry with respect to hamstring length can make one susceptible to hamstring strains (45). Moreover, when posture is viewed as a kinetic chain, stretching to symmetry only makes good sense.

Validity and Reliability. Kippers and Parker (46) found that FTF distance was a good indicator of hip flexion but not of vertebral flexion in young adult subjects of both sexes. Comparable findings were noted for the SR (two legs extended) when it was administered to teen-age young women (47) and college-age women (48); we found the same results when we administered the SR (one leg extended) test to young adults of both sexes (49). Both the FTF and the SR tests can be used to measure hamstring length, particularly if the tester is familiar with nuances concerning each; furthermore, both are very reliable measures. However, neither is a good measure of low back mobility. Because the FTF is seldom used other than as part of a Schober test, this discussion will concentrate on the nuances of the SR.

The usefulness of the SR has also been challenged because disproportionate body lengths may cloud true ROM. For example, if individuals have long arms and short legs, they could be expected to do well on the SR; conversely, if their arms were short and their legs were long, they would be expected to do poorly (50). Although Wear (51) found that the excess of trunk and arm length over leg length significantly affected SR scores in college-age men, Simoneau (48) did not find this to be a factor in his study with both sexes. Hopkins and Hoeger (52) developed a test in which the reach distance is first measured with the subject's back against a wall (or other vertical surface); after this number is recorded, the individual bends forward and the second reach measure is taken. The first measure is then subtracted from the second for the net score. The net reach score is a more precise measure of hamstring length because the arm-to-leg length discrepancy is controlled.

The position of the ankles can also affect performance on the SR test, regardless of whether one or two legs are extended. In our research, we have found that asymptomatic male and female subjects could reach approximately 5 cm and 2 cm better, respectively, on the SR with the ankles in passive plantar flexion as opposed to the dorsiflexed position usually required in test administration (53) (Fig. 2-16). Gajdosik et al. (54) noted that subject performance on the SLR was significantly greater when the ankle was permitted to plantar flex passively as opposed to being fixed in dorsiflexion. These investigators attributed this difference to tightness in the fascial connections between the gastrocnemius and the hamstrings and to tension on the sciatic nerve; fascial connections in particular would also logically explain the differences that we saw.

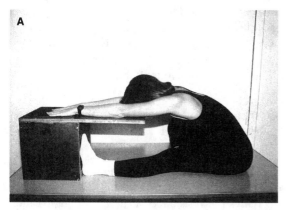

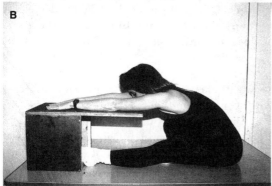

Fig. 2-16 Different sit-and-reach tests. **(A)** The sit-and-reach test with a measuring box. **(B)** In the Tennessee sit-and-reach test, there is a removable foot plate, so that the range of motion can be measured with the foot in fixed dorsiflexion and in passive plantar flexion (53).

Testers using the SR as a primary test of hamstring length should always consider the quality of the movement. One quality point to check is the angle of the sacrum. If the SR is the measurement, then the "sacral angle" should be 80 or more degrees with the floor; a book or other object with a 90-degree angle placed next to the sacrum provides a good criterion (Fig. 2-17). This angle will be less than 80 degrees in individuals with tight hamstrings. Using an inclinometer placed on the sacrum, Cornbleet and Woolsey (55) concluded

that the final position of the hip joint (i.e., sacral angle) was a better indicator of hamstring length than the position of the fingers in the SR test. Kendall et al. (7) believed that the SR could be used as a double check for the SLR measurement if sacral angle is the primary criterion of performance. Martin et al. (50) provide a comprehensive review of SR research.

Repeatability of Measurements

High correlation coefficients for trunk and hip joint ROM reliability have been reported when intratester variability was studied (56). Conversely, very low correlation coefficients have been reported when intertester variability was studied (20). In estimating reliability across several trials, as previously discussed, intraclass correlation coefficients are more stringent than Pearson coefficients and thus are preferred (31). Several different factors can adversely affect reliability of repeated measures; a few will be discussed in the next sections.

Instrument Placement   Mayer et al. (57) studied the variances seen in the measurement of sagittal

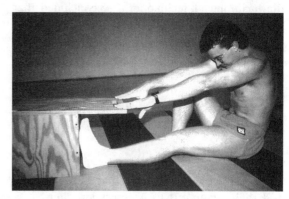

Fig. 2-17 Perhaps the most important key reference point in the sit-and-reach test is the sacral angle (not the number of centimeters reached) because it is a good indicator of hamstring length. This subject demonstrates tight or shortened hamstrings; his sacral angle is only 60–70 degrees.

spine ROM across examiners, subjects, and instruments. The instruments that they used were the fluid inclinometer, kyphometer, and the electronic inclinometer. In their complex analysis, they isolated variance due to subject inconsistency, differences among instruments, and interrater and intrarater reliabilities. They concluded that the cause of error in determining a subject's ROM was more often due to differences in the tester's placement of the instrument on the subject (e.g., variability in locating bony landmarks) rather than in the instrumentation per se.

Diurnal Variation   Diurnal variation is also a factor that should be considered when taking repeated measurements of flexibility. Ensink et al. (15) found that measurement repeatability often depended on the test. In other words, some testing protocols are more affected than others by diurnal variation. For example, these researchers found that mean flexion LROM increased more than 10 degrees from morning to evening when using an inclinometer technique. The same investigators noted that LROM as measured by the modified Schober technique also increased significantly. However, because the change was not as great as that noted when using the inclinometer technique, they concluded that the skin distraction techniques were not as valid as their inclinometer ones. It would appear that, despite the protocol used to measure LROM, the time of the day that measurements are taken must be considered and that diurnal variation affects some testing protocols more than it does others.

IMPROVING ROM

To move body segments, the antagonistic muscles and their tendinous tissue must lengthen sufficiently. Shortened, or tight, musculature refers to the entire musculotendinous unit, not just to the contractile elements. Because of reciprocal inhibition, the contractile elements of the antagonist muscle group typically relax as the agonist muscle group actively contracts. Therefore, it is usually the series elastic components of tendons (the tendon

proper being the foremost) and then the parallel elastic components (i.e., epimysium, perimysium, and endomysium connective tissue sheaths that enclose individual muscle fibers or groups of muscle fibers) that preclude ROM.

Neurologic and Mechanical Aspects of Improving ROM

Although ROM can be improved by increasing the strength of the antagonistic muscle or group of muscles, more often a strategy is chosen that decreases the resistance of the target (tight) musculature. The latter can be done by (a) decreasing its contractile activity and (b) increasing the length of its connective tissue. Each of these topics will now be discussed.

Muscle Relaxation   When a muscle such as a flexor contracts and causes a movement on one side of a joint, reciprocal inhibition typically causes a relaxation in its extensor antagonist. In such a scenario, reciprocal inhibition not only eases the action of the agonist but also decreases the chance of injury to the antagonist. Conversely, if a muscle is stretched quickly, the antagonist muscle contracts to resist rapid lengthening; thus, it provides a protective mechanism against overstretching. This phenomenon, which can oppose or reduce the desired stretch in dynamic and ballistic flexibility exercises, is the myotatic or stretch reflex. The proprioceptor responsible for the stretch reflex is the muscle spindle. The muscle spindle, its different sensory endings, its afferent and efferent component parts, and its relationship to the entire muscle, are delineated in Fig. 2–18.

Connective Tissue Lengthening   Assuming the contractile elements of the target muscle are relaxed, the tendon and its associated connective tissue are the major deterrents to good ROM. Tendons and all biologic tissue show viscoelastic behavior (58). Before elaborating on techniques of connective tissue lengthening, a brief discussion on viscoelasticity and the mechanics of length change in a tendon is presented.

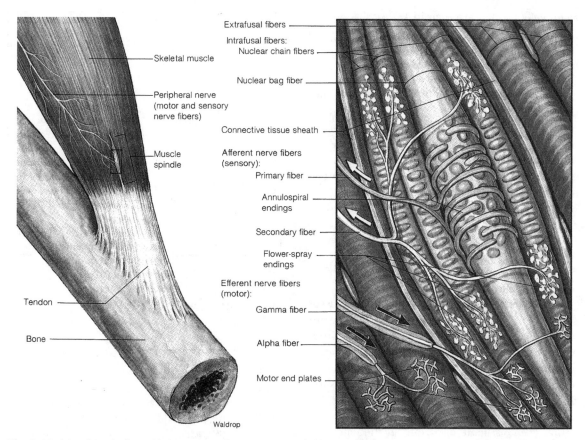

Fig. 2-18 Muscle spindle, with its component parts, namely the annulospiral and flower spray endings. (From Fox, SI. *Human Physiology.* © 1999. Reprinted with permission from the McGraw-Hill Companies, Inc.)

Viscoelasticity. Viscoelasticity may be defined as the time-dependent characteristic of a material displayed as it reacts to an outside force (e.g., tension) (58,59). A rubber band behaves in a manner analogous to the viscoelasticity displayed by the connective tissue of a tendon. A moderate stretching stress increases its "stiffness" and, assuming the stress is neither maintained long enough nor of sufficient magnitude to damage it, the elasticity of the rubber band will enable it to return to its resting length once the stretching stress ceases. However, if the same rubber band were slowly stretched two to three times its resting length, placed stretched around an object and then kept in that position for

an extended period, its length would be permanently increased because its molecular make-up would change. In other words, its viscous (plastic) characteristics have been changed.

In tendinous tissue the elastic property permits recoverable springlike behavior and allows the musculotendinous unit to return to its original length after a brief and nonsustained stretch. Because the tissue is returned to its normal ROM, moderate dynamic activities would typically not be expected to affect ROM. Moreover, in sporting activity, elastic energy as described is often harnessed by forcibly stretching a musculotendinous unit just before maximal muscle contraction;

examples of its use are seen in (a) the back swing just before striking a ball and (b) crouching just before jumping for height. Elastic energy is a major factor in eccentric and plyometric exercises.

By convention, applied force on a tissue (per unit area) is called *stress*, and the resulting deformation is called *strain* (5,12,58,59). When tissues are strained longitudinally, the stress is called *tension*; other stresses to which tissues might be subjected include compression, shear, and torsion. The stress-strain curve of collagen (a major constituent of tendinous material) is presented in Figure 2-19. At rest, collagen fibers are typically convoluted or crimped; when some tensile-stress of short duration (e.g., <1 s) is applied to collagen, the crimp straightens. During this process, no chemical bonds are broken; when the tension is released, the crimp returns as the tissue shows its elasticity.

The viscoelastic nature of connective tissue causes it to react to different stresses in specific ways; how it reacts is dependent on the magnitude and duration of the stress. For example, a tendon would display elasticity coupled with stiffness (i.e., a resistance to deformation) to high force, short duration stretching. However, low force, long duration stretching can enhance permanent elongation (i.e., plastic deformation). If the tendinous tissue is overloaded into its linear phase and stretched 4 to 6% beyond its resting length, macro-failure or rupture could logically occur (60). If lengthening through plastic deformation is the goal, then the strain must result in a controlled debonding of the molecular make-up of the tendinous material; one way to achieve this is by placing the tissue on a low stress of long duration.

The viscoelastic behavior of biologic materials is often depicted by the spring-dashpot model from engineering; one such model is depicted in Figure 2-20. The spring represents the ability of elastic materials to reverse themselves to their original length (e.g., as with the rubber band). The dashpot is analogous to a hydraulic piston; however, in biologic tissues such as a tendon, it represents the displacement of intracellular viscous fluids that provide the resistance to movement. Similar types of resistance behavior are exemplified in the

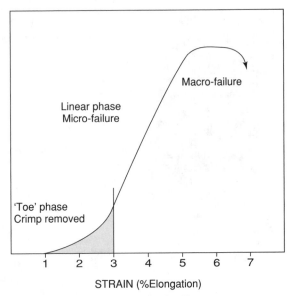

STRAIN (%Elongation)

Fig. 2-19 Stress-strain curve of collagen.

action of a syringe, a hydraulic door closer, and in certain accommodating resistance training equipment that uses hydraulic principles as its basis. In these examples, the size of the orifice through which the hydraulic fluid passes governs the speed or ease with which the resistance can be moved;

MODEL

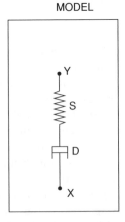

Fig. 2-20 The dashpot-spring model represents the viscoelastic nature of connective tissue such as tendon.

this explains why quick movements are much more difficult than slow ones. Similarly, lengthening connective tissue with a low force of long duration is easier than lengthening with high force of short duration; this time-dependent property of connective tissue is an example of its viscoelasticity.

Stress Relaxation and Creep   If tendinous (or any viscoelastic) material is stretched safely below its linear phase (see Fig. 2-19) and then held at its new length, the stress (i.e., force per area) required to hold it at that length diminishes; this reduction in stretching force needed is called *stress relaxation* (58,59,61). This decline in tension takes place because of the changes in the tendon's viscoelastic structure that occur with each stretch as it lengthens.

In addition to stress relaxation, creep is phenomenon associated with the lengthening of connective tissue. In a creep test, the stress is kept constant but below the linear region of the stress-strain curve (12,58). For example, a creep response in the facet joints of the lumbar spine occurs if prolonged loading in flexion exceeds 10 min or more (58). A creep response may occur in certain occupational groups such as brick-layers, factory workers at a conveyor belt, and typists; all these individuals are susceptible to "creep" in flexion. Another example of creep would be in the slight diminishment in height from getting up in the morning to retiring in the evening; in this example, however, creep is temporary and height is regained while recumbent (5).

Stretching Regimens

The general categories of ROM, or flexibility, improvement regimens include the traditional types of stretching exercises, namely dynamic stretching, static stretching (SS), and proprioceptive neuromuscular facilitation (PNF) techniques. In recent years, some newer techniques have come on the scene. They draw primarily from SS and PNF techniques.

Dynamic Stretching   These techniques are sometimes referred to as *dynamic-ballistic stretching*. These

protocols were once very popular. Although research has suggested that they are as effective as SS in improving ROM (62), there is now perceived to be a greater chance of injury in their use, especially if movements are ballistic and exceed end ROM. It should be understood that some dynamic exercises do not require ballistic elements and thus may never exceed the elastic stretch phase; therefore, each exercise should be judged on its own merit. However, although ballistic stretching activities may have the potential to improve both active and passive ROM, because of concern for injury their use is limited primarily to an adjunct in the training of competitive athletes for sports that have ballistic elements (e.g., those seen in jumping and throwing events).

Static Stretching   Static stretching is probably the most often used ROM improvement regimen. In SS the target muscle is typically lengthened to the point of slight discomfort by increasing the distance between the muscle's origin and insertion; when this point is reached, the position is usually held 10 to 30 s or more and then repeated at least two to three times per exercise session.

Static stretching can be effective in improving and maintaining ROM; it is usually contended that it seldom results in injury or causes muscle soreness (63), although soreness has been reported (64). Although SS regimens have been effective in increasing musculotendinous length through plastic deformation (61), significant improvements are not always seen (65).

How long should static stretches be held? The research is quite equivocal on the exact length of static stretch that should be taken. Although stretches of 10 to 20 s are common, stretching periods from 30 to 60 s have been recommended (66). However, in SS research with animal models, it was found that the stress relaxation occurring in the first 12 to 16 s of stretch was significantly greater than that occurring after this time (58); the same researchers reported that the greatest changes occurred in the first four stretches. Although Taylor et al. (58) found that the most stress relaxation occurred in the first

15 s, Magnusson et al. (67) found that stress relaxation may occur up to 45 s. In those studies that contrasted SS with PNF training, most individual stretches were held for less than 15 s and the stress relaxation that occurred was not measured.

Proprioceptive Neuromuscular Facilitation Unfortunately, the terms and acronyms used in describing PNF exercises lack standardization. For example, some may use the term *reversals* to describe a technique in which the target muscle (i.e., the muscle deemed short) is contracted and then relaxed just before the contraction of its antagonist starts; however, the ordering of agonist or antagonist contraction and relaxation could be altered, but action might still be called *reversals*. Because the terms used by Moore and Hutton (63) may be those most reported in the research literature, they are used in the chapter; their PNF terms are *contract relax* (CR) and *contract-relax agonist-contract* (CRAC).

Research on SS and PNF Stretching Techniques

The efficacy of the different PNF and SS techniques appears equivocal; in part this is due to the variance in terminology and protocols used in the research conducted in this area. Etynre and Lee (65) and Etynre and Abraham (68) found that those PNF protocols that include active contraction of the agonist (e.g., the CRAC technique) appear to produce better results than either the CR or the SS protocols; they attributed the difference to a greater degree of reciprocal and autogenic inhibition.

Contraction of the target muscle before its lengthening theoretically enhances autogenic inhibition; the CR and the CRAC techniques both provide this inhibition. However, after contracting the target muscle in CRAC protocols, the subject actively contracts the target muscle's antagonist and moves the limb to active end ROM. When the latter point is reached, the therapist or trainer moves the limb to passive end ROM. Conversely, in the CR technique, there is no active contraction of the antagonist, and the entire movement is passive

and is directed by the therapist or trainer. In the CRAC technique, contracting the agonist during the stretching of the target muscle is theoretically enhanced because of reciprocal inhibition; this aspect is not present in either the SS or CR technique. It is also possible that the stretching regimens that included only passive stretching might cause an increase of the active inadequacy zone (i.e., the difference between passive and active ROM). Such an increase could theoretically make the individual more susceptible to joint injury because less muscle control is available during the movement.

Role of Reciprocal/Autogenic Inhibition Some research done in this area reports that PNF CRAC training produces at least as good, if not better, results than PNF CR training and that PNF CR training produces at least as good, if not better, results than SS training (68). Nevertheless, questions have been raised concerning autogenic inhibition in both SS and PNF training. Moore and Hutton (63) found that, although their subjects who participated in PNF CRAC training experienced the greatest ROM increases in hip flexion, this group also had more hamstring electromyographic (EMG) activity than did either the SS or the PNF CR group. Subsequently, other researchers, using a different protocol, found that PNF training following a modified CRAC protocol generated about twice the EMG activity in the hamstrings as the SS and PNF CR groups (69). Somewhat paradoxically, the subjects following the PNF CRAC technique produced 9 to 13% greater extension ROM gains than did the subjects following the other techniques. Etynre and Lee (65) contended that the EMG activity seen in the target musculature by some researchers may have resulted from intermuscle cross talk that would not be manifest if needle electrodes rather than surface electrodes had been used. However, research by Taylor et al. (58) suggests that a muscle's adaptation to a stretching regimen is not influenced much by reflex effects because denervation did not affect results in their investigation.

Sullivan et al. (70) compared a slight modification of the PNF CRAC training protocol (a second contraction of the target muscle group was included, which theoretically provided a greater degree of autogenic inhibition) with SS training. In their protocol they (a) examined the effect of pelvic positioning (i.e., anterior pelvic tilt versus posterior pelvic tilt) and (b) had one limb participate in static stretching and the contralateral limb in PNF CRAC training. They found that the anterior pelvic tilt position was more important than either stretching technique for increasing hamstring muscle length. This finding suggests that the anterior pelvic tilt position may have placed more tension on the musculotendinous unit and that the type of training was unimportant. However, Grady and Saxena (71) found that training paradigms such as this can produce training effects in the contralateral limb serving as the control; thus, in the study by Sullivan et al. (70), neural learning may have contaminated the findings.

Other ROM Improvement Programs As stated previously, there are other stretching programs that have used aspects of the dynamic/ballistic, SS, or PNF programs. These programs will now be discussed; however, it must be stressed that very little research has been reported on these programs.

Nonballistic Active Knee Extension. Webright et al. (39) compared the effect of nonballistic AKE with that of SS on hamstring flexibility in healthy university students; the dependent variable was performance on the AKE test. In their study, 40 subjects were randomly assigned to a nonballistic training group, an SS training group, or a control group. The AKE group performed 30 AKE repetitions from the neural slump position daily, and the SS group performed a 30-s stretch twice daily from a modified hurdler's stretch position while attempting to maintain a neutral spine. At the end of 6 weeks of training, both the AKE and the SS groups improved significantly over the control group. Although greater gains were made by those in the AKE group, the differences were not statistically significant. From a time efficiency perspective, the SS regimen required less than 25% of the time required for the AKE regimen.

Dynamic Range of Motion Training (DROM). Bandy et al. (72) stated that the originators of this training speculated that this technique enhances reciprocal inhibition and more closely simulates movement. In DROM training, a slow contraction of the muscle antagonistic to the target muscle is made (e.g., 4 to 5 s for an active SLR movement from the supine position, with the hip and knee joints at 90 degrees) until active end ROM is reached; then the limb is slowly returned (also 4 to 5 s) to the neutral position with eccentric contraction (72). Their 60 subjects performed five repetitions of this exercise (i.e., 30 s of stretching), a 30-s static stretch, or were in a control group. The experimental groups trained 5 days each week for 6 weeks. Both experimental groups increased their ROM, but the SS group's 11.5-degree mean increase was more than double the increase experienced by the DROM group.

Active Isolated Stretching. In part in an attempt to avert the stretch reflex contraction in target muscle during PNF training, as noted by Moore and Hutton (63) and Osternig et al. (69), a form of stretching called active isolated stretching (AIS) was devised (73). Active isolated stretching has similarities to the DROM training with regard to hamstring lengthening (72). However, AIS differs from DROM in that, after end ROM is reached, the subject pulls the leg (by means of a rope looped around the foot) to the point of light irritation; this position is then held for up to 2 s (73). In this technique, as discussed by Mattes (73), active contraction of the antagonist to the target musculature is performed slowly to active end ROM, and then the limb is moved farther passively to end ROM and held in this position for only 1 to 2 s (Fig. 2-21). Mattes (73) contended that this technique uses reciprocal inhibition as the limb is actively moved to end ROM. If the passive end–ROM that follows this is held no more than 2 s, Mattes purports that the reflex contraction often resulting when a muscle is stretched will not occur (61,69). His rationale is that, if the passive end ROM position is held only for 2 s or less, the threshold of the

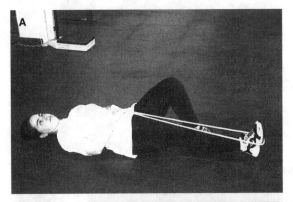

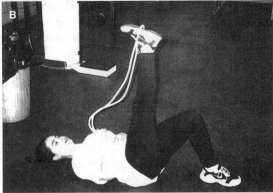

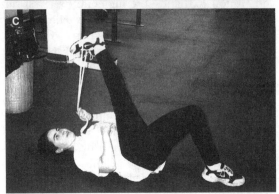

Fig. 2-21 Active isolated stretching. To use this form of stretching for the hamstrings, with one knee bent a rope is looped around the foot of the extended leg (**A**). This leg is slowly raised to end range of motion (**B**); after this point is reached, the patient pulls with the rope until passive end range of motion is reached and holds this position for only 1 to 2 s (**C**). The leg is returned to the starting position, and then the procedure is repeated 9 to 11 times at 2-s intervals.

flower spray ending of the muscle spindle will not be reached.

We attempted to determine whether AIS was as effective as SS in improving hip joint extension ROM in the nondominant leg in normally active male and female university students (38). Subjects were stratified randomly and 10 each (five men and five women) were assigned to the SS, AIS, or control group. An active SLR was the dependent measure, and subjects participated in a nine-treatment session protocol over a 3-week period. The AIS group performed 15 repetitions of this exercise in each training period, and the SS group performed one 30-s stretch in each training period by following the protocol used by Sullivan et al. (70). Both training groups significantly improved their flexibility from pretest to posttest; post hoc analysis showed that the AIS group improved significantly more than the SS group. At face value, the training differences seen were quite convincing, but these results must be qualified by the fact that the morphology of the SLR test used as the dependent variable had similarities to the AIS training.

Clinical Relevance Increases in ROM can be attained through several different training programs if the technique induces stress relaxation. Stress relaxation seems to depend on how much tension can be generated in the training, which can be affected by several variables. Neither time-dependent stress relaxation nor creep could be responsible for any gain in ROM with ballistic stretching techniques because the movement is too quick for tissue fluid movement at the cellular level. Thus, if increases in ROM are found after ballistic training regimens, these increases may be due to strain extending into the linear phase (see Fig. 2-19). In other words, a microtrauma of insufficient magnitude to preclude compensatory adaptation may be responsible for the increase in ROM.

Ballistic ROM programs incorporate both concentric and eccentric contractions. However, eccentric contraction could be used in regimens that do not incorporate ballistic movement. Because eccentric contraction can place more tension on the musculotendinous unit, this type of training could have potential for the improvement of ROM, but it has not been adequately researched.

Because ballistic training cannot be recommended for improving ROM, ramifications of the SS and PNF techniques may be the best options. Although either the SS or PNF technique can be effective, their effectiveness may be more dependent on the quality of the training regimen than on the specific technique employed, as suggested by the research of Sullivan et al. (70). However, the issue may even be more complex. According to Halbertsma and Goeken (74), an increase in hamstring extensibility can be achieved by either a change in the stiffness of the muscles or an increase in pain (or stretch) tolerance. Their testing protocol included determinations of the muscle moment of the hamstrings (e.g., resistance). As the leg was mechanically raised in their stretching protocol, subjects intervened when the stretch-pain reached a point at which the subjects were too uncomfortable. The maximum moment that could be applied markedly increased in trained subjects; however, they attributed this increased tolerance to an increase in stretch (pain) tolerance (75).

General ROM Considerations

For best results, stretching exercises should be done daily. Although stretching during the warm-up phase of an exercise bout is usually thought to be important, the temperature of the muscle and connective tissue should be considered. For example, if lengthening connective tissue is the objective, then it is most important that the temperature of this tissue be raised sufficiently before subjecting it to extreme demands despite the stretching regimen to be employed. However, if the planned activity is nothing more than a jog or a run, a stretching regimen may not be necessary, and the warm-up may be limited to the activity itself. Because connective tissue temperature should be elevated at the end of the work-out, this would be a most appropriate time to work on improvement in ROM.

For limb stretching, a unilateral stretching regimen is advocated for the lower extremities in particular. If the body is thought of as a "biomechanical chain," any asymmetry between functional units can obligate both superior and inferior joints to make compensatory adjustments. These adjustments will affect the biomechanics of the joint (or joints), and they may result in uneven wear of articular surfaces and potentially exacerbate the extant problem. If such adjustments lead to uneven wear on paired facet joints, it could lead to problems at this site.

CONCLUSIONS

When low back problems are the consideration, ROM measurements can play critical roles in prevention, diagnosis, and rehabilitation. Even though most of the measurement protocols discussed are valid, if the individual taking the measurements is not skilled in their use, any given technique can be worthless. Therefore, it is imperative that anyone using a test be familiar with its nuances and understand its limitations. Because variance in testing results can be a function of locating bony landmarks (57) and diurnal variation (15), these factors also should be considered when reevaluations are done.

There are many variations in the techniques that can be used to improve scores on ROM tests. What is less clear is the reason some techniques work more for some individuals than they do for others. More research is needed to determine what happens at the tissue level. Also unclear is the role that stretch (pain) tolerance plays in ROM score improvement.

REFERENCES

1. Biering-Sorensen, F. Physical measurements as risk indicators for low-back trouble over a one-year period. *Spine* 1984, 9(2): p. 106–119.
2. Cady, L.D., Bischoff, D.P., O'Connell, E.R., et al. Strength and fitness and subsequent back injuries in firefighters. *J Occup Med* 1979, 21(4): p. 269–272.
3. Mellin, G. Correlations of hip mobility with degree of back pain and lumbar spinal mobility in chronic low-back pain patients. *Spine* 1988, 13: p. 668.
4. Lindh, M. Biomechanics of the lumbar spine, in *Biomechanics of the Musculoskeletal System*,

M. Nordin, and V.H. Frankel, editors. 1989, Lea & Febiger: Philadelphia. p. 183–207.

5. White, A.A., and M.M. Panjabi. *Clinical Biomechanics of the Spine,* 2nd ed. 1990, Philadelphia: Williams & Wilkins. p. 722.

6. Bogduk, N. *Clinical Anatomy of the Lumbar Spine and Sacrum.* 3rd ed. 1998, London: Churchill Livingstone. p. 261.

7. Kendall, F.P., McCreary, E.K., Provance, P.G. *Muscle Testing and Function.* 1993, Baltimore: Williams & Wilkins.

8. Feldman, D., Shrier, I., Rossignol, M., et al. Adolescent growth is not associated with changes in flexibility. *Clin J Sport Med* 1999, 9(1): p. 24–29.

9. McKenzie, R. *The Lumbar Spine-Mechanical Diagnosis and Therapy.* 1981, Waikanae, New Zealand: Spinal Publications. p. 164.

10. Sullivan, M.S., Dickinson, C.E., Troup, J.D.G. The influence of age and gender on lumbar spine sagittal plane range of motion-a study of 1126 healthy subjects. *Spine* 1994, 19(6): p. 682–686.

11. Hasten, D.L., Lea, R.D., Johnston, F.A. Lumbar range of motion in male heavy laborers on the Applied Rehabilitation Concepts (ARCON) system. *Spine* 1996, 21(19): p. 2230–2234.

12. Twomey, L., and J. Taylor. Flexion creep deformation and hysteresis in the lumbar vertebral column. *Spine* 1982, 7: p. 116–122.

13. McGregor, A.H., McCarthy, I.D., Hughes, S.P. Motion characteristics of the lumbar spine in the normal population. *Spine* 1995, 20(22): p. 2421–2428.

14. Youdas, J.W., Garrett, T.R., Harmson, S. Lumbar lordosis and pelvic inclination of asymptomatic adults. *Phys Ther* 1996, 76(10): p. 1066–1081.

15. Ensink, B.B.M., Saur, P.M.M., Frese, K., et al. Lumbar range of motion: influence of time of day and individual factors on measurements. *Spine* 1996, 21(11): p. 1339–1343.

16. Buchalter, D., Parnianpour, M., Viola, K., et al. Three-dimensional spinal motion measurements. Part 1: a technique for examining posture and functional spinal motion. *J Spinal Disord* 1989, 1: p. 279–283.

17. Fitzgerald, G.K., Wynveen, G.K., Rheault, W., et al. Objective assessment with establishment

of normal values for lumbar spinal range of motion. *Phys Ther* 1983, 63: p. 1776–1781.

18. Twomey, L.T., and J.R. Taylor. Lumbar posture, movement and mechanisms, in *Physical therapy of the low back,* L.T. Twomey and J. Taylor, editors. 1987, New York: Churchill Livingstone. p. 51–84.

19. MacRae, I., and V. Wright. Measurement of back movement. *Ann Rheum Dis* 1969, 28: p. 584.

20. Williams, R., Binkley, J., Bloch, R., et al. Reliability of the modified-modified Schober and double inclinometer methods for measuring lumbar flexion and extension. *Phys Ther* 1993, 73: p. 26.

21. Mayer, T.G., Tencer, A.F., Kristoferson, S., et al. Use of noninvasive techniques for quantification of spinal range-of-motion in normal subjects and chronic low-back dysfunction patients. *Spine* 1984, 9: p. 588–595.

22. Dubravica, M., Liemohn W., Martin, S. *Pouzdanost izabranih nacina ispitivanja opsega kretnji u lumbalnoj kraljesnici medu ispitivacima.* Fiz Med Rehabil 1994, 11(3).

23. Mayer, T.G., and R.J. Gatchel. *Functional Restoration for Spinal Disorders: The Sports Medicine Approach.* 1988, Philadelphia: Lea & Febiger. p. 321.

24. Keeley, J., Mayer, T.G., Cox, R., et al. Quantification of lumbar function-part 5: reliability of range-of-motion measures in the sagittal plane and an in vivo torso rotation measurement technique. *Spine* 1986, 11: p. 31–35.

25. Miller, M.A., Liemohn, W., Haydu, T., et al. A biomechanical analysis of pelvic tilt control and trunk muscle activity during isometric and dynamic lifting, *J Athletic Training* 2000, 35(2) Suppl., p. 32.

26. Saur, P.M., Ensink, F.B., Frese, K., et al. Lumbar range of motion: reliability and validity of the inclinometer technique in the clinical measurement of trunk flexibility. *Spine* 1996, 21(11): p. 1332–1338.

27. Breum, J., Wiberg, J., Bolton, J.E. Reliability and concurrent validity of the BROM II for measuring lumbar mobility. *J Manipul Physiol Ther* 1995, 18(8): p. 497–502.

28. Madson, T.J., Youdas, J.W., Suman, V.J. Reproducibility of lumbar spine range of motion

measurements using the back range of motion device. *J Orthop Sports Phys Ther* 1999, 29(8): p. 470–477.

29. Salisbury, P.J., and R.W. Porter. Measurement of lumbar sagittal mobility: a comparison of methods. *Spine* 1987, 12: p. 190–193.

30. Thomas, J.R., and J.K. Nelson. *Research Methods in Physical Activity.* 1990, Champaign, IL: Human Kinetics.

31. Baumgartner, T.A. Estimating reliability when all test trials are administered on the same day. *Res Q,* 1969. 40(1): p. 222–225.

32. Liemohn, W., and B. Moore. Measurement of lumbar rotation range of motion. *Med Sci Exerc Sport* 1997, 29(5): p. S166.

33. Youdas, J.W., Suman, V.J., Garrett, T.R. Reliability of measurements of lumbar spine sagittal mobility obtained with the flexible curve. *J Orthop Sports Phys Ther* 1995, 21(1): p. 13–20.

34. Mellin, G., Kiiski, R., Weckstrom, A. Effects of subject position on measurements of flexion, extension, and lateral flexion of the spine. *Spine* 1991, 16: p. 1108.

35. Donelson, R. The McKenzie method, in *Conservative Care of Low Back Pain*, A.H. White and R. Anderson, editors. 1991, Baltimore: Williams & Wilkins. p. 97–104.

36. Saal, J.S., and J.A. Saal. Strength training and flexibility, in *Conservative Care of Low Back Pain*, A.H. White and R. Anderson, editors. 1991, Baltimore: Williams & Wilkins. p. 65–77.

37. Gajdosik, R., and C. Lusin. Hamstring muscle tightness: reliability of an active knee extension test. *Phys Ther* 1983, 63: p. 1085.

38. Liemohn, W., Mazis, N., Zhang, S. Effect of active isolated and static stretch training on active straight leg raise performance. *Med Sci Sports Exerc* 1999, 31(5): p. S116.

39. Webright, W.G., Randolph, P.J., Perrin, D.H. Comparison of nonballistic active knee extension in neural slump position and static stretch techniques on hamstring flexibility. *J Orthop Sports Phys Ther* 1997, 26(1): p. 7–13.

40. Worrell, T.W., Sullivan, M.K., DeJulia, J.J. Reliability of an active-knee-extension test for determining hamstring muscle flexibility. *J Sport Rehabil* 1992, 1: p. 181–187.

41. Cailliet, R. *Low Back Pain Syndrome.* 1988, Philadelphia: F.A. Davis Co.

42. Nachemson, A.L. The lumbar spine-an orthopaedic challenge. *Spine* 1976, 1: p. 59–71.

43. Adams, M.A., and W.C. Hutton, The mechanical function of the lumbar apophyseal joints. *Spine* 1983, 8: p. 327–330.

44. Liemohn, W., Sharpe, D.L., Wasserman, J.F. Lumbosacral movement in the sit-and-reach and in Cailliet's protective-hamstring stretch. *Spine* 1994, 19: p. 2127– 2130.

45. Liemohn, W. Factors related to hamstring strains. *J Sports Med* 1978, 18: p. 71–76.

46. Kippers, V., and A.W. Parker. Toe-touch test-a measure of its validity. *Phys Ther* 1987, 67: p. 1680.

47. Jackson, A.W., and A.A. Baker. The relationship of the sit and reach test to criterion measures of hamstring and back flexibility in young females. *Res Q Exerc Sport* 1986, 57: p. 183–186.

48. Simoneau, G.G. The impact of various anthropometric and flexibility measurements on the sit-and-reach test. *J Strength Cond Res* 1998, 12(4): p. 232–237.

49. Liemohn, W., Sharp, G., Wasserman, J. Criterion-related validity of the sit-and-reach test. *J Strength Cond Res* 1994, 8: p. 91–94.

50. Martin, S.B., Jackson, A.W., Morrow, J.R., et al. The rationale for the sit and reach test revisited. *Measure Phys Educ Exerc Sci* 1998, 2(2): p. 85–92.

51. Wear, C.L. Relationship of flexibility measurements to length of body segments. *Res Q* 1963, 34: p. 234–238.

52. Hopkins, D.R., and W.W.K. Hoeger. A comparison of the sit-and-reach test and the modified sit-and-reach test in the measurement of flexibility for males. *J Appl Sport Sci Res* 1992, 6: p. 7–10.

53. Liemohn, W., Martin, S.B., Pariser, G. The effect of ankle posture on sit-and-reach test performance in young adults. *J Strength Cond Res* 1997, 11: p. 239–241.

54. Gajdosik, R.L., LeVeau, B.F., Bohannon, R.W. Effects of ankle dorsiflexion on active and passive unilateral straight leg raising. *Phys Ther* 1985, 65: p. 1478–1482.

55. Cornbleet, S.L., and N.B. Woolsey. Assessment of hamstring muscle length in school-aged children using the sit-and-reach test and the inclinometer measure of hip joint angle. *Phys Ther* 1996, 76(8): p. 850–855.

56. Boline, P.D., Keating, J.C., Haas, M., et al. Interexaminer reliability and discriminant validity of inclinometric measurement of lumbar rotation in chronic low-back pain patients and subjects without low-back pain. *Spine* 1992, 17(3): p. 335–338.

57. Mayer, R.S., Chen, I.H., Lavender, S.A., et al. Variance in the measurement of sagittal lumbar spine range of motion among examiners, subjects, and instruments. *Spine* 1995, 20(13): p. 1489–1493.

58. Taylor, D.C., Dalton, J.D., Seaber, A.V., et al. Viscoelastic properties of muscle-tendon: the biomechanical effects of stretching. *Am J Sports Med* 1990, 18: p. 300–309.

59. McHugh, M.P., Magnusson, S.P., Gleim, G.W., et al. Viscoelastic stress relaxation in human skeletal muscle. *Med Sci Sports Exerc* 1992, 24: p. 1375–1382.

60. Carlstedt, C.A., and M. Nordin. Biomechanics of tendon and ligaments, in *Basic Biomechanics of the Musculoskeletal System*, M. Nordin and V.H. Frankel, editors. 1989, Philadelphia: Lea & Febiger. p. 59–74.

61. Gajdoski, R.L. Effects of static stretching on the maximal length and resistance to passive stretch of short hamstrings. *J Orthop Sport Phys Ther* 1991, 14: p. 250–255.

62. deVries, H. Evaluation of static stretching procedures for improvement of flexibility. *Res Q Exerc Sport* 1962, 33: p. 222.

63. Moore, M.A., and R.S. Hutton. Electromyographic investigation of muscle stretching techniques. *Med Sci Sports Exerc* 1980, 12: p. 322.

64. Smith, L.L., Brunetz, M.H., Chenier, T.C., et al. The effects of static and ballistic stretching on delayed onset muscle soreness and creatine kinase. *Res Q Exerc Sport* 1993, 64(1): p. 103–107.

65. Etynre, B.R., and J.L. Lee. Chronic and acute flexibility of men and women using three different stretching techniques. *Res Q Exerc Sport* 1988, 59: p. 222–228.

66. Bandy, W.D., and J.M. Irion. The effect of time on static stretch on the flexibility of the hamstring muscles. *Phys Ther* 1994, 74(9): p. 845–852.

67. Magnusson, S.P., Simonsen, E.B., Aagaard, P., et al. Viscoelastic response to repeated static stretching in the human hamstring muscle. *Scand J Med Sci Sports* 1995, 5: p. 342–347.

68. Etynre, B.R., and L.D. Abraham. Antagonistic muscle activity during stretching: a paradox reassessed. *Med Sci Sports Exerc* 1988, 20(3): p. 285–289.

69. Osternig, L.R., Robertson, R.N., Troxel, R.K., et al. Differential responses to proprioceptive neuromuscular facilitation (PNF) stretch techniques. *Med Sci Sports Exerc* 1990, 22(1): p. 106.

70. Sullivan, M.K., DeJulia, J.J., Worrell, T.W. Effect of pelvic position and stretching method on hamstring muscle flexibility. *Med Sci Sports Exerc* 1992, 24: p. 1383.

71. Grady, J.F., and A. Saxena. Effects of stretching the gastrocnemius. *J Foot Surg* 1991, 30(5): p. 465–469.

72. Bandy, W.D., Irion, J.M., Briggler, M. The effect of static stretch and dynamic range of motion training on the flexibility of the hamstring muscles. *J Orthop Sports Phys Ther* 1998, 27(4): p. 295–300.

73. Mattes, A.L. *Active Isolated Stretching*. 1995, Sarasota, FL: Aaron L. Mattes.

74. Halbertsma, J.P.K., and L.N.H. Goeken. Stretching exercises: effect on passive extensibility and stiffness in short hamstrings of healthy subjects. *Arch Phys Med Rehabil* 1994, 75: p. 976–981.

75. Halbertsma, J.P.K., von Belhuis, A.K., Goeken, L.N.H. Sport stretching: effect on passive muscle stiffness of short hamstrings. *Arch Phys Med Rehabil* 1996, 77: p. 688–692.

PART II

EPIDEMIOLOGY AND DIAGNOSIS

CHAPTER 3

FUNCTIONAL PHYSICAL ASSESSMENT FOR LOW BACK INJURIES IN THE ATHLETE

Joseph P. Zuhosky

Jeffrey L. Young

INTRODUCTION

Low back pain is a ubiquitous problem in modern industrialized culture. Lifetime prevalence has been estimated to be anywhere from 60 to 90%, with an annual incidence of 5% (1–3). Despite their generally superior aerobic conditioning as compared with the general population, athletes have not escaped the grasp of this disabling condition. The challenge for health care professionals in treating these athletes is to identify the underlying source of pain and dysfunction in a timely fashion so as to minimize impact on performance, training time lost, and absence from competition. Compounding matters, the recurrence rate after an episode of acute low back pain has been estimated at 60% in the first year alone (4,5). Thus, the aim in assessment of these patients is not only to identify and remedy the acute dysfunction but also to identify those underlying factors that may predispose the athlete to recurrent injury.

At the outset this may appear to be a daunting task, given the complexity of the anatomic structures involved in low back disorders. In theory, all of the innervated structures within the low back are potential pain generators and sources of lumbar dysfunction. These would include the annulus of the intervertebral disc, periosteum of the vertebral body, anterior and posterior longitudinal ligaments, nerve root epineurium, zygapophyseal joints, erector spinae musculature, and various other ligaments including the mamillo-accessory ligament and posterior superior and intertransversus ligaments but not the ligamentum flavum (6–10). Of these, the most likely culprits are the intervertebral disc and zygapophyseal joint (11,12).

With that being said, it is still true that most lumbar spine injuries are not due to disc herniations or discernable zygapophyseal joint injury but rather to segmental dysfunction. Segmental dysfunction encompasses a spectrum of injuries to one or more segmentally related structures, with compensatory changes (13). These changes include multifidus atrophy, decreased tissue compliance, and a decreased pain threshold, which is manifest as tenderness. These changes result in articular dysfunction with altered segmental motion that contributes to muscular imbalances and ultimately segmental facilitation of the levels above and below the level of dysfunction to preserve functional movement. There may also be concomitant loss of proprioceptive feedback, all of which may act in a vicious cycle to perpetuate low back pain and dysfunction. A lack of resolution of this segmental dysfunction and in particular multifidus atrophy has been theorized as one of the potential contributing factors to the high recurrence rate after an acute low back pain episode (14).

Currently, the most widely accepted theory for the pathophysiology of low back pain and dysfunction is the degenerative cascade model of Kirkaldy-Willis (15). In short, this theory is based on the concept of a motion segment and the three-joint complex, which is composed of the intervertebral discs and the paired zygapophyseal joints at each level. It is theorized that injury and cumulative trauma lead to changes in the integrity of the intervertebral disc, the zygapophyseal joints and the associated supporting ligamentous structures, and the vertebral body endplates to create lumbar dysfunction and ultimately low back pain.

Stage I is described as the stage of dysfunction (Fig. 3-1). This is manifest at the zygapophyseal joints as joint synovitis, subluxation, and early cartilage degeneration. Within the intervertebral disc, there is breakdown of the annulus, with radial and linear tears and subsequent release of inflammatory mediators. Local ischemia results, and surrounding musculature responds with sustained segmental hypertonicity, which ultimately strains the ligamentous supporting structures. Within the concept of this degenerative cascade, most adolescent and young adult athletes presenting with low back pain would best be characterized as within this stage I of dysfunction. However, by no means does this exclude more advanced injuries in this population such as frank disc herniation or stress overload of the articular arch, which may ultimately manifest as spondylolysis.

Stage II is described as the stage of instability (Fig. 3-2). At the zygapophyseal joints, increased cartilage

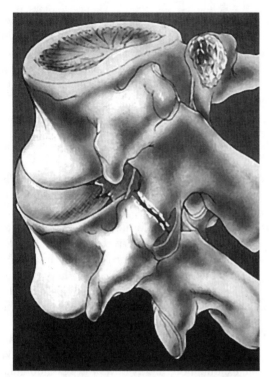

Fig. 3-1 Degenerative cascade: stage of dysfunction. (Reproduced with permission from D. Selby and J.S. Saal. *Degenerative Series.* Camp International.)

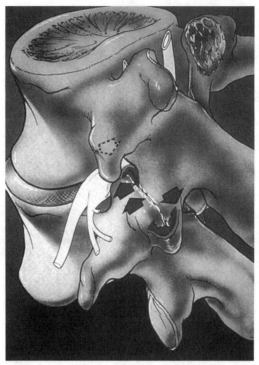

Fig. 3-2 Degenerative cascade: stage of instability. (Reproduced with permission from D. Selby and J.S. Saal. *Degenerative Series.* Camp International.)

degeneration and capsular laxity is seen, with resultant increased rotational movement. Within the intervertebral disc there is an increased frequency of annular tears with coalescence. There may also be nuclear and annular disruption and frank disc herniation. These changes lead to increased annular laxity, which result in increased translational forces and yet more stress placed on the intervertebral disc and zygapophyseal joints.

Stage III, or the stage of stabilization (Fig. 3-3), is marked by rather typical changes of osteoarthritis within the zygapophyseal joints including loss of joint surface cartilage, joint space narrowing, fibrosis, hypertrophy, and osteophyte formation. This may contribute to both central and foraminal stenosis. Within the intervertebral discs, there is further nuclear deterioration with changes in collagen type, disc resorption and fibrosis, and resultant loss of disc space height. At the vertebral endplates, there is also typically osteophyte formation. All of these changes may contribute to further central and foraminal stenosis. Epidemiologically, this model explains in large part the relative peaks in incidence of spine syndromes. Discogenic sources for pain are seen most commonly in the fourth and fifth decades (stages of dysfunction and instability), whereas central and foraminal stenosis represent the primary underlying pain generators in the sixth and seventh decades (stage of stabilization). As athletes continue to compete at older and older ages, health care professionals need to maintain a higher index of suspicion for both central and foraminal stenosis as an etiology of low back and refined lower limb pain in the senior population.

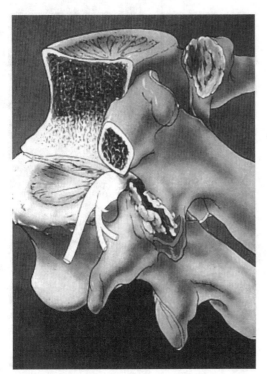

Fig. 3-3 Degenerative cascade: stage of stabilization. (Reproduced with permission from D. Selby and J.S. Saal. *Degenerative Series.* Camp International.)

FUNCTIONAL PHYSICAL ASSESSMENT

The purpose of this chapter is to provide a framework of reference for functional physical assessment for athletes presenting with low back pain. As always, the physical examination is only one piece of the puzzle, and it must be correlated with the patient's stated history of injury, past medical history, and family history. Electrodiagnosis and advanced imaging technologies also provide invaluable assistance in the diagnosis of spine disorders. Although this chapter focuses on the role of physical assessment, a word of caution regarding imaging technology is in order. Although magnetic resonance imaging and computed tomography can certainly aid in our diagnostic acumen, recent literature suggests there is a high rate of false positive results for both of these imaging studies (16,17). Imaging findings should always be carefully correlated with the patient's history and physical examination. Advanced imaging technology is not a substitute for a detailed history and physical assessment.

Standing Examination

Physical assessment ideally begins the instant the patient walks into the office. The clinician initially observes the patient's gait to determine whether it is antalgic. Position transfers, especially transitioning from a seated to standing posture, which tends to preferentially load the intervertebral disc (18–20), may yield clues as to whether there is a discogenic source for the patient's pain. It is also important to note whether the patient exhibits any pain behaviors, such as grimacing or overly guarded movements, which may give the clinician a first clue as to whether there is any psychological overlay. Gait should also be assessed formally within the context of the examination for any obviously weak musculature, such as a Trendelenburg gait belying gluteus medius weakness. Performance of both heel and toe walking provides a rough assessment of strength in the L5 and S1 myotomes, respectively. The gastrocnemius and soleus strength is best assessed in the standing position with single limb stance heel raises. The examiner evaluates for both the symmetry of excursion between limbs and the number of repetitions before fatigue. Single limb stance can also provide information regarding proprioceptive balance loss.

Examination for symmetry of bony landmarks is also performed best in the standing position. A few key landmarks are important to keep in mind in the overall musculoskeletal assessment. The vertebral prominence at the junction of the cervical and thoracic spines represents the spinous process of the seventh cervical vertebrae. The scapular spines in general reside at the third thoracic vertebrae, whereas the tip of the scapula corresponds with the seventh thoracic vertebrae. The iliac crests are at the level of the fourth lumbar vertebra. Assessment of bony landmarks should be made only after the patient's stance has been standardized. The patient is asked to place the arch of each of the feet on either side of the examiner's foot, fully extend their knees, and assume an otherwise neutral posture. Assessment begins at the shoulder heights of the patient. The shoulder of the dominant hand is generally found to be slightly lower than that of the nondominant hand. The heights of the tips of the scapula, iliac crests, posterior superior iliac spines (PSIS), greater trochanters, and anterior superior iliac spines (ASIS) are normally symmetric. If both an iliac crest and greater trochanter height are lower ipsilaterally, one should suspect a true leg length discrepancy and consideration should be given to further radiographic assessment. Assessment at this time is also made for any varus or valgus deformity at the hips or knees, the presence of pes planus, and positioning of the talar and subtalar joints. Abnormalities within the ankle,

knee, or hip joints invariably affect the kinetic chain and may ultimately manifest as low back or referred pain at any of a number of points along the kinetic chain.

In the standing position, palpation of the posterior elements, paravertebral soft tissues, iliolumbar ligaments, and piriformis should also be performed. In addition, the PSIS is examined by palpation. Tenderness here may represent underlying sacroiliac joint dysfunction (21), but in our experience, this is a very common site of referred pain from underlying L5 or S1 nerve root irritation. The greater trochanter and associated bursa are also palpated for tenderness, as is the sciatic notch.

Lumbosacral range of motion is also performed in a standing position, with assessment of not only the quantity but also the quality of movement made (Fig. 3-4). In lumbosacral flexion, the lumbar spine should be fully rounded out. Maintenance of a

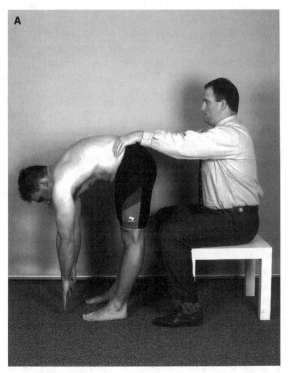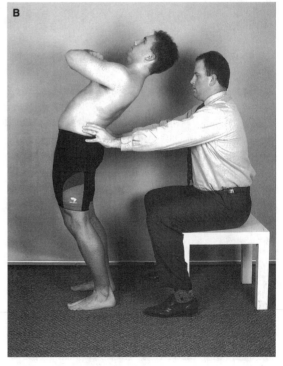

Fig. 3-4 Assessment of lumbosacral range of motion. **(A)** Lumbosacral flexion. **(B)** Lumbosacral extension.

lumbar lordosis in a fully flexed position is an example of poor quality of motion within the lumbar segments. As one assesses lumbosacral range of motion, it is important to keep in mind a few biomechanical concepts (22). The lowest lumbar segments, those being L4–L5 and L5–S1, account for 80 to 90% of available motion in the sagittal plane. The first 60 degrees of lumbar flexion is achieved predominantly at these two levels, with the next 25% of lumbar flexion resulting from hip rotation. These movements are thus coupled, and it is important to recall that this coupling of movement results in pelvic extension when the lumbar spine flexes and in pelvic flexion when the lumbar spine extends. At the muscular level, in lumbosacral flexion, there is eccentric activation of the gluteus maximus and erector spinae, whereas in lumbosacral

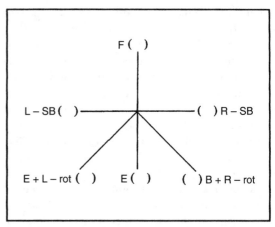

Fig. 3-6 STAR diagram to record assessment of lumbosacral range of motion: 1 = 25% limitation, 2 = 50% limitation, 3 = 75% limitation, 4 = 100% limitation. Use one to three dash lines for patient's report of pain severity on a specific motion: - represents mild pain, = represents moderate pain, ≡ represents severe pain. (Reproduced with permission from M.C. Geraci and J.T. Alleva. Physical examination of the spine and its functional kinetic chain, in *The Low Back Pain Handbook: A Practical Guide for the Primary Care Physician*, A.J. Cole and S.A. Herring, editors. 1997, Philadelphia: Hanley and Belfus.)

extension, there is concentric activation of the gluteus maximus and erector spinae. The most powerful spine extensors are in fact the hip extensors and not the erector spinae. In theory, forward flexion maximally loads the intervertebral disc, whereas extension loads the zygapophyseal joints, with ipsilateral rotation and extension maximally loading the zygapophyseal joint. In adolescent and young adult athletes, especially those in high-risk sports such as gymnastics or football, one-legged hyperextension testing serves as an additional screen for acute spondylolysis (Fig. 3-5).

When assessing lumbosacral range of motion, a STAR diagram is used and movement is described in 25th percentiles of normal (Fig. 3-6). Typically, one would describe a lumbosacral movement as

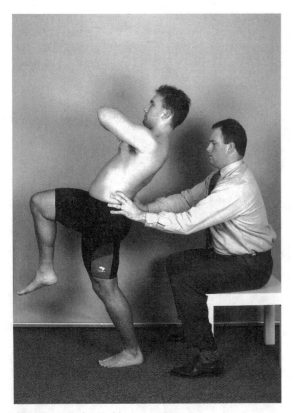

Fig. 3-5 One-legged hyperextension.

lacking 25, 50, 75, or 100% of the normal range in flexion, extension, or right or left lateral side bending as determined on examination. Lateral side bending also provides a rough assessment of quadratus lumborum range of motion. In general, side bending can be considered of normal range when the posterior axillary fold contralateral to the direction of movement falls in line with the lumbosacral junction in the mid-line (Fig. 3-7) (23).

Although not within the lumbar spine per se, the sacroiliac joints have been recognized as a common cause of low back and extremity pain. Multitudes of tests for sacroiliac joint assessment have been proposed (24–28). However, recent literature suggests there may be a considerable false positive rate with these tests (29). Using injection of the sacroiliac joint with provocation as the gold

standard, these clinical tests, when taken singly or in combination, were neither sensitive nor specific in identifying when the sacroiliac joint is a significant pain generator (30). Given these restrictions, it is nevertheless important to include an assessment of the sacroiliac joints in the examination of patients with low back or extremity pain. The evaluation begins with the standing assessment of bony landmark heights, which are often asymmetric in patients with sacroiliac joint dysfunction (Fig. 3-8). For example, one may see a unilateral elevation of the right PSIS and iliac crest with an associated diminished height of the ASIS height compared with the corresponding landmarks on the left. Many conventions have been set forth to describe such asymmetries within the pelvis. For the example given, this may be described as an anterior rotation

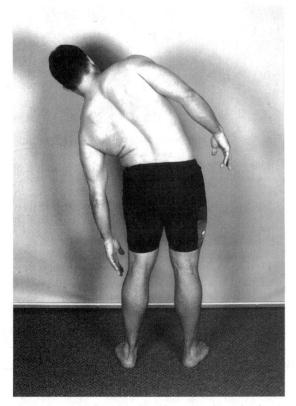

Fig. 3-7 Lumbosacral range of motion, lateral side bending.

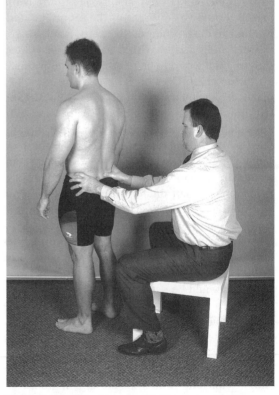

Fig. 3-8 Standing assessment of bony landmark heights.

of the right innominate or a right pelvic mutation. A right posterior innominate or countermutation of the pelvis would thus describe findings of a lower iliac crest and PSIS height coupled with an elevated ASIS height on the right versus corresponding landmarks on the left. We prefer a description of these asymmetries in terms of anterior or posterior innominates because this is a more descriptive designation of the underlying asymmetry. It should be recognized that this convention does oversimplify the biomechanics of this region because it assumes that the sacrum is fixed and movement of the ilium or innominate is relative to this fixed point. Although it is not critical how one describes the underlying dysfunction, it is important to be consistent in the use of this terminology in the description of underlying asymmetries. By convention, the abnormalities are also described on the basis of which side is symptomatic.

We prefer Gillet's test, otherwise known as the march test, for assessment of the sacroiliac joint in the standing position (Fig. 3-9). Each side is assessed individually. With a standardized stance, the patient is asked to bend each knee individually up to the chest. On the right side, the examiner places his or her right thumb over the PSIS and left thumb over the sacrum at the same height. In a normal examination, with flexion at the hip and knee as the patient raises the knee to the chest, on the right the movement of the thumb circumscribes an "L-shaped" movement. On the left side, the examiner's left thumb is placed over the PSIS and the right thumb over the sacrum, with a normal movement of the sacroiliac joint circumscribing a "backward L." Once again, the abnormalities are described on the basis of the symptomatic side. For example, if the patient is having left-sided pain, this would be described as "the left sacroiliac joint is hypo- or hypermobile as compared with the right sacroiliac joint."

If one suspects an underlying ankylosing spondylitis, Schober's test should be performed. As discussed in Chap. 2, the points of reference should elongate by 5 cm or more in lumbosacral flexion and should shorten a minimum of 2.5 cm with extension.

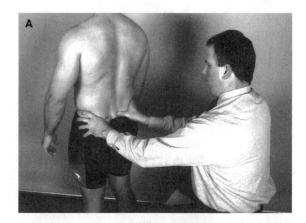

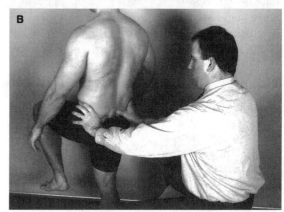

Fig. 3-9 Gillet's testing. **(A)** Localization of bony landmarks. **(B)** Assessment of posterior superior iliac spine movement with flexion of the hip and knee.

Seated Examination

With the leg dangling, sensation for both light touch and pin prick is assessed by dermatome (Fig. 3-10). Dermatomes L1 through S2 are routinely examined. Muscle stretch reflexes provide additional information about potential lumbosacral nerve root involvement. Stretching of the quadriceps at the patellar tendon assesses lumbar roots 3 and 4 primarily. The gastrocnemius and soleus reflexes are tested at the Achilles tendon and reflect the first sacral nerve root. Medial hamstring reflex corresponds with the fifth lumbar nerve

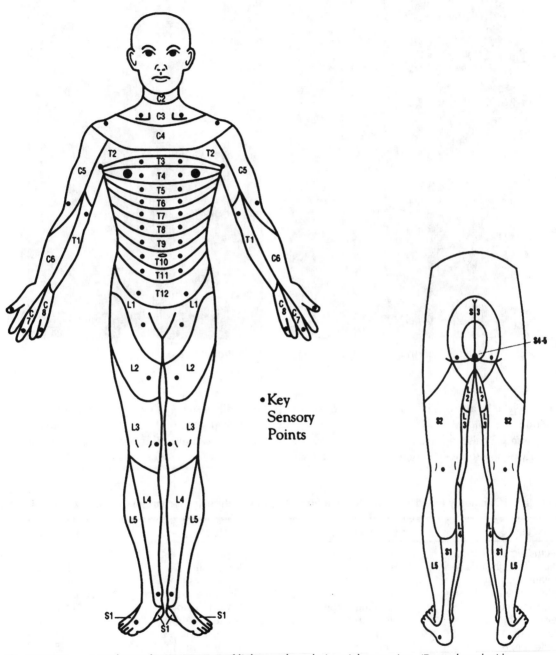

Fig. 3-10 Dermatomal map for assessment of light touch and pin prick sensation. (Reproduced with permission from *International Standards for Neurological and Functional Classification of Spinal Cord Injury, Revised 1992.* 1994, Chicago: American Spinal Injury Association.)

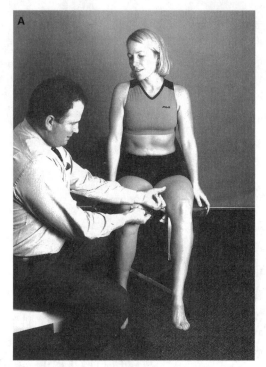 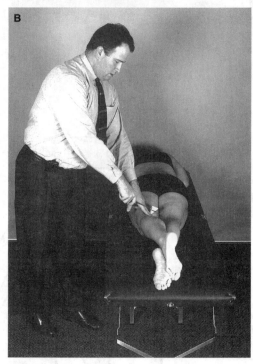

Fig. 3-11 Medial hamstring reflex. **(A)** Seated position. **(B)** Prone position.

root and can be assessed in either a seated or prone position (Fig. 3-11).

Strength is also assessed with attention to the underlying myotome. Myotomes L1 through S2 can be readily tested (Table 3-1). Strength is graded on an Oxford scale of 0 to 5 (31–34) (Table 3-2). The Babinski response and testing for clonus at both ankles serve as screens for an upper motor neuron

Table 3-1 Commonly Tested Muscles During a Strength Exam with their Mechanism of Action and Myotome(s)

MUSCLE	POSITION TESTED	ACTION	MYOTOME(S)*
Rectus femoris/iliopsoas	Seated	Hip flexion	(L1), L2, L3, (L4)
Quadriceps femoris	Seated	Knee extension	L2, L3, L4
Tibialis anterior	Seated	Ankle dorsiflexion	L4, L5
Extensor hallucis longus	Seated	Great toe extension	L5
Gastrocsoleus	Standing on one leg	Plantar flexion	(L5), S1, S2
Peroneal muscles	Side-lying	Ankle eversion	L5, S1
Hamstrings	Prone	Knee flexion	L5, S1
Gluteus maximus	Prone	Hip extension	L5, S1, (S2)
Gluteus medius/minimus	Side-lying	Hip abduction	L5, S1, (S2)

*The myotomes in parentheses indicate anatomic variations depending on source used.

(Modified with permission, Geraci MC, Alleva JT: Physical examination of the spine and its functional kinetic chain, in Cole AJ, Herring SA (eds.): *The Low Back Pain Handbook: A Practical Guide for the Primary Care Physician.* Philadelphia, Hanley and Belfus, 1997.)

Table 3-2   Oxford Scale of Strength Assessment and Grading

NUMERIC GRADE	DESCRIPTION
0	Total paralysis
1	Palpable or visible contraction
2	Active movement, full range of motion (ROM) with gravity eliminated
3	Active movement, full ROM against gravity
4	Active movement, full ROM against moderate resistance
5	(Normal) active movement, full ROM against full resistance
NT	Not testable

The strength of each muscle is graded on a six-point scale.

(Modified with permission, *International Standards for Neurological and Functional Classification of Spinal Cord Injury, Revised 1992.* Chicago, American Spinal Injury Association, 1994.)

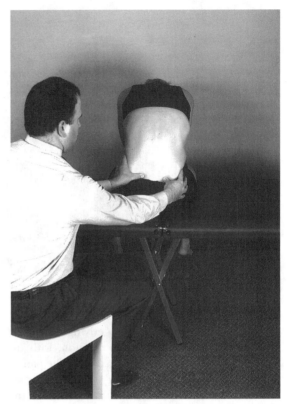

Fig. 3-12 Seated assessment of sacroiliac joint mobility and symmetry.

lesion. In addition, distal pulses of both the posterior tibial and dorsalis pedis arteries are palpated as a screen for a vascular etiology for low back and lower limb pain.

The quality and symmetry of sacroiliac joint movement can also be examined in a seated position by observing the excursion of the posterior superior iliac spines with seated forward flexion (Fig. 3-12).

A multitude of tests have been described as provocative of dural tension and, by supposition, indicative of underlying disc disorders and nerve root irritation (35–40). These tests have their roots in a search for physical signs of meningitis, as described initially by Lasegue (41) and subsequently by Kernig and Brudzinski, with minor deviations (42–45). These tests of dural tension have been examined biomechanically in cadavers and were found to impart true tension on the dura mater (46,47). In our estimation, the slump sit test as described by Butler is the most sensitive screen for dural tension and lower lumbar and sacral nerve root irritation (48) (Fig. 3-13). The patient is asked

to place his or her hands behind the back with palms up. The patient assumes a "slumped" posture by bringing the chin to the chest, rounding the shoulders and flexing at the waist. The examiner then passively extends the knee. Ankle dorsiflexion is added to increase the dural tension. Reproduction of radicular pain into the limb represents a positive test. This test also passively stretches the hamstrings and may produce pain, which can be difficult to differentiate from radicular symptoms because this is a common site of discogenic referred pain for both the L5 and S1 nerve roots. Several points of differentiation may prove helpful. Pain at the popliteal fossa is more consistent with dural tension because stretching of the hamstring tends to produce more discomfort within the belly of the muscle. Side-to-side comparison can also be helpful because hamstring length and pain with passive stretch is typically

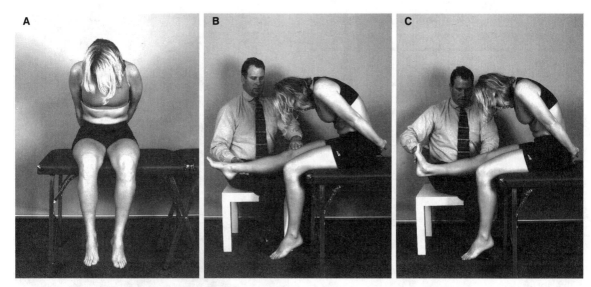

Fig. 3-13 Slump sit test. **(A)** "Slumped" posture. **(B)** Passive extension of the knee. **(C)** Addition of ankle dorsiflexion.

symmetric in the absence of underlying nerve root irritation. In the fully slumped position, with the knee extended and the ankle dorsiflexed, the patient is asked to fully extend the neck alone while otherwise maintaining the slumped posture. Although this does not change the effective length of the hamstrings and thus their pain with passive stretch, it does reduce the tension on the dural structures and may relieve radicular pain.

Supine Examination

The modern day champion for the role of muscular imbalance as it relates to low back pain and dysfunction has been Janda (49,50). In theory, muscles with restricted range of motion, especially the lumbopelvic musculature, impart biomechanical changes and restricted motion. These shortened muscles tend to maintain their hypertonicity, whereas their antagonists are maintained in a more stretched position. Over time, although true atrophy may not develop, these muscles have been described by Janda as "inhibited" and exhibiting "pseudoparesis." All of this feeds back in a vicious cycle to perpetuate the biomechanical changes that ultimately lead to segmental and lumbopelvic dysfunction. The literature has long recognized a

relation between restricted hamstring range of motion and spondylolisthesis (51). More recently, two prospective studies in athletes have demonstrated an increased risk of low back injury when imbalances of strength and flexibility are noted on preparticipation screening (52,53).

The hamstrings, especially in young athletes, are perhaps the most important muscles to assess. When there is restriction of hamstring range of motion, a relative posterior pelvic tilt is created, with resultant flexion in the lumbar spine given

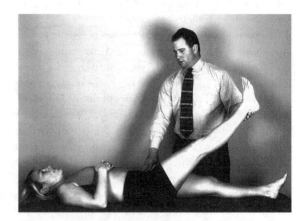

Fig. 3-14 Hamstring range of motion with estimation of pelvis engagement.

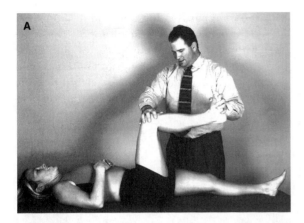

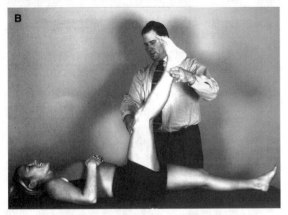

Fig. 3-15 Hamstring range of motion with estimation of popliteal angle. **(A)** Hip flexion to 90 degrees. **(B)** Passive knee extension with estimation of popliteal angle.

popliteal angle. These techniques have also been presented in great detail in Chap. 2.

The piriformis should also be assessed in a supine position (Fig. 3-16). It is a unique muscle

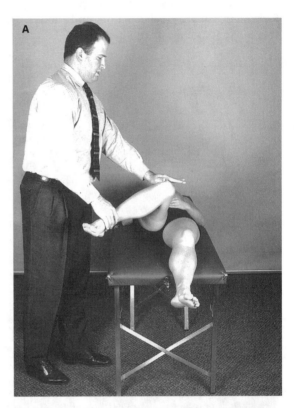

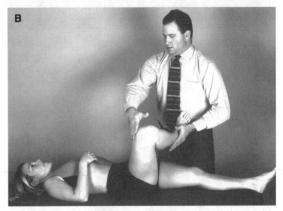

Fig. 3-16 Piriformis range of motion. **(A)** Assessment below 90 degrees of hip flexion. **(B)** Assessment above 90 degrees of hip flexion.

their coupled movements. This tends to increase intradiscal pressures and may exacerbate underlying discogenic pain and perhaps predispose athletes to the development of disc degeneration. Hamstring length can be assessed by passively raising the fully extended limb and estimating the degrees at which the pelvis engages to allow continued hip flexion (Fig. 3-14). Perhaps the most reproducible and clearest assessment is to flex the knee and flex the hip to 90 degrees and passively extend the knee while maintaining a neutral spine posture (Fig. 3-15). Hamstring length is then described by the measurement of the resultant having different activities depending on the amount of hip flexion present. Below 90 degrees of hip flexion, it is an external rotator and abductor of the hip; therefore, its range and motion should be tested with hip internal rotation and femur adduction. Above 90 degrees of hip flexion, the piriformis is an internal rotator and adductor; therefore, its range of motion should be tested

with hip external rotation and femur abduction. Although we have found true piriformis syndrome (54) with entrapment neuropathy of the sciatic nerve to be quite rare, findings of tenderness and reproduction of symptoms on stretching of the muscle itself are not uncommon. In our experience, most cases labeled as "piriformis syndrome" on further inspection are found to have L5 nerve

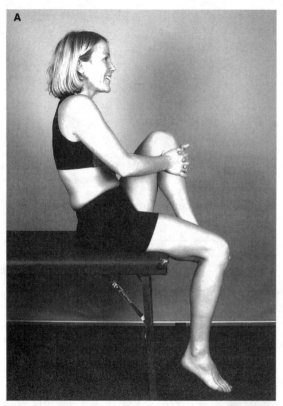

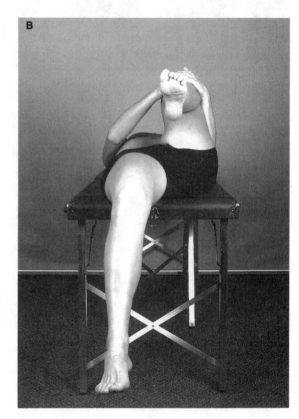

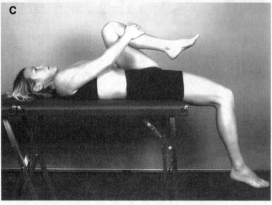

Fig. 3-17 Modified Thomas test. **(A)** Initial seated position. **(B)** Assessment of tensor fasciae latae tightness. **(C)** Supine position with lateral vantage point allows assessment of the range of motion of both the iliopsoas and rectus femoris.

root irritation as the underlying etiology. Hip internal and external rotation range of motion should also be assessed at this time.

Perhaps the most efficient test of lumbopelvic musculature range of motion is the modified Thomas test, which has also been described in detail and illustrated (Fig. 2-11) in Chap. 2 (Fig. 3-17). When performed appropriately, this allows one to assess the range of motion of the iliopsoas, rectus femoris, and tensor fasciae latae. The patient begins in a seated position and fully flexes one hip and knee while holding the knee tight to the chest. The patient then assumes a supine position and is asked to maintain a posterior pelvic tilt. From a lateral vantage point, the examiner can measure how many finger breadths the popliteal fossa remains above the supporting surface. This provides a functional and reproducible measure of iliopsoas range of motion. From this perspective, the amount of passive knee flexion present provides a means of assessing the length of the rectus femoris. In normal patients, the popliteal fossa should lay flush with the table and the knee should passively flex to 90 degrees. Moving to the foot of the examination table, the positioning of the femur is noted. Deviation laterally from the plane of the trunk is indicative of tensor fasciae latae tightness.

Performance of pelvic clocks, as has been described in Chap. 7, is an excellent way both qualitatively and quantitatively to assess lumbopelvic rhythm, and they provide a dynamic assessment of lumbopelvic musculature. Abdominal muscle strength can also be assessed in the supine position, but it is difficult to objectively quantify. The abdominal muscles, acting in concert with the thoracolumbar fascia, play a crucial role in stabilizing the lumbar spine (55,56). Thus, irrespective of any findings on physical examination, targeted strengthening of the abdominals as a group and of the lower abdominal musculature in particular should be part of any rehabilitation program for patients with lumbar dysfunction. A gross assessment of abdominal strength (57) can be achieved by having the supine patient maintain a posterior pelvic tilt and then lower fully extended knees from 70 to 30 degrees and then to 10 degrees of hip flexion (Fig. 3-18). As the limb is lowered from

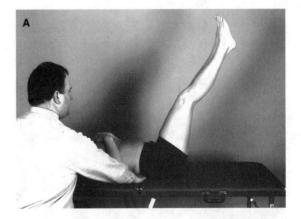

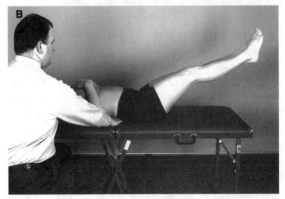

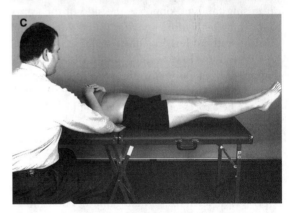

Fig. 3-18 Assessment of abdominal muscle strength. **(A)** Seventy degrees of hip flexion. **(B)** Thirty degrees of hip flexion. **(C)** Ten degrees of hip flexion.

70 to 10 degrees of hip flexion, there is greater and greater eccentric load placed especially on the lower abdominals. The inability to maintain a pos-

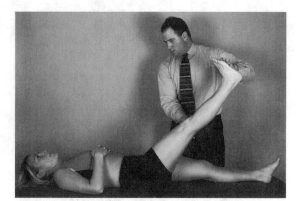

Fig. 3-19 Straight-leg raise test.

terior pelvic tilt is indicative of lower abdominal weakness.

In terms of provocative testing in the supine position, the classically described straight-leg raise test (58), as described in Chap. 2, can also be performed as an adjunct to the slump sit test (Fig. 3-19). This should be performed in both lower limbs with close attention to the anatomic distribution of symptoms provoked. It has been suggested that a positive contralateral straight-leg raise (defined as provocation of the patient's usual lower limb pain on raising the limb opposite the side of the symptoms) may be a more specific indicator of dural tension and underlying disc prolapse (59). Reproduction of lower limb symptoms below 70 degrees of hip flexion with the knee fully extended is considered positive for dural tension, and findings can be expressed in the degrees of hip flexion at which radicular symptoms occur.

Gaenslen's maneuver serves as an additional screen for sacroiliac joint dysfunction (Fig. 3-20). The contralateral leg is fully flexed at the hip and knee and is held firmly to the chest by the patient. A posterior pelvic tilt is maintained. The limb to be assessed is then hung over the side of the table, with the leg dangling. The test can be modified with overpressure applied to the side being tested, producing additional hip extension. Reproduction of the patient's buttock or groin symptoms, especially if this is a usual symptom pattern, is deemed a positive test. Patrick's and Faber's testing can also

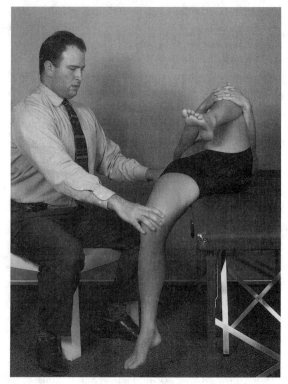

Fig. 3-20 Gaenslen's test.

be performed and may be provocative of either underlying hip pathology (typically groin pain) or sacroiliac joint dysfunction (generally buttock or lateral hip pain) (Fig. 3-21).

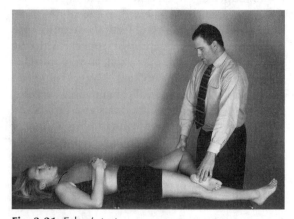

Fig. 3-21 Faber's test.

Side Lying Examination

In addition to modified Thomas testing, the range of motion of the tensor fasciae latae can also be assessed by using Ober's test (60) (Fig. 3-22). It is very important to maintain the pelvis in a neutral position and perpendicular to the examination table to standardize this test. The pelvis is in neutral position and square to the table when a plane connecting the PSIS lies perpendicular to the table. Tensor fasciae latae length is then described as the number of finger breadths the medial femoral condyle remains elevated from the supporting surface. This then serves as an objective means of comparison for future evaluation. The strength of the gluteus medius, which is an important pelvic stabilizer, should also be assessed (Fig. 3-23). The patient is asked to maintain neutral pelvic posture perpendicular to the table and actively abduct the hip against

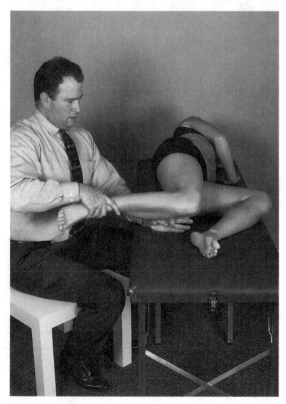

Fig. 3-22 Ober's test.

resistance. The examiner should look for signs of substitution of the tensor fasciae latae (produces internal rotation at the hip) or quadratus lumborum (may result in lateral flexion and extension of the trunk) in the presence of gluteus medius weakness.

Prone Examination

The spring test is performed over the spinous process of each of the lumbar vertebrae (Fig. 3-24). The examiner places the palm and pisiform bone over the patient's spinous process and exerts a downward force. At normal levels, there should be a "spring" of the segment back up into the examiner's hand, with no pain elicited. Findings of pain and an absence of spring may be indicative of underlying disc, zygapophyseal joint, or segmental dysfunction. A prone press-up (Fig. 3-25) with maintenance of the pelvis against the examination table can also provide both quantitative and qualitative information regarding segmental mobility of the lumbar segments. If the patient has difficulty maintaining the pelvis against the examination table, the palms of the hands may be moved forward to reduce the hyperextension and eliminate motion from the pelvis.

The length of the rectus femoris can also be assessed in the prone position by fully flexing the knee and is described as the number of finger breadths the heel remains from the buttock (Fig. 3-26). In this position, the femoral nerve is also stretched, and dural tension may result (61,62). A femoral nerve stretch can also be achieved by extending the hip with the knee flexed (63) (Fig. 3-27). This may eliminate the potential false positive result of pain on passive stretch of a tight rectus femoris; however, it still places the iliopsoas on stretch. Careful attention should be paid to where the patient complains of pain with this maneuver because multiple nerve roots are placed on tension (L2, L3, and L4), not to mention the iliopsoas and psoas major muscles. Pain referred to the medial femoral condyle is generally considered more consistent with an L3 nerve root origin, whereas referral into the anterior tibialis region is considered more indicative of the L4 nerve root.

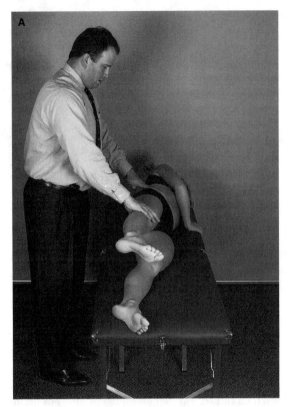

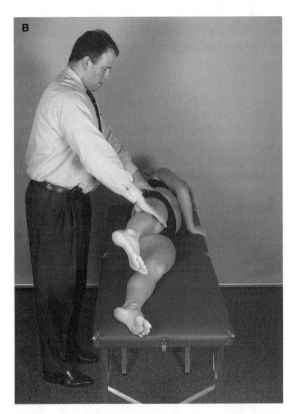

Fig. 3-23 (A) Assessment of gluteus medius strength. **(B)** Substitution of the tensor fascia latae. Note the hip internal rotation.

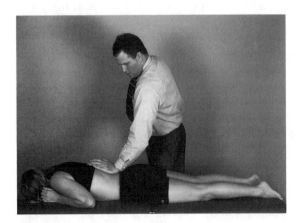

Fig. 3-24 Spring test.

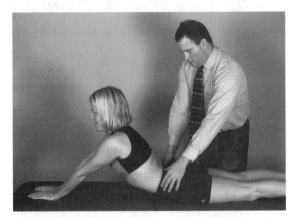

Fig. 3-25 Prone press-up.

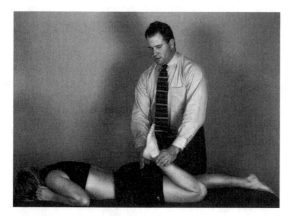

Fig. 3-26 Assessment of rectus femoris range of motion.

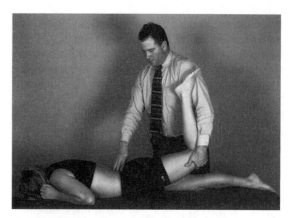

Fig. 3-27 Femoral nerve stretch test.

EVALUATION OF PSYCHOLOGICAL OVERLAY

Spine care practitioners have long recognized the contribution of secondary gain issues and psychological overlay in certain patient populations. Although much less common in athletes, the contribution of psychological overlay should not be ignored. A number of objective signs and assessments have been described to identify patients in whom psychological overlay may be a component of their symptomatology (64–67). However, a word of caution is necessary in the potential overinterpretation of these findings. The presence of signs or symptoms of psychological overlay do not rule out underlying pathology. Although their presence should encourage an investigation of potential secondary gain issues, findings of psychological overlay do not obviate the need for further medical work-up and treatment.

The most widely used measures of potential psychological overlay or secondary gain are the five nonorganic physical signs in low back pain as described by Waddell (68). These include both subjective assessments on the part of the examining clinician and objective physical examination tests. An initial indication for a possible nonorganic component to a patient's symptoms is the presence of regional disturbances, that is, complaints of pain in the entire right side of the body or globally in one lower limb or both lower limbs. Patients with potential nonorganic contribution may also demonstrate superficial or nonanatomic tenderness, that is, pain or marked tenderness reported with even light touch and nonpainful stimulus. These patients may also demonstrate overreaction with exaggerated grimacing, withdrawal from examination, and moving the examiner's hand away. Two objective physical examination maneuvers are also described. In simulation testing, the examiner applies an axial load over the cranium or axially rotates the hips, pelvis, and lumbar spine, all as one segment. A positive simulation test is noted when these maneuvers reproduce low back pain. The final test is the test of distraction, where the examiner performs a distracted seated straight-leg raise and a supine straight-leg raise. A positive test is reproduction of extremity pain only in the supine position.

Nonorganic physical signs in the athletic population should lead the clinician to ask additional questions to try to identify potential secondary gain issues. These may also represent a manifestation of underlying conflict with coaches or trainers and, in the adolescent population, conflict with parents.

CONCLUSION

Low back pain is a common presenting complaint in both athletes and the general population. As outlined in this chapter, the potential pain generators are numerous, and the complexity of the anatomy in the lumbar spine is unmatched in any other region of the body. However, if the clinician takes the time to obtain a detailed history and complete a functional physical assessment of the lumbar spine, a specific working diagnosis can quite often be achieved. Adjunctive imaging and electrodiagnostic studies can also provide additional information to further corroborate or clarify the clinical picture. However, the physical assessment remains the critical component in terms of individualizing the rehabilitation prescription. A specific diagnosis coupled with a specific treatment remains the key to early return of the athlete to the field of play and optimization of their performance.

REFERENCES

1. Grazier, K.L., et al., editors. *The Frequency of Occurrence, Impact, and Cost of Musculoskeletal Conditions in the United States.* 1984, Chicago: American Academy of Orthopaedic Surgeons.
2. Frymoyer, J.W., et al. Risk factors in low back pain: an epidemiological survey. *J Bone Joint Surg* 1983, 65A: p. 213–218.
3. Frymoyer, J.W., and W.L. Cats-Buril. An overview of the incidences and cost of low back pain. *Orthop Clin North Am* 1991, 22: p. 263–271.
4. Berquist-Ullman, M., and U. Larsson. Acute low back pain in industry: a controlled prospective study with special reference to therapy and confounding factors. *Acta Orthop Scand* 1977, 170(suppl): p. 1–117.
5. Troup, J.D.G., et al. Back pain in industry: a prospective survey. *Spine* 1981, 6: p. 61–69.
6. Bogduk, N. The innervation of the lumbar spine. *Spine* 1983, 8: p. 286–293.
7. Bogduk, N., and L.T. Twomey. *Clinical Anatomy of the Lumbar Spine,* 2nd ed. 1991, Melbourne: Churchill Livingstone.
8. Bogduk, N. The lumbar disc and low back pain. *Neurosurg Clin North Am* 1991, 2: p. 791–806.
9. Cavanaugh, J.M. Neural mechanisms of lumbar pain. *Spine* 1995, 20: p. 1804–1809.
10. Sinclair, D.C., et al. The intervetebral ligaments as a source of segmental pain. *J Bone Joint Surg* 1948, 30B: p. 515–521.
11. Kuslich, S.D., et al. The tissue origin of low back pain: a report of pain response to tissue stimulation during operations on the lumbar spine using local anesthesia. *Orthop Clin North Am* 1991, 22: p. 181–187.
12. Schwarzer, A.C., et al. The relative contribution of the disc and zygapophyseal joint in chronic low back pain. *Spine* 1994, 19: p. 801–806.
13. Cole, A.J., et al. Clinical presentations and diagnostic subsets, in *The Low Back Pain Handbook: A Practical Guide for the Primary Care Physician,* A.J. Cole and S.A. Herring, editors. 1997, Philadelphia: Hanley and Belfus. p. 71–96.
14. Hides, J.A., et al. Multifidus muscle recovery is not automatic after resolution of acute, first-episode low back pain. *Spine* 1996, 21: p. 2763–2769.
15. Kirkaldy-Willis, W.H. Three phases of the spectrum of degenerative disease, in *Managing Low Back Pain,* 3rd ed, W.H. Kirkadly-Willis and C.V. Burton, editors. 1992, New York: Churchill-Livingstone. p. 105–119.
16. Boden, S.D., et al. Abnormal MRI of the lumbar spine in asymptomatic subjects. *J Bone Joint Surg* 1990, 72A: p. 403–408.
17. Wiesel, S.W., et al. A study of computer-assisted tomography. I. The incidence of positive CAT scans in an asymptomatic group of patients. *Spine* 1984, 9: p. 549–551.
18. Nachemson, A. The influence of spinal movement on the lumbar intradiscal pressure and on the tensile stresses in the annulus fibrosus. *Acta Orthop Scand* 1963, 33: p. 183–207.
19. Nachemson, A. The effect of forward leaning on lumbar intradiscal pressure. *Acta Orthop Scand* 1965, 35: p. 314–328.
20. Nachemson, A. In vivo discometry in lumbar discs with irregular nucleograms: some differences in stress distribution between normal and moderately degenerated discs. *Acta Orthop Scand* 1965, 36: p. 418–434.
21. Fortin, J.D., and F.J. Falco. The Fortin finger test: an indicator of sacroiliac pain. *Am J Orthop* 1997, 26: p. 477–480.
22. White, A.A., and M.M. Panjabi, editors. *Clinical Biomechanics of the Lumbar Spine,* 2nd ed. 1990, Philadelphia: Lippincott-Raven. p. 1–125.

23. Geraci, M.C., and J.T. Alleva. Physical examination of the spine and its functional kinetic chain, in *The Low Back Pain Handbook: A Practical Guide for the Primary Care Physician*, A.J. Cole and S.A. Herring, editors. 1997, Philadelphia: Hanley and Belfus. p. 49–70.

24. Bernard, T.N., Jr., and J.D. Cassidy. The sacroiliac joint syndrome: pathophysiology, diagnosis and management, in *The Adult Spine: Principles and Practice*, J.W. Frymoyer, editor. 1991, New York: Raven Press. p. 2107–2130.

25. Greenman, P.E. Principles of diagnosis and treatment of pelvic girdle dysfunction, in *Principles of Manual Medicine*, P.E. Greenman, editor. 1989, Baltimore: Williams & Wilkins. p. 225–270.

26. Laslett, M., and M. Williams. The reliability of selected provocation tests for sacroiliac joint pathology. *Spine* 1994, 19: p. 1243–1249.

27. Russell, A.S., et al. Clinical examination of the sacroiliac joints: a prospective study. *Arthrit Rheum* 1981, 24: p. 1575–1577.

28. Walker, J.M. The sacroiliac joint: a critical review. *Phys Ther* 1992, 72: p. 903–916.

29. Dreyfuss, P., et al. Positive sacroiliac screening tests in asymptomatic adults. *Spine* 1994, 19: p. 1138–1143.

30. Dreyfuss, P., et al. The value of medical history and physical examination in diagnosing sacroiliac joint pain. *Spine* 1996, 21: p. 2594–2602.

31. *Aids to Investigation of Peripheral Nerve Injuries. Medical Research Council War Memorandum*, 2nd ed., rev. 1943, London: HMSO.

32. Brunnstrom, F., and M. Dennen. Round table on muscle testing, in *Annual Conference of American Physical Therapy Association*. 1931, New York: Federation of Crippled and Disabled, Inc. p. 1–12.

33. Daniels, L., and C. Worthingham. *Muscle Testing: Techniques of Manual Examination*, 3rd ed. 1972, Philadelphia: WB Saunders.

34. Lovett RW. *The Treatment of Infantile Paralysis*, 2nd ed. 1917, Philadelphia: P. Blackiston's Son. p. 136.

35. Butler, D., and L. Gifford. The concept of adverse mechanical tension in the nervous system. *Physiotherapy* 1989, 75: p. 622–636.

36. Cram, R.H. A sign of sciatic nerve root pressure. *J Bone Joint Surg* 1953, 35B: p. 192.

37. Dyck, P. The stoop-test in lumbar entrapment radiculopathy. *Spine* 1979, 4: p. 89–92.

38. Mierau, D., et al. Low back pain and straight leg raising in children and adolescents. *Spine* 1989, 14: p. 526–528.

39. Scham, S.M., and T.R.F. Taylor. Tension signs in lumbar disc prolapse. *Clin Orthop Rel Res* 1970, 75: p. 197.

40. Woodhall, R., and G.J. Hayes. The well-leg-raising test of Fajersztajn in the diagnosis of ruptured intervertebral disc. *J Bone Joint Surg* 1950, 32A: p. 786.

41. Wilkins, R.H., and I.A. Brody. Lasegue's sign. *Arch Neurol* 1969, 21: p. 219–220.

42. Brody, I.A., and R.H. Wilkins. The signs of Kernig and Brudzinski. *Arch Neurol* 1969, 21: p. 215–216.

43. Brudzinski, J. A new sign of the lower extremities in meningitis in children. *Arch Neurol* 1969, 21: p. 217.

44. Kernig, W. Concerning a little noted sign of meningitis. *Arch Neurol* 1969, 21: p. 216.

45. Wartenberg, R. The sign of Brudzinski and Kernig. *J Pediat* 1950, 37: p. 679–684.

46. Breig, A., and D.G. Troup. Biomechanical considerations in the straight-leg-raising test: cadaveric and clinical studies of the effects of medial hip rotation. *Spine* 1979, 4: p. 242–250.

47. Goddard, M.D., and J.D. Reid. Movements induced by straight leg raising in the lumbo-sacral roots, nerves and plexus and in the intrapelvic section of the sciatic nerve. *J Neurol Neurosurg Psychiatry* 1965, 28: p. 12–18.

48. Butler, D. *Mobilization of the Nervous System*. 1991, New York: Churchill Livingstone. p. 139–146.

49. Janda, V. *Muscle Function Testing*. 1983, London: Butterworths.

50. Janda, V. Muscle weakness and inhibition (pseudoparesis) in back pain syndromes, in *Modern Manual Therapy of the Vertebral Column*, G.P. Grieve, editor. 1986, London: Churchill Livingstone. p. 197–201.

51. Barash, H.L., et al. Spondylolisthesis and tight hamstrings. *J Bone Joint Surg* 1970, 52A: p. 1319–1328.

52. Knapic, J.T., et al. Preseason strength and flexibility imbalances associated with athletic injuries in female collegiate athletes. *Am J Sports Med* 1991, 9: p. 76–81.

53. Nadler, S.F., et al. Low back pain in college athletes: a prospective study correlating lower

extremity overuse or acquired ligamentous laxity with low back pain. *Spine* 1998, 23: p. 828–833.

54. Retzlaff, E.N., and A. Berry. The piriformis muscle syndrome. *J Am Orthop Assoc* 1974, 73: p. 799–807.

55. Bogduk, N., and J.E. Macintosh. The applied anatomy of the thoracolumbar fascia. *Spine* 1984, 9: p. 104–110.

56. Tesh, K.M., et al. The abdominal muscles and vertebral stability. *Spine* 1987, 12: p. 501–508.

57. Kendall, F.P., et al. Trunk muscles, strength tests and exercises, in *Muscles Testing and Function*, 4th ed., F.P. Kendall et al., editors. 1993, Baltimore: Williams & Wilkins. p. 131–176.

58. Urban, L.M. Straight leg raise: a review. *J Orthop Sports Phys Ther* 1981, 2: p. 117.

59. Hudgins, W.R. The crossed-straight-leg-raising test. *N Engl J Med* 1977, 279: p. 1127.

60. Ober, F.R. Relation of the fascia lata to conditions of the lower part of the back. *JAMA* 1937, 109: p. 554–555.

61. Dyck, P. The femoral nerve traction test with lumbar disc protrusion. *Surg Neurol* 1976, 6: p. 163.

62. Estridge, M.N., et al. The femoral stretching test: a valuable sign in diagnosing upper lumbar disc herniations. *J Neurosurg* 1982, 57: p. 813–817.

63. Herron, L.D., and H.C. Pheasant. Prone knee-flexion provocation testing for lumbar disc protrusion. *Spine* 1980, 5: p. 65–67.

64. Archibald, K.C., and F. Wiechec. A re-appraisal of Hoover's test. *Arch Phys Med Rehabil* 1970, 51: p. 234.

65. Arieff, A.J., et al. The Hoover sign: an objective sign of pain and/or weakness in the back or lower extremities. *Arch Neurol* 1961, 5: p. 673.

66. Hoover, C.F. A new sign for the detection of malingering and functional paresis of the lower extremities. *JAMA* 1980, 51: p. 746.

67. Waddell, G., et al. Clinical assessment and interpretation of abnormal illness behavior in low back pain. *Pain* 1989, 39: p. 41–53.

68. Waddell, G. Non-organic physical signs in low back pain. *Spine* 1980, 5: p. 117–125.

CHAPTER 4

AEROBIC CONDITION AND LOW BACK FUNCTION

Wendell Liemohn

Gina Pariser

Julie Bowden

INTRODUCTION

Physical activity has been recognized as an important factor in the prevention and treatment of low back pain (LBP), at least since 1904 (1). The benefits that can be gleaned from physical activity can be deduced in part by considering the detrimental effects of immobilization or inactivity on articular cartilage (2,3), specifically on the tissues of the spine (1,3–6). Inactivity is considered a primary risk factor for cardiovascular disease (7); in recent years, parallels have been drawn about the benefits of aerobic exercise for LBP (8).

The term *aerobics* was coined by Kenneth Cooper (9); he, more than anyone else, is responsible for the "aerobics craze" that subsequently swept the United States in the last third of the 20th century. It has been a boon to the fitness industry, including health clubs and manufacturers of sporting equipment; moreover, it is a craze that shows no signs of diminishing.

BENEFITS OF AEROBIC ACTIVITY

Although aerobic condition is usually associated with cardiorespiratory condition, its effects are not limited to this facet of health. In this chapter, several aspects of aerobic condition will be mentioned, and the aspects of aerobic activity relating specifically to the spine will be emphasized.

Aerobic Activity and the Heart

In 1992 the American Heart Association Scientific Council stated that inactivity is a risk factor for coronary artery disease. The benefits of aerobic activity cited in their statement included:

- increase in cardiac output
- decrease in myocardial oxygen demand (for same work levels)
- beneficial changes in hemodynamic, hormonal, metabolic, neurologic, and respiratory function
- favorable alteration of lipid and carbohydrate metabolisms (7).

Even though the importance of aerobic condition to cardiovascular function has been known at least since 1968 (9,10), this declaration by the American Heart Association has added to the credibility of the aerobics movement.

Aerobic Activity and Low Back Pain

The most frequently cited research in this area is the prospective study by Cady et al. (11). They examined the performance of 1652 firefighters on five strength and fitness protocols and then assigned their subjects to a high, middle, or low fitness group. The physical fitness items on which the firefighters were tested included (a) back-leg isometric strength, (b) spinal rotation range of motion, (c) work output on a bicycle ergometer at a heart rate of 160 beats per minute, (d) diastolic blood pressure response during bicycle ergometer exercise, and (e) heart rate recovery 2 min after cessation of the bicycle ergometer test. Based on these data, the firefighters were placed into the least fit group (the lowest 16th percentile, $n = 266$), the middle fit group (the middle 68th percentile, $n = 1127$), and the most fit group (the upper 16th percentile, $n = 259$). Subsequently, the firefighters' back injuries and associated worker compensation costs were analyzed in relation to the three fitness groups to which the 1652 firefighters were assigned. It was found that the least fit group sustained approximately 10 times as many back injuries as the most fit group. Moreover, the cost per claim for those 19 firefighters sustaining back injuries in the least fit group was 13% higher than the cost for the 36 firefighters sustaining back injuries in the much larger middle fit group. Cady et al. concluded that physical fitness and conditioning were important considerations in the prevention of back injuries. In part, because three of the five tests in this study were cardiovascular in nature, there has been a particular interest in the relationship between aerobic condition and LBP.

BENEFITS OF AEROBIC ACTIVITY TO THE SPINE

Although Cady et al. (11) presented a strong argument for the role aerobic conditioning and general physical fitness play in reducing the incidence of LBP, this benchmark study did not delineate the reason aerobic condition was beneficial to the functioning of the spine. Theoretically, aerobic fitness could serve to decrease the chances of becoming symptomatic to LBP in several ways; the rest of this chapter will be devoted to an examination of some of the research done in this area. Before beginning this discussion, some more relevant points of the intervertebral disc will be reviewed because the disc is so important to this topic.

Review of Biomechanics of the Disc

Some researchers contend that most cases of acute LBP in mature adults are caused by damage of some sort to the intervertebral disc (4,5,12,13). If the homeostasis of a disc is affected, its pivotal responsibility as a shock absorber of the spine and an integral part of a motion segment can be diminished. An analogy can be drawn between a damaged disc and a radial tire that is low in air pressure; neither will provide the stability that they did when they were at their optimum working condition. When the disc is damaged, its increased mobility can influence nociceptive endings in the annulus and nerve roots in the intervertebral foramen. As the motion segment becomes further compromised, instability increases; with increased instability, abutting or overriding of the adjacent facet joints can also occur. This is just one scenario of what can happen if disc integrity is affected. The point stressed is that the disc is an important element in maintaining a healthy back free from symptomatology. If any significant biomechanical or chemical changes occur to the disc, the spine will be compromised. It makes sense, therefore, that the circulatory and mechanical mechanisms that provide nutrition to the disc and its contiguous structures are important considerations in the prevention and treatment of LBP.

Obesity and Spine Health

Because it is unlikely that an aerobically fit individual would be obese, obesity could be a marker for lack of aerobic fitness. Heliovaara (12) found that obesity was related to lumbar disc herniation. Others have indicted obesity as a condition that affects spine biomechanics and thus places one at risk for having LBP (4,5,13–15).

Deyo and Bass (14) found a substantial increase in back pain prevalence in those subjects falling into the highest quintile in each of the following: (a) subscapular skin fold thickness, (b) triceps skinfold thickness, and (c) body mass index. When the sexes were examined separately, the association for body mass index was stronger for women than for men. Similarly, Han et al. (16) found a greater association between anthropometric measures and LBP in women than in men. Although Deyo and Bass (14) assumed that the obesity was a predisposing cause of LBP, they also raised the possibility that LBP could decrease activity levels to the point that obesity could be the result.

It should be apparent that increased weight increases the compressive loads on discs (12,17). However, perhaps more importantly, the incumbent anterior displacement of the center of gravity with obesity obligates the extensor muscles of the spine (e.g., erector spinae and multifidus) to counterbalance this turning moment (4,5). Because of their short force arms (18), the dorsal muscles of the spine must contract forcibly to maintain equilibrium; this puts even greater pressure on the intervertebral discs (Fig. 4-1).

Obesity could also cause an increase in the lordotic curve and a concomitant increase in tilt of the sacrum and pelvis. Because shear force is directly related to the sine of the sacral angle (19), the posterior elements would be obligated to absorb more stress in the obese individual than in one who was not overweight.

Muscle Endurance and Spine Health

An aerobically fit individual would be expected to have a high level of muscle endurance. Being aerobically fit would decrease the chance of being obligated to assume biomechanically compromising postures at the end of a work day as muscle groups become fatigued (1,4,13). The landmark study by Cady et al. (11) surmised this and established a research focus on the effect of aerobic condition

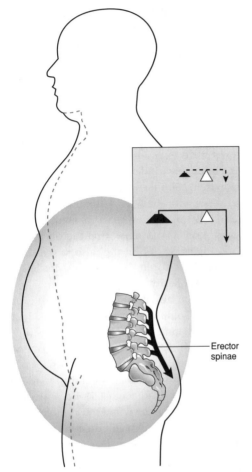

Erector
spinae

Fig. 4-1 The dotted line represents an athletic individual; the center of gravity is very close to the spine. The solid line represents an overweight individual; note how the center of gravity is shifted anteriorly. The important point is that regardless of the distance of the anterior shift of the center of gravity, the force vectors (i.e., leverage) of the erector spinae and multifidus musculature remain essentially the same. Thus, these muscles would be obligated to contract with increased force to balance the load when an individual adds weight anteriorly; this as well as the increased load itself, can place compromising compressive stresses on intervertebral discs. (Adapted from White, A.A., and Panjabi, M.M., *Clinical Biomechanics of the Spine, 2nd ed.* 1990, Philadelphia: JB Lippincott, p. 461).

on back function; this led to studies by others on the relationships between LBP and related factors such as disc nutrition, endorphin levels, and pain tolerance. Nicolaisen and Jorgensen (20) found that individuals experiencing serious low back problems, when compared with those who had not, had similar strength but less endurance capacity in their trunk extensor muscles.

AEROBIC FITNESS AND LOW BACK PAIN

In this section, the causal relationship between aerobic fitness and LBP will be discussed. This will be followed by a discussion on the use of aerobic activities in the prevention and rehabilitation of individuals who have LBP.

Disc Nutrition

Because the disc is avascular (21), it is dependent on diffusion for its nutrition. Diffusion is helped by imbibition as movement occurs in the spinal column; movement promotes an exchange of nutrients from the vertebral endplates and the annuli fibrosi to the avascular disc. The training effect resulting from physical activity could also affect the tissues surrounding the disc by increasing the capillary network of all contiguous areas.

Disc nutrition was examined in a classic study that Holm and Nachemson (2) conducted with canines. In previous research, Holm and Nachemson had noted that (a) a 2-h exercise period did not enhance disc nutrition more than a 30-min period, and (b) only two exercise periods per week did not produce significant training effects. The purpose of the study with canines was to examine the effects of three different intensities of exercise on disc lactate concentration. Twenty-one Labrador dogs were assigned to one of three training programs; each training program included a daily 30-min exercise session for a period of 3 months. The training programs were (a) moderate exercise (i.e., easy jogging on flat ground), (b) "violent exercise" (i.e., hard speed running, including going over obstacles and up steep slopes), and (c) specific spinal motion (i.e., jumping over fences and crawling under obstacles). At the end of 3 months of training, the animals were sacrificed. Although there was no significant difference in disc lactate concentration reduction between the violent and moderate exercise groups, lactate concentration in these two groups was much lower than in the spinal motion group. Holm and Nachemson concluded that aerobic exercise stimulates solute and metabolite transport, which in turn enhances disc nutrition.

Aerobic Exercise in Prevention and Rehabilitation

Others have endorsed the idea that aerobic exercise is an important factor not only in the prevention of LBP but also in the treatment of this condition (6,13,22–24). Statements made by Nutter and by Nachemson may aptly present the majority opinion: (a) "Though not a panacea, aerobic exercise should be a part of the treatment for virtually all causes of low back pain" (1), and (b) "The success of such activity programs in randomized studies for acute, subacute, and chronic patients clearly speaks in favor of the fact that exercise and fitness are likely the most important factors in the overall treatment of patients with low-back pain"(25). In the next section, the research done in this area will be discussed.

Role of Aerobic Exercise in LBP Prevention

Brennan et al. (26) compared aerobic capacity in patients with disc herniations with age- and sex-matched controls. They found that the mean maximal aerobic power (maximal aerobic power was predicted from a submaximal bicycle ergometer test) of the patient group was significantly less than that of the control group. Although no causal relationship can be drawn from this cross-sectional study, the investigators noted that the reduced aerobic fitness may be related to decreased exercise frequency and duration and to changes in type of exercise activity after the onset of back pain. Furthermore, they suggested that there may be a need for aerobic exercise training to enhance cardiorespiratory fitness in individuals with LBP.

Leino (27) studied the effect of leisure time physical activity on the development of LBP in employees in government-owned metal factories in Finland during a 10-year period. Purposive sampling techniques controlled for the variance in work tasks of the employees. Leisure time physical activity and low back symptoms over the 10-year study period were assessed with questionnaires and interviews. Subjects also received a physical therapy assessment of their low back at the beginning and end of the study period. Increased exercise during leisure was associated with decreased low back symptomatology in the male employees but not in the female employees. The investigators suggested that the lower proportion of female employees who participated in leisure time physical activity was the reason for this sex difference.

In a prospective study conducted in Europe comparable to that by Cady et al. (11), Harreby et al. (28) examined 580 subjects at 14 years of age and then at 38 years of age. Their subjects completed a report of LBP history, and a low back radiologic examination was done on each subject. The results showed that subjects who regularly engaged in physical exercise during leisure time reported fewer incidences of LBP over the 25-year follow-up period. However, no relationship was seen between radiographic changes, decreased leisure time physical activity in adulthood, and LBP over the 25-year follow-up period.

In summary, the studies done by Leino (27) and Harreby et al. (28) suggest that there may be an association between low physical activity and an increased incidence of LBP. Low physical activity will lead to decreased muscular and cardiovascular fitness over time. However, a cause-and-effect relationship cannot be determined from these studies because one cannot be sure if decreased physical activity caused LBP or if decreased activity were a consequence of back pain.

Role of Aerobic Exercise in LBP Rehabilitation

Rehabilitation programs typically include a variety of exercises for improving muscle strength, muscle endurance, joint flexibility, and cardiovascular fitness. The use of multiple modes of physical activity makes it difficult to determine the efficacy of a single form of exercise in preventing or alleviating LBP, and consequently, very few studies have focused specifically on the merits of aerobic conditioning. In one study subjects with and without a prior history of LBP were assigned to either an aerobic exercise group or a control group (29). The treatment group participated in two 1 h aerobic exercise sessions per week; one weekly training session was supervised and the other was unsupervised. At a 1.5 year follow-up, no significant improvements in maximal aerobic capacity were achieved by either group, but the exercise group did report less back pain and took fewer sick days compared with the control group. The investigators noted that intensity of exercise was not monitored and suggested that the lack of an increase in aerobic capacity may have been due to insufficient intensity.

Brennan et al. (30) found that after microdisectomy the patient group that was assigned to participate in a walking program made significant gains in aerobic fitness and were able to do so without enduring increases in back pain. In concurrence with this finding, guidelines for treating LBP, established in 1994 by the Agency for Health Care Policy and Research (31), stated that aerobic exercises that minimally stress the back, such as walking, biking and swimming, should be started during the first 2 weeks for most patients with acute LBP to prevent deconditioning due to inactivity and thereafter to help patients return to their highest possible level of functioning. Protas (32) reviewed the research in this area and noted that significant improvements in aerobic capacity were documented in the majority of studies that examined changes in aerobic condition as a result of multimodal rehabilitation programs for individuals with LBP.

There are, however, other considerations that relate to this issue. Because it has been accepted that aerobic condition enhances disc nutrition, some causes that potentially alter nutrition to the disc have been examined; smoking is one such variable.

Effect of Smoking on Aerobic Condition and Spine Health

Even though smoking is not likely to be a factor with athletic populations, the research conducted in this area may have some generic relevance in addition to being relevant for the nonathlete. In animal models, it has been reported that nicotine and exposure to smoke reduce solute transport into the disc (33). In recent years, smoking has been considered a marker for poor aerobic condition when the latter variable has been studied in relation to LBP. Many studies have indicated smoking as a mechanism that can compromise the nutritional pathway to the disc.

Deyo and Bass (14) reported on the incidence of LBP in a sample of 27,801 subjects. Among the subjects who smoked three or more packs a day, 25.1% reported a presence of LBP; among the nonsmokers, only 9.6% reported having LBP. Deyo and Bass concluded that the effects of smoking on the disc were mediated through (a) cough symptoms in their subjects (e.g., smoking tends to increase cough incidence; coughing in turn could increase intradiscal pressure) and (b) circulatory changes. Research conducted previously to the latter study (33) and subsequently (17) have pointed out how smoking can diminish disc nutrition.

Battie (6) led a study that examined the effects of smoking on disc degeneration in identical twins who were highly discordant for cigarette smoking. The smokers and nonsmokers in their data pool showed similar distributions of possible muddling factors, including similar exposure to occupational insults (e.g., lifting, vibration, etc.). Although most from both groups were apt to exercise regularly, interestingly the smokers participated more in team sports, whereas the nonsmokers participated more in aerobic sports such as running, suggesting that personality differences also existed. Magnetic resonance imaging techniques were used as the dependent variable to determine whether disc degeneration could be differentiated. The data showed a significantly greater mean degeneration in the spine of the smoking twin than in the spine of the nonsmoking twin; moreover, the effect was present throughout the lumbar spine, suggesting a mechanism acting systematically. Because there was no interaction between smoking and degeneration at different spinal levels, the investigators did not feel that smoking was a marker for another factor causing disc degeneration.

Further indictments against smoking have been noted in postsurgical healing (34). Investigators examined the effect of smoking on patients who had a spinal fusion from L4 to S1. Almost without exception the smokers had lower blood gas levels than the nonsmokers. Moreover, the difference in the incidence of pseudoarthrosis (surgical nonunion) between nonsmokers and smokers was striking. Four of the 50 nonsmokers (8%) had a pseudoarthrosis, whereas 20 of the 50 smokers (40%) in the study had a pseudoarthrosis. These investigators deduced that inadequate oxygenation of blood flow to the graft site was the major cause of the surgical nonunion; however, they did allow that mechanical factors, such as increased coughing associated with smoking, could have contributed to the variance.

Deyo and Bass (14) and Leboeuf-Yde et al. (35) investigated whether cessation of smoking resulted in a reduction of LBP. Both groups of investigators found that smoking was associated with an increased prevalence of LBP, with Leboeuf-Yde et al. showing a positive association between smoking and recurrent low pain and LBP of long duration. Deyo and Bass (14) found that the prevalence of LBP was the same in current smokers and ex-smokers who had quit for fewer than 10 years. However, ex-smokers who had stopped for 10 years or more had a prevalence of LBP similar to that of nonsmokers. However, Leboeuf-Yde et al. (35) did not find a reduction in LBP symptomatology with cessation of smoking, and, furthermore, this was the case regardless of the time since smoking had stopped.

The evidence against smoking with respect to its deleterious effect on the low back is substantial. Other factors may confuse this issue. Education level, occupation, and socioeconomic status are also factors related to smoking; their contribution to this variance is not clear. Other psychosocial vari-

ables also have been found to have an impact on this issue; Jamison et al. (36) found maladaptive pain behaviors (e.g., decreased physical activity, reliance on medication) to be greater in smokers than in nonsmokers.

EFFECT OF AEROBIC CONDITION ON PAIN AND DEPRESSION

Because of the benefits cited from being aerobically fit, it might be assumed that deconditioning would have significant consequences for the individual with LBP. For example, it has been contended that (a) individuals with chronic LBP have diminished endorphin levels in the cerebral spinal fluid, and (b) aerobic exercise increases endorphin production (23). This could suggest that aerobically fit individuals may have a higher pain tolerance because of increased endorphin levels. Although this contention is not supported by much definitive research, Raithel (3) presented an interesting question about this issue. When patients become physically active and exercise, does their pain perception change because of endorphins or because of increased self-confidence resulting from the fact that they can exercise?

In addition to improving fitness levels with the goal of preventing reinjury, aerobic exercise training in rehabilitation programs may help prevent depression. McQuade et al. (23) administered a battery of psychological disability assessments and physical assessments including tests of strength, flexibility, and aerobic capacity to 96 people with chronic LBP. They reported that lower overall fitness was significantly correlated with increased LBP symptomatology and symptoms of depression. The combined measures of fitness accounted for 17% of the variance in depression, and strength contributed more than flexibility or aerobic capacity to the observed relationship. More studies exploring the relationships between the various modes of exercise and mental health with LBP are needed. Given that participation in all major modes of exercise is needed to optimize overall physical fitness, it seems plausible that a comprehensive exercise program would also have the most beneficial effect on mental health.

SUMMARY

There appears be a link between physical activity, aerobic fitness, and LBP because individuals with back symptomatology tend to have reduced physical activity levels and reduced cardiovascular fitness. Although it is at times difficult to determine whether decreased physical activity and cardiovascular deconditioning are causal factors or the consequence of LBP, low impact aerobic exercise training seems to improve cardiovascular fitness in the population with LBP without risking exacerbation. However, the exact mechanism by which aerobic exercise affects spine function is less certain. For example, although aerobic exercise can improve nutrition to the disc, it can also increase capillary density in skeletal muscle. If the latter happens, there could be better perfusion of the skeletal muscle; this in turn could reduce ischemia and pain. Even though more research on this topic is needed, aerobic exercise appears to be a safe and an important adjunct to most any program designed to protect and rehabilitate the spine.

REFERENCES

1. Nutter, P. Aerobic exercise in the treatment and prevention of low back pain. *Occup Med State Art Rev* 1988, 3: p. 137–145.
2. Holm, S., and A. Nachemson. Variations in the nutrition of the canine intervertebral disc induced by motion. *Spine* 1983, 8: p. 866–873.
3. Raithel, K.S. Chronic pain and exercise therapy. *Phys Sports Med* 1989, 17: p. 203–209.
4. Reilly, K., Lovejoy, B., Williams, R., et al. Differences between a supervised and independent strength and conditioning program with chronic low back syndromes. *J Occup Med* 1989, 31: p. 547–550.
5. White, A.A. and M.M. Panjabi. *Clinical Biomechanics of the Spine,* 2nd ed. 1990, Philadelphia: Williams & Wilkins. p. 722.
6. Battie, M.C. Aerobic fitness and its measurement. *Spine* 1991, 16: p. 677–678.
7. American Heart Association. Statement on exercise. *Circulation* 1992, 86: p. 340–344.
8. Hurri, H., Mellin, G., Korhonen, O., et al. Aerobic capacity among chronic low-back-pain patients. *J Spinal Disord* 1991, 4(1): p. 34–38.
9. Cooper, K.H. *Aerobics.* 1968, New York: Bantam Books, p. 513.
10. Blair, S.N., Kohl, H.W., Goodyear, N.N. Rates and risks for running exercise injuries: studies in three populations. *Res Q Exerc Sport* 1987, 58(3): p. 221–228.
11. Cady, L.D., Bischoff, D.P., O'Connell, E.R., et al. Strength and fitness and subsequent back injuries in firefighters. *J Occup Med* 1979, 21(4): p. 269–272.
12. Heliovaara, M. Body height, obesity and risk of herniated lumbar intervertebral disc. *Spine* 1987, 12: p. 469.
13. Mayer, T.G. Discussion: exercise, fitness, and back pain, in *Exercise, Fitness, and Health,* C. Bouchard, et al. editor. 1990, Champaign, IL: Human Kinetics. p. 541.
14. Deyo, R. and J. Bass. Lifestyle and low-back pain. The influence of smoking and obesity. *Spine* 1989, 14: p. 501–506.
15. Griffith, C.J. Low back pain—clinical presentation, diagnosis, and treatment. *Phys Assist* 1992, 16: p. 86–99.
16. Han, T.S., Schouten, J.S., Lean, M.E., et al. The prevalence of low back pain and associations with body fatness, fat distribution and height. *Int J Obesity* 1997, 21: p. 600–607.
17. Waddell, G. Simple low back pain: rest or active exercise? *Ann Rheum Dis* 1993, 52: p. 317–319.
18. Bogduk, N. and J.E. Macintosh. The applied anatomy of the thoracolumbar fascia. *Spine* 1984, 9: p. 164–170.
19. LeVeau, B.F. *Williams & Lissner's Biomechanics of Human Motion,* 3rd ed. 1992, Philadelphia: W.B. Saunders. p. 326.
20. Nicolaisen, T. and K. Jorgensen. Trunk strength, back muscle endurance and low-back trouble. *Scand J Rehabil Med* 1985, 17: p. 121–127.
21. Bogduk, N. and L.T. Twomey. *Clinical Anatomy of the Lumbar Spine.* 1987, Edinburgh: Churchill Livingstone. p. 166.

22. Palmoski, M.J., Colyer, R.A., Brandt, K.D. Joint motion in the absence of normal loading does not maintain normal articular cartilage. *Arthrit Rheum* 1980, 23: p. 325–334.

23. McQuade, P.T., Turner, J.A., Buchner, D.M. Physical fitness and chronic low back pain. *Clin Orthop Rel Res* 1988, 233: p. 198–204.

24. Borenstein, D. Epidemiology, etiology, diagnostic evaluation, and treatment of low back pain. *Curr Opin Rheumatol* 1992, 4: p. 226–232.

25. Nachemson, A.L. Exercise, fitness, and back pain, in *Exercise, Fitness, and Health*, C. Bouchard et al., editor. 1990, Champaign, IL: Human Kinetics. p. 533.

26. Brennan, G.P., Ruhling, R.O., Hood, R.S., et al. Physical characteristics of patients with herniated intervertebral lumbar discs. *Spine* 1987, 12: p. 699–702.

27. Leino, P.I. Does leisure time physical activity prevent low back pain disorders? *Spine* 1993, 18: p. 863–871.

28. Harreby, M., Hesselsoe, K.J., Neergaard, K. Low back pain in leisure time in 38-year old men and women: a 25-year prospective cohort study of 640 school children. *Eur Spine J* 1997, 6: p. 181–186.

29. Kellett, K.M., Keller, D.A., Nordholm, L.A. Effects of an exercise program on sick leave due to low back pain. *Phys Ther* 1991, 4: p. 283–293.

30. Brennan, G.P., Shultz, B.B., Hood, R.S., et al. The effects of aerobic exercise after lumbar microdisectomy. *Spine* 1994, 19: p. 735–739.

31. Agency for Health Care Policy and Research. *Clinical Practice Guidelines for Acute Low Back Pain.* 1994, Rockville, MD: Agency for Health Care Policy and Research.

32. Protas, E.J. Aerobic exercise in the rehabilitation of individuals with chronic low back pain: a review. *Crit Rev Phys Rehabil Med* 1996, 8: p. 283–295.

33. Holm, S., and A. Nachemson. Nutrition of the intervertebral disc: acute effects of cigarette smoking: an experimental study. *Int J Microcirc Clin Exp* 1984, 3: p. 406.

34. Brown, C., Iorme, T., Richardson, H. The rate of pseudoarthrosis (surgical nonunion) in patients who are smokers and patients who are nonsmokers: a comparison study. *Spine* 1986, 11: p. 942.

35. Leboeuf-Yde, C., Kyvik, K.O., Brunn, N.H. Low back pain and lifestyle. Part I: smoking. Information from a population-based sample of 29,424 twins. *Spine* 1998, 23(20): p. 2207–2213.

36. Jamison, R.N., Stetson, B.A., Parris, W.C.V. The relationship between cigarette smoking and chronic low back pain. *Addict Behav* 1991, 16: p. 103.

CHAPTER 5

LOW BACK PAIN INCIDENCE IN SPORTS

Wendell Liemohn

Marisa A. Miller

INTRODUCTION

From an epidemiologic perspective, the highest incidence of low back pain (LBP) is seen in adults in their third and fourth decades of life. When LBP is seen in athletes who are typically younger, it would appear that the interplays between the magnitude of forces and their frequency of application are factors responsible for the early age onset. Before discussing these age-related differences, a quick review of the motion segment model presented in Chap. 1 is in order (Fig. 1-5). An intimate linkage exists between the anterior disc joints and the posterior facet (zygapophyseal) joints. Kirkaldy-Willis (1) described how trauma at a facet joint has an impact on the disc and how trauma or degenerative disease at the disc affects the facet joints. Similarly, a stress fracture of the pars interarticularis, one of the major causes of LBP in teenagers, could eventually be expected to affect disc function. However, the discogenic pain that is more prevalent in adults is still seen in young athletes (2); although it may not initially affect the pars interarticularis per se, it could eventually affect the facet joints. Sports that heavily involve trunk rotation create torsion stress on various segments of the spine, with the potential for producing injury.

In younger athletes, injuries are more often in the posterior part of the motion segment (i.e., pars interarticularis and facet joints); the injury can result in conditions such as spondylolysis and spondylolisthesis. Frequency of spondylolysis is higher among athletes who do movements involving repetitive flexion and extension of the spine than in the nonathletic population (3). Saal (4) contended that spondylolysis and spondylolisthesis are often seen in gymnastics, weight lifting, football, dance, rowing, and wrestling (5). Torsion forces around the long axis of the spine with load-bearing hyperextension are common causative factors; it has been theorized that this can cause a unilateral stress reaction in the pars interarticularis (6).

Most who study causal relationships of spondylolysis see it as an overuse injury rather than some innate pedicle defect (7). Thus, both disc and pars defects are most likely caused by repetitive microtrauma, defined as cycles of trauma that go unnoticed until their additive result presents symptoms. However, other factors enter the equation when LBP is seen in athletes. Although the types of LBP problems seen in sport are not necessarily very different from the types seen in other walks of life, the frequency and age of occurrence can vary. For example, in a study in which investigators examined spondylolysis in individuals younger than 19 years, all but 5 of the 185 cases seen were in youth who were active in sport (8). Although individuals between the ages of 8 and 14 (i.e., the adolescent growth spurt) are at the greatest risk for spondylolisthesis, Weir and Smith (6) estimated that half the patients with spondylolisthesis are asymptotic. According to their data, disc disease accounts for fewer than 10% of the cases of LBP.

Because the types of injuries are fewer than the sporting activities that can prompt their occurrence, an overview of the typical injuries seen in sport is presented first. Injuries are presented as one of two categories: the posterior or anterior element sectors of spine motion segments. The chapter is then divided into sections alphabetically by sport or sport grouping (e.g., racquet sports). Such division permits presentation of the incumbent stresses in each sport independently; however, the reader should keep in mind that the stresses presented in different sports may be very similar, even though the activities that caused the trauma may be different.

POSTERIOR ELEMENT INJURY

It has been estimated that 10 to 15% of chronic back pain in the general population originates in the facet joints. The occurrence is projected to be higher in athletes because of sports-related rotational components (9). The pars interarticularis is the site of spondylolysis and spondylolisthesis (Fig. 5-1). In spondylolysis, there is a stress fracture or pseudoarthrosis in the pars interarticularis; little support exists for congenital etiology because spondylolysis is so uncommon in infant autopsy studies (10). Spondylolysis is believed to be caused by repetitive, sudden loading in hyperextension with torsion. It is typically a unilateral injury; however, if it occurs on both sides, spondylolysis may lead to spondylolisthesis. In the type of spondylolisthesis prevalent in sports, a bilateral frank fracture of the pars interarticularis is seen. The common clinical pattern is back pain that is not incapacitating but that worsens after specific activity; however, it can lead to a frank fracture of the pars interarticularis (6).

In addition to repeated stresses in hyperflexion and hyperextension, rapid rotation movement is thought to contribute to fatigue fractures of the pars interarticularis (11). If the loading is symmetrical, damage is more apt to occur bilaterally to the pars interarticularis; not surprisingly, asymmetrical loading could logically damage one side more than the other. Damage to the pars interarticularis can occur in other aspects of training such as in the weight room; moreover, some contend that most

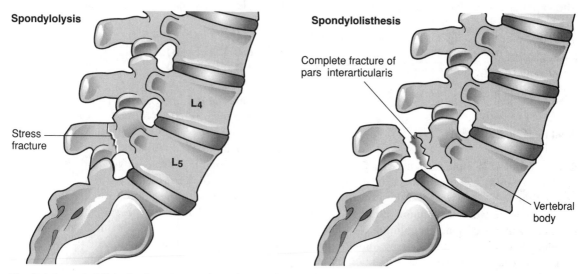

Fig. 5-1 In spondylolysis, there is a unilateral stress fracture of the pars interarticularis. In the spondylolisthesis typically seen, there is a bilateral frank fracture of the pars accompanied by an anterior displacement of the vertebral body. (From Pansky B. *Review of Gross Anatomy.* © 1996. Reprinted with permission from the McGraw-Hill Companies, Inc.)

low back problems in athletes emanate from improper weight-lifting technique (4,12,13) and the improper use of weight training equipment (14).

There is also a degenerative form of spondylolisthesis. This type is more often seen in elderly women and L4 slips over L5, with no frank fracture of the pars interarticularis. Recent research suggests that this form of spondylolisthesis is related to facet joint morphology (15). No research has been found linking "athletic spondylolisthesis" to facet joint morphology.

The bilateral frank fracture of the pars interarticularis seen in spondylolisthesis can lead to slippage of the damaged vertebral body over the vertebra immediately below it. In sport the most frequent site for its occurrence is at the L5-S1 level. Because the amount varies that the damaged vertebra may slip, spondylolisthesis is categorized by degrees of slipping. In first-degree spondylolisthesis, the superior vertebra slips up to 30% of the diameter of the inferior vertebra; in second-degree spondylolisthesis, the slippage is 30 to 50%; in third-degree spondylolisthesis, the slippage is 50 to 75%, and in fourth-degree spondylolisthesis, the vertebra slips completely over the inferior vertebra (12). Athletes with spondylolysis or spondylolisthesis who experience less than 50% slippage may be restricted from activity until healing, typically a minimum of 3 months. Individuals with persistent back pain, greater than 50% slippage, and who fail to respond to treatment may be candidates for surgical intervention (16).

ANTERIOR ELEMENT INJURY

Saal and Saal (17) estimated that the site of back pain problems in 85% of the cases in the general population is the intervertebral disc; they furthermore contended that a common initiator of the problem is forward flexion combined with lateral rotation. They believed that these combined movements could produce peripheral tears of the annulus fibrosis or the cartilaginous endplate and that this could lead to a weakening and tearing of the internal annular fibers to the point that the nucleus pulposus is extruded.

Therefore, it is possible that rotational and torsional stresses may damage the disc and its supporting ligaments instead of the pars interarticularis. As previously stated, the disc is particularly at risk when the spine is subjected to bending and turning moments that occur quickly and are coupled with extreme amounts of exertion. In mature adults, disc damage is the predominant cause of LBP. Although disc injury may be seen in young athletes, its incidence rate is lower than that to the posterior portion of the motion segment, as just discussed (e.g., facet damage, spondylolysis, and spondylolisthesis) (18).

Saal and Saal (17) reported that golf, tennis, and weight training represent the sport activities that are most frequently associated with disc problems, with a common causal mechanism of inadequately controlled trunk rotation. They also contended that disc injury susceptibility increases with deficits in spinal mobility, spinal balance, lower extremity flexibility, trunk strength, muscle endurance, sport matched fitness level, dynamic stabilization ability, and peripheral joint biomechanics (i.e., foot, ankle, knee, hip, and shoulder). They also identified the warm-up, cool-down, equipment, preparticipation fitness, and technique and instruction as common sports deficits related to these types of injuries (17).

GENERAL REHABILITATION CONSIDERATIONS

Two fundamental principles have been identified with regard to rehabilitation that are relevant to prevention: (a) control the lumbar spine through all movements and (b) develop the necessary strength to control these movements. Basic to attaining muscular control of spine movements is at least adequate range of motion (ROM) of the trunk and its adjacent peripheral joints (see Chap. 2). This is particularly important in the athletic realm, where extremes of motion (voluntary or involuntary) are inherent (19).

Sport-specific skills must be modified to ensure "spine-safe" movements; these may be met with hesitation and resistance by athletes in particular because they have achieved success in doing it their own way (19). For example, athletes may need to learn to move more through their lower extremity joints rather than through the lumbar spine. Forward bending at the hip joint (hip hinging) can replace some lumbar flexion, pivoting on a peripheral joint can replace some rotation and twisting movements, and hip abducting can replace side bending (19). These skills can then be incorporated into daily activities and ultimately into sport-specific activities.

SPECIFIC SPORTS

For purposes of convenience, identical headings are presented under most sections. An introductory section in which epidemiology is briefly discussed is followed by sections on the respective roles of *mechanics* (including roles of a disc, facet joint, and neural arch), followed by *strength and flexibility* considerations.

Baseball

Studies examining the incidence and distribution of baseball injuries are limited, despite the popularity and large number of participants at all levels. (Although no relevant reports have been found with regard to softball and although pitching differs markedly between these two sports, the mechanics of batting and other throwing would be the same.) Spine injuries in baseball may result from head-first slides, sudden twists, improper swing mechanics, or sudden bursts of muscular activity (20). McFarland and Wasik (21) investigated the injury incidence, onset, location, type, and severity for a single collegiate baseball team. The incidence of injury to the trunk or back was 15%, accounting for 17% of the total time lost from injury; these injuries included diagnoses to the upper back, spine, low back, ribs, sternum, and coccyx. The most common diagnoses were back muscle strains and spondylolysis. In their 3-year analysis, 12 players were treated for LBP and six lost time from their sport. The investigators stated that defining injury as time lost or as altered participation underestimates the actual occurrence of injury.

General Mechanical Considerations Both batting and throwing can create rotation forces that may compromise the integrity of the lumbar disc and posterior elements (Fig. 5-2). There is also a concern of producing a cascading effect in which adjacent structures may become susceptible to injury (19). Novice pitchers and batters may be particularly vulnerable to these injuries because their trunk musculature may not have been adequately trained to decelerate the rotational forces transmitted through the lumbar spine.

Hitting Mechanics. Watkins (20) recorded electromyographic activity of the trunk musculature of professional baseball players while they batted. The muscle demonstrating maximum intensity in generating power from the legs to the trunk in the preswing and early swing phases was the gluteus maximus of the rear leg. Although the abdominal muscles were active throughout the swing, the erector spinae exhibited greater intensity in the later swing phases. The oblique abdominal muscles were identified as the most important of the torque-transferring muscles of the trunk. Actually, the mechanics of hitting begin with the coordination of the eye muscles; if the athlete is not adequately seeing or misjudges the pitch, the hips may open too early, with the bat and upper body lagging behind the lower body; this produces sudden torsion stress on the lumbar spine (20).

Pitching (Baseball) Mechanics. Watkins (20) contended that, during the cocking phase of pitching, the degree of trunk extension that occurs could produce posterior element injury if the abdominal musculature is not adequately developed and recruited to control this motion. He noted that some rookie pitchers lacked the coordination needed to prevent fatigue and maintain a reproducible throwing pattern and that, once fatigue ensued, the degree of lumbar lordosis increased. With increased lordosis, the body would be behind the point that it should be in the throw; thus, the arm would also be behind and logically result in a high pitch (20). If the abdominal muscles were stronger and had greater endurance, pelvic position would be easier to control.

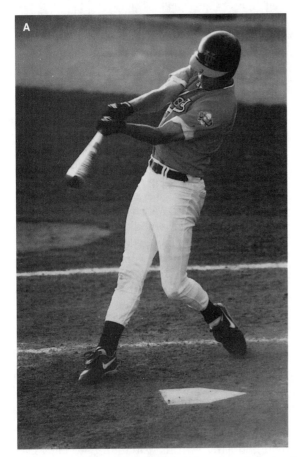
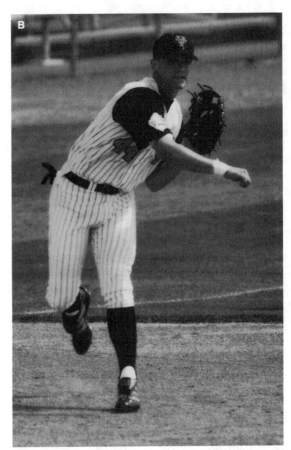

Fig. 5-2 Torsional stresses can be placed on the spine in both **(A)** batting and **(B)** throwing. (Courtesy of the *Vol Sports Information Office*, University of Tennessee, TN.)

Fielding Mechanics. Repetitive bending, standing bent over in ready position, and relative periods of inactivity are common occurrences for these position players. To reduce turning moments as in biomechanically correct lifting techniques, the fielders should bend at the knees and keep the glove and ball in close to the body. Infielders in particular are susceptible to disc injury from repetitive flexion, particularly if they bend at the waist rather than at the knees (19). Emphasis on good posture will help control injuries of this sort; however, controlling other stresses that are apt to be encountered is much more difficult. For example, fielders must commonly go into sudden extreme torsion and twisting motions of the lumbar spine

as they attempt to field the ball or make the throw (20). Also, fielding a fly ball off balance or above the head may produce acute hyperextension of the lumbar spine, predisposing the posterior elements to injury.

Flexibility and Strength Batting requires a considerable amount of hip rotation to accommodate the ROM needed for the wind-up and swing phases. Developing strong lower extremity muscles can help to ensure an increased use of the legs and theoretically reduce the need for excessive force by the trunk muscles. Hip hinging rather than trunk flexion will place the hip extensors in the optimal position to achieve this goal; by emphasizing full motion and strength of the hip extensors and hip rotators, more power can be derived for the swing and at the same time excessive lumbar rotation can be reduced (19).

For pitching and throwing, muscle coordination and trunk strength should be the focus of preventive and injury management training (20). Trunk, hip, and thigh strength facilitate a synchrony of motion between the upper and lower extremities and the controlled unwinding of the trunk during rotation motions. Emphasizing full external rotation of the throwing arm to be able to achieve the entire throwing motion with minimal lumbar extension is important. Because there is a need to reverse quickly out of an eccentric contraction to a concentric contraction to begin the throw, Garges et al. (19) stressed the importance of strong abdominal muscles. They recommended medicine ball training starting in the supine position and progressing toward standing. From the supine position, athletes assume a partial sit-up position as they throw the ball overhead to their partner. This position is maintained as they catch the ball overhead with eccentric control during the deceleration to the starting supine position. The key is a quick reversal from eccentric contraction to concentric contraction as the ball is tossed again, while maintaining a neutral spine posture (19). As good control is developed, the same activity can be performed from the standing position.

Learning to use the feet and hips to pivot rapidly promotes a quick directional change that may enable one to roll up from a diving catch or make a quick throw from a knee without losing the neutral spine position. A plyometric strength program is also recommended to train players how to land appropriately while balanced and off-balanced. In this case, emphasis is placed on eccentric hip, knee, and ankle control (19).

Preventive training for infielders and outfielders includes learning to squat to gather a ground ball as opposed to bending over at the waist with the knees straight. Comparable to lifting techniques, it is recommended that the athletes bend at the knees and keep the glove and ball in close to the body; this simple maneuver can serve to pro-tect the spine (20). However, the ability to work in a forward bend position requires the development of greater proportional strength in the quadriceps muscle group; otherwise, the back will be unduly stressed if the legs are weak (20).

Basketball

Herskowitz and Selesnick (16) contended that back injury is one of the commonest injuries in basketball players. A rudimentary analysis suggests that basketball requires running, cutting, jumping, landing, twisting, and physical contact (Fig. 5-3). Minkoff et al. (22) noted that in players in the National Basketball Association for the season of 1989 and 1990, knee and ankle injuries ranked number one and two, respectively; injuries to the low back ranked number three and accounted for about 7% of all injuries that occurred. In the season of 1990 and 1991, Minkoff et al. noted that low back injuries accounted for nearly 9% of the injuries.

In a 5-year retrospective study of female basketball athletes at the Australian Institute of Sport, Hickey et al. (23) found that injuries to the lumbar spine was the second most frequently occurring injury (11.7%). Mechanical and facet joint-related LBP accounted for 6.3% of all of the injury diagnoses and 53.8% of all low back diagnoses. The second most frequently occurring diagnosis was disc-related pain (11.5%). The researchers suggested that the high incidence of low back injury occurring in this study might be due to the elite nature of the squad and the emphasis placed on weight and strength training.

Tall and DeVault (24) cited a longevity study of 325 professional basketball players during the season of 1984 and 1985 of the National Basketball Association. In this study, the center and forward positions are identified as being at increased risk for back injury; the increased height of these position players could be one reason for this finding.

General Mechanical Considerations From a purely mechanical perspective, a mesomorphic individual with a disproportionate amount of total height due to axial skeleton length would have a greater turning moment above his or her center of gravity than an individual who was more "arms and legs." Overall, taller individuals have more LBP than do shorter individuals.

Posterior Element Injuries. Pars interarticularis defects may produce unilateral pain, with the greatest severity occurring in hyperextended postures (Fig. 5-3); however, symptoms may increase with rotational motion (16). Herskowitz et al. (25) contended that spinal stenosis occurs more fre-

quently in taller athletes than in the general population; sometimes these are accompanied by radicular symptoms.

Anterior Element Injuries. Some particularly tall individuals may have assumed "slouched postures" in their youth because of their height. Nachemson (26) showed how these postures can place stress on the discs of the lumbar spine. Brady et al. (14) believed that improper use of the Leaper (Strength/ Fitness Systems, Independence, MO) was responsible for some low back injuries in young basketball players. These researchers contended that compression-type stresses are placed on the spine if the shoulder harness does not maintain contact with the shoulders. As with most other sports, improper use of the equipment or improper lifting techniques in the weight room also may be responsible for some low back problems.

Flexibility and Strength   Hyperlordotic and hypolordotic posturing can result from tight hip flexors and tight hamstrings, respectively. As emphasized in Chap. 2, good ROM at the iliofemoral joint can be an important safeguard against having LBP. As in any rehabilitation program, it behooves the basketball player to have strong lateral abdominal muscles to enable him or her to brace the trunk and counteract rotational stresses. This is not to suggest that the muscles of the spine are not important; on the contrary, it has been contended that back strengthening is often ignored in basketball players (25).

Football

The game of American football presents many opportunities for different types of injuries to the lumbar spine. Repetitive flexion, extension, and torsion stresses to the lumbar spine predispose the football athlete to injury (9). Moreover, the collision nature of this sport can result in impacts and stresses from a variety of directions; therefore, the type of lumbar spine injury is dependent on not only the point of impact but also the direction

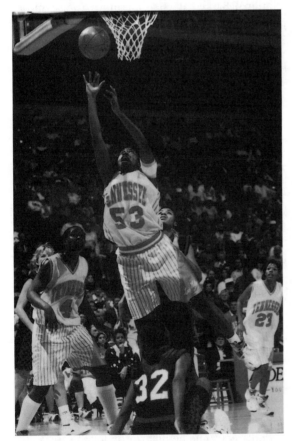

Fig. 5-3 In basketball, the spine is subjected to stress in a number of different ways. In this figure, the offensive player is in hyperextension as she goes up for the shot. (Courtesy of the *Lady Vol Media Relations Office*, University of Tennessee, TN.)

and magnitude of force. It has been estimated that up to 30% of football players lose playing time because of LBP (4).

General Mechanical Considerations   Mechanical factors inherent to the position played suggest that interior linemen are the most prone to having low back problems (9,12,27). For example, to be successful on offense or defense, the lineman must overpower his opponent. The spine of the individual losing these bouts is often put in a compromising position (Fig. 5-4). If the loading is symmetrical, the incumbent extension jamming can lead to facet joint pain and stress on the neural arch. The repetitive loading of the posterior elements in rising from the low starting position to the blocking posture creates a predisposing risk of injury for linemen (9). By the very nature of the sport, asymmetrical loading is more apt to occur; thus, some degree of torsion stress will also be a factor.

There are other scenarios in the sport that place athletes at risk. Garges et al. (19) proposed that attempting to catch a pass while an opponent placed a hit might force the spine into sudden hyperextension when it is most vulnerable. This position finds the abdominal musculature at near peak eccentric length, rendering the athlete incapable of protecting and stabilizing the lumbar spine from additional extension. If the abdominal muscles are weak, the problem may be compounded.

Posterior Element Injury.   It has been estimated that spondylolysis occurs in up to 50% of interior linemen (28). McCarroll et al. (29) believed that the genesis of the problem occurs in adolescence. Use of the blocking sled is believed by some to be a cause of spondylolysis (7). It is also possible that poor technique in lifting weights may be an initial prompter of the problem. Theoretically, a low back problem may be the result of the stresses occurring in a single play; however, it would be more likely to be the result of repetitive stresses occurring over time, with a single play exacerbating an already damaged structure. In spondylolysis and spondylolisthesis, the structure is the pars interarticularis. This portion of a vertebra (Fig. 5-1)

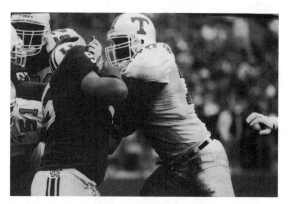

Fig. 5-4 A lineman in football may be forced into hyperextension if he cannot neutralize the force imposed by his opponent. (Courtesy of *Football Time in Tennessee.*)

can be at risk in forceful hyperextension and rotation movements.

Anterior Element Injury.   Returning to our offensive lineman scenario, if his spine is forcibly hyperextended by the defensive man who he is trying to block, a large shear force must be absorbed. Because the weakest link in the spinal column is the vertebral endplate, in sports such as football, Barber (12) hypothesized that disc problems evolve when a shearing force separates the cartilaginous endplate from its vertebral attachment. When the endplate is damaged, material from the nucleus pulposus enters the body of the adjacent vertebra. As the disc loses nuclear material, it becomes less stable, and annular fissures occur. Additional stress placed on the damaged annulus leads to further weakening of its walls, followed by increased instability. What started as a vertebral endplate fracture leads to an unstable motion segment that will continue to degenerate. Blocking sled use was cited as a causative factor in posterior element injury (7); however, it would also appear to present the same type of problem experienced by basketball players using the Leaper (14). In sled use, the problem may be related to how much mobility or give that the sled allows. An improper three-point stance, eliminating lumbar lordosis and producing shoulder flexion when hitting an opponent, has been implicated in magnifying intradiscal pressure, with the potential of causing disc disruption (19).

Flexibility and Strength   Flexibility is a significant consideration in the prevention of injuries to the low back for the football player and can be important to rehabilitation. To reemphasize a point stressed throughout this book, if either the hip flexors (e.g., psoas and iliacus) or the hip extensors (e.g., hamstrings) are tight, the trunk musculature cannot control the attitude of the pelvis. Thus, if a player has tight hamstrings, he can be operating near end ROM for posterior pelvic rotation; in such a scenario, there would be very little give in his hip joint musculature to rotate the pelvis anteriorly should an overwhelming stress occur. Returning to our example of the blocking guard or tackle, if the defensive player overpowers an offensive tackle with tight hamstrings, something must absorb the energy of this stress. If the musculotendinous structures crossing the hip joint do not give, the soft tissue structures of the spine (e.g., facet joint capsules, supraspinous ligaments) may be obligated to absorb these stressors; obviously, this would not be desirable.

The main goal of a preventive or rehabilitation program is to "attain adequate musculoligamentous control of lumbar spine forces to eliminate repetitive injury to the intervertebral discs, facet joints, and related structures" (9, p. 145). The emphasis is on training with specific lumbar stabilization exercises incorporating muscle fusion to protect the motion segments from repetitive microtrauma and excessive loads (9). *Muscle fusion* is another term that is sometimes used to describe what occurs as agonist and antagonistic muscles of the trunk co-contract to brace and stabilize the spine.

Day et al. (30) contended that training schedules often do not place enough emphasis on strengthening the abdominal muscles and stretching the low back area. Ideally, off-season strength programs will prepare the athlete for the types of stresses that are apt to be incurred. Other things being equal, the individual who can exert more power (e.g., good technique and strength) than the opposition will absorb forces more effectively and be less apt to sustain a low back injury.

The extremity muscles that might be thought of as the most important for football players would include the leg, hip, and all the muscles of the shoulder girdle and arm. However, extremity power and speed stem from a strong core that includes the spinal flexors and extensors. Although the lateral abdominal muscles would doubtfully be overlooked, it is contended that they are particularly important. For example, the large moment arms of the external and internal obliques and the transversus abdominis enable these muscles to exert strong antirotation moments that can help the athlete resist rotational and shearing stresses. These types of stresses are particularly endemic in line play. From a perspective of mechanics, the connections of the lateral abdominal muscles to the thoracolumbar fascia also enable these muscles to play a key role in the stabilization and splinting of the spine and resisting forces in all planes; the specific mechanics of this were described in Chap. 1. However, the more effectively the player can stabilize the spine and prevent excessive hyperextension, shearing, and torsion stresses, the less chance that injury will occur. This obviously relates to the football player's strength. Two exercises for strengthening the lateral abdominal muscles are presented in Figs. 5-5 and 5-6.

The skills wanted for baseball (throwing, catching, directional changes, and diving) are also essential for football; however football requires greater stability for blocking and hitting and for absorbing both expected and unexpected contact forces (19). The medicine ball can be used to design a progressive momentum-absorbing program in which the momentum of the ball is absorbed by bracing the spine in a neutral position. The lower extremities also receive simultaneous eccentric loading during these drills. Changing the direction from which the ball is thrown at the body or catching it while airborne can increase the challenge. Directional change, sideways movement, and blocking and diving should emphasize using a neutral spine posture (19).

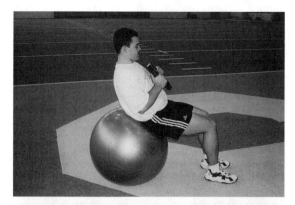

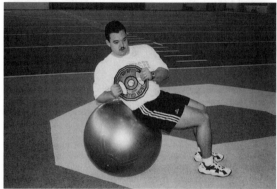

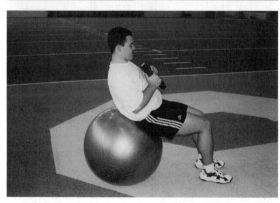

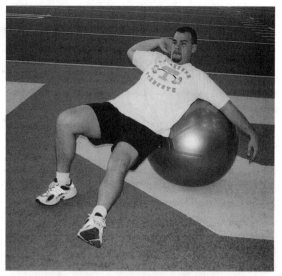

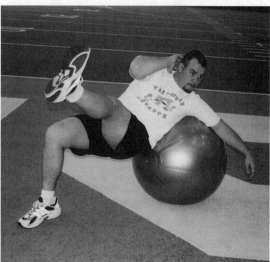

Fig. 5-6 This oblique curl exercise requires even more proprioception than the exercise depicted in Figure 5-5. This exercise also develops core strength.

Fig. 5-5 Lifting weights while balancing on a therapy ball requires good proprioception to stabilize trunk and would appear to be more specific to some of the requirements of football and other sports. This trunk rotation exercise is good for core strength development.

An underlying point should be emphasized concerning the dynamics of football. Although an analysis can be made of the different demands that could be placed on the spine, and training programs could be designed to meet these stresses, performance on the field is a complete process that can defy simple fragmentation. In other words, although the requirements of different positions could be analyzed and weight training tasks designed to counter the stresses faced, this training should merely be part of the strategy to follow in the football player's strength development. It would appear that those training activities that have the highest degree of specificity to the stresses encountered on the field of play would provide the most insurance against injury.

Golf

Low back pain is a common golf-related injury in amateurs (31,32). In a survey of 461 amateur golfers, Batt (33) reported that back problems accounted for nearly half of all ailments. Low back pain is also the most common area of complaint among male golfers in the Professional Golf Association; Duda (34) reported that 90% of professional golfers' tour injuries involve the cervical or lumbar spine. In the Ladies Professional Golf Association (LPGA), injury to the spine ranked second, with injury to the wrist as the most prevalent injury (35). It should be noted, however, that stress fractures of the ribs in golfers may sometimes be incorrectly diagnosed as back strain (36).

General Mechanical Considerations   Gracovetsky (37,38), in describing his "spinal engine" notion, showed how a man without legs and walking on his ischial tuberosities showed essentially the very same movement patterns in the spine as a man with legs. The spinal engine concept is most relevant to the golf swing because it relies on a tightly coiled body to store power for maximum club head acceleration at impact (35). For example, a good golfer may generate a club head speed of approximately 100 miles per hour in less than two-tenths of a second (39); this obviously could subject the lumbar spine to rapid, complex, and intense loads. However, professional golfers are usually more efficient and consistent in their swing patterns, which decreases the forces placed on their trunks (40). Because of poor swing mechanics, amateurs often develop higher loads in the lumbar spine than professional golfers (33,35). Batt (41) found that amateurs attempt to generate more power with their arms, whereas professionals generate power with their hips and legs by shifting their body weight. This would support the contention that professional golfers have greater club speed than amateurs but that it is not at the expense of increased spinal loads (42).

The back swing is where many problems begin with regard to injury. It consists of a turning, twisting, and tension-producing motion. Starting at the ankle and moving up the kinetic chain, twists and turns occur in different directions. Uniform acceleration is recommended where momentum is gradually created through the joints; stopping the follow-through too abruptly is another source of injury (43).

Ideally, the golf swing should be completed with the spine in a neutral position (i.e., neither flexed nor extended too much). A common error is using spinal flexion rather than hinging at the hip joint to position the body over the ball (Fig. 5-7). This disrupts the neutral spine position, changing the center of gravity, and limiting the amount of available trunk rotation (40). Moreover, if the spine is flexed too much, greater distraction occurs between the superior and inferior articular processes; this sets the stage for facet joint sprains and annular tears of the disc. However, when a proper hip joint hinging and neutral spine are used, the center of gravity remains stable and the compressive forces are transferred to the feet. This maximizes balance, spinal mobility, and provides a good foundation from which to swing the club (40).

Strength, balance, proper posture, and flexibility are the essential components of a mechanically sound golf swing. The power is generated in the trunk, and the hip and trunk muscles transmit this power and speed. The previously taught reverse-C swing is harmful and biomechanically inefficient because it places the golfer off-balance and reduces the power obtained by the trunk and hips (20). Using the large trunk muscles to provide the needed power and speed and support the lumbar spine in a neutral position or range throughout the swing not only maximizes power but also reduces stress on the lumbar spine (20).

Posterior Element Injury.   Although LBP in the golfer may develop secondarily to the rotation of

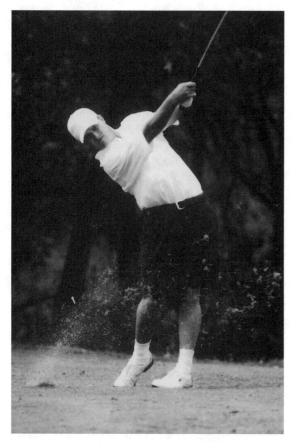

Fig. 5-7 In this figure, a small bend in the knees and hips necessitates a greater bend in the spine that can increase torsional stress. Ideally, the spine should remain in a more neutral position than presented in this figure. (Courtesy of the *Vol Sports Information Office*, University of Tennessee, TN.)

the lumbar spine at the top of the back swing, it is often the subsequent uncoiling and hyperextension through the forward swing and follow-through that causes the problem (35). A high and complete follow-through is often deemed desirable, but, to achieve this reversed-C position, the lumbar spine must rotate while in hyperextension; this can induce posterior element stress and degenerative changes (41). Overuse and poor mechanics during the follow-through phase are the most probable

causes of lumbar facet injury to the golfer; with repetitive swings and incorrect form, the lumbar facet joints bear the abnormal forces being placed in the lumbar region (36). Trunk control is easier with a compact swing, and cutting down on the back swing and follow-through are two ways to achieve this goal. However, the tradeoff is that, although stress on the spine is decreased, power and distance are diminished.

Anterior Element Injury. Torsion increases intradiscal pressure; if rotation is carried beyond normal ROM limits, circumferential tears in the annulus can result. In putting, the posture is often "hunched over," with negligible if any lordotic curve in the lumbar spine. Nachemson (26) graphically showed how intradiscal pressures increase in the bent standing posture; therefore, a lengthy putting session could be particularly stressful to the spine. The golfer who picks up the ball out of the cup with straight legs may be adding stress to the spine.

Wallace and Reilly (44) showed that simulated golf play induced greater spinal shrinkage (loss of intervertebral disc height) than a control condition designed to mimic walking the course. Their findings related the extent to which additional physical and physiologic loadings are incurred due to carrying clubs during a simulated round of golf of more than nine holes. However, it was suggested that compressive loading was not a major source of strain in recreational golfers.

Flexibility and Strength Flexibility and stability must be increased to allow for the ROM and efficient muscle firing, which are needed to complete a safe and effective swing (40). Exercises that would appear to help golfers the most would be those that enable them to maintain their spines in the neutral position. However, before the neutral spine can be attained, the golfer must have adequate ROM at the hip joint. Full ROM in the back, hips, hamstrings, and shoulders and strengthening of the back, hips, legs, shoulders and wrists allow for more explosive shots over a longer period without fatigue (36). Once full ROM is attained, exercises that strengthen the muscles of the trunk, with emphasis on the muscles that rotate the trunk, should be emphasized. The focus is to strengthen the key muscles responsible for trunk control (internal and external obliques, transverse abdominis, multifidus, erector spinae, quadratus lumborum, and psoas major). These muscles provide an antitorsion moment to counter the rotational forces. The net effect is a decrease of the shearing forces on the spine in the golf swing (40). Flexibility and strength development in the upper extremities are also important.

Other Considerations Muscle endurance and aerobic condition may often be overlooked in the golfer (31,33,36,42,45). Fatigued muscles take longer to adapt to changes in loading; this leads to compensation and can lead to poor posture, with increased abnormal loadings on the spine (36). Because the emphasis in golf is placed more on skill and finesse than on fitness, the high low back injury rate in golfers could often relate to their degree of general physical fitness and aerobic condition (45).

Gymnastics

In a prospective study conducted by Caine et al. (46), it was found that the body part most frequently injured in competitive female gymnasts was the wrist; however, the second most frequently injured body part was the lower back. Most of these gymnastic injuries were classified as repetitive stress or overuse injuries. According to Michelli and Wood (2), periods of rapid growth make the athlete particularly vulnerable to this type of injury. Although football and wrestling at the high school and collegiate levels have been viewed as "high risk" sports, gymnastic injury rates have consistently approached this level (47). Moreover, Snook (48) believed that gymnastics should be classified as a hazardous sport because it has been estimated that the incidence of LBP in female gymnasts may be as high as 75%. Although most of the research in gymnastics concerns LBP in females rather than in males, one study reported that male gymnasts had twice as much disc degeneration as male control subjects (49).

Floor exercises are responsible for most of the injuries in women's gymnastics, followed by the balance beam, uneven bars, and vaulting (50). However, not factored in this equation are the time spent practicing on each event and the event's level of difficulty. Elite gymnasts have a higher injury rate than do gymnasts with less skill (47,51,52); however, (a) they would be expected to practice more than the non-elite would, and (b) it stands to reason that the elite gymnast would practice more risky stunts than the non-elite gymnast would. Thus, the window of opportunity for exposure to injury is greater than for the non-elite as far as hours practiced, as is the risk factor of the stunts done. The epidemiologic data support this notion because it has been reported that United States Gymnastics Federation class I gymnasts have almost 5, 11, and 25 times as many injuries as class II through IV gymnasts, respectively (49). Moreover, Caine et al. (46) found that elite gymnasts practice 5.36 days per week for an average of 4 to 5 h per day. Although Tsai and Wredmark (53) reported that the elite gymnasts that they studied did not have more back problems than age-matched control subjects, their subjects practiced only 10 h per week.

General Mechanical Considerations The stresses to which the spine is subjected in gymnastics may be many. The stresses may be event-specific or may occur in several events.

Posterior Element Injury. One major type of stress to the spine is the gymnastic routine that typically calls for extension into hyperlordosis, such as that seen in dismounts. This shifts the load from the stronger anterior portion of the motion segment (i.e., disc and vertebral body) to the weaker posterior portion (i.e., pars interarticularis and the facet joints). Stress to the pars interarticularis may also result from the routine flexion and hyperextension maneuvers seen in back and front walkovers and in vaults (Fig. 5-8). In gymnastics, the repetitive flexion, extension, and hyperextension of the lumbar spine can predispose athletes to a fatigue fracture of the pars interarticularis (8); the adolescent growth spurt (8 to 14 years of age) is a particularly critical period for this injury (46,49). Repeated trauma such as this could very

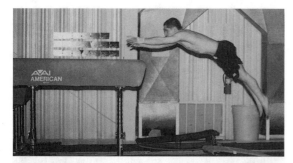

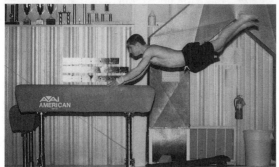

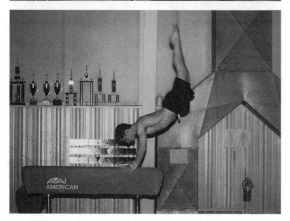

Fig. 5-8 The spines of gymnasts are often subjected to extreme stresses. Forceful hyperextension in vaults could lead to problems such as spondylolysis or spondylolisthesis. (Courtesy of *Knoxville Gymnastics Training Center*, Knoxville, TN.)

well be responsible for the nearly four to five times greater prevalence of spondylolysis in female gymnasts than is the norm for white females (47,52). Ohlen et al. (54) found a significant relationship between lordosis and LBP complaints, and they noted an increased risk of overloading the spine in maximal extension with lordosis.

Anterior Element Injury. This type of injury can result from vertical impact with a reduced lordosis; this places the stress on the strong anterior elements of the motion segment in activities such as landing. Although the anterior elements are stronger than the posterior elements, microfractures may occur to vertebral endplates that could disrupt their normal growth (55); this could also lead to an expulsion of nuclear material into an adjacent vertebra.

Flexibility and Strength   The traditional role of flexibility may be unimportant as a cause of LBP in gymnasts because they typically have an exceptional amount of flexibility. Nevertheless, reduction in flexibility due to pathology such as spondylolysis or spondylolisthesis would be symptomatic of a problem. Hamstring tightness, the most common symptom, is found in up to 50% of gymnasts with spondylolysis or spondylolisthesis (10). The deep pike position requires flexibility in the hamstrings, buttocks, and lower back muscles and strength in the trunk flexors and hip flexors (56).

A gymnast must be prepared for the many hours of practicing movements to achieve a skilled and safe performance (56). An improvement in core strength can help splint the spine and prevent or reduce rotational and torsional stresses. Exercises recommended for the development of strength in the abdominal and iliopsoas groups are various bent hip and knee curl-ups and leg raises from a hanging position, respectively. For the leg raises, the gymnast can begin by lifting with bent knees to half position and from there begin to extend one leg at a time and then progress to lifting with straight legs (56).

Racquet Sports

The occurrence of LBP and injury in racquet sports differs depending on the sport in question. The least injurious racquet sport to the lower back is racquetball (57), followed by badminton (58), and then squash (59). Of the racquet sports, back pain is the most common in tennis, with a reported incidence as high as 43% (60). In a 6-year study of the United States Tennis Association Boys' Championships (i.e., for age 18 years and younger), 16% of the injuries were to the back (61).

Saraux et el. (62) found little evidence that linked tennis with an increased risk of LBP; however, their subjects were recreational rather than competitive tennis players, the sample size was small, and the findings were based on subjective interviews rather than on an objective physical examination.

General Mechanical Considerations   Most low back injuries sustained in racquet sports are intrinsic in nature, occurring while moving to the ball or performing some strokes (58,60). The simple act of repetitive bending to pick up the ball or awaiting the next volley poised on the balls of the feet, with the trunk flexed to the point that the shoulders are hanging over the toes, can place significant demands on the lumbar spine.

Although the stroke mechanics are about the same in all racquet sports, the time between the strokes and the court distance to be covered differ (61). Knowledge of stroke mechanics and their impact on the spine is essential for understanding the nature and mechanisms of low back injury in racquet sports. In tennis Saal (63) believed that the greatest low back stress occurs during the serve or overhead motion (Fig. 5-9). If, when serving, the ball toss occurs behind the shoulder of the server, the player must rotate and hyperextend the spine to contact the ball; with ball impact, there is a rapid reversal of spine rotation. For the right-handed server, the spine shifts rapidly from hyperextension and from counterclockwise rotation to clockwise rotation and hyperflexion (63). This combination of hyperextension and rotation in the overhead hit or serve, followed by the flexion and rotation necessary to complete the stroke, can place excessive stress on the disc (60). The spinal rotation seen in tennis can place high torsion stresses on the disc; this can result in fatigue-related disruption or microtrauma of the posterior annulus. The position of the ball in relation to the

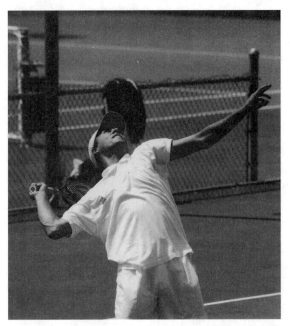

Fig. 5-9 One of the greatest low back stresses occurs during the serve or overhead motion. In serving, the stress can be magnified if (a) the ball is not thrown far enough in front of the server or (b) the shoulders and pelvis do not rotate as a coupled unit. (Courtesy of the *Vol Sports Information Office*, University of Tennessee, TN.)

body can also magnify the stresses applied to the back. A ball in front of the body, or baseline, in a serve will decrease the amount of lumbar hyperextension, whereas a ball behind the body, or baseline, will increase hyperextension needed to execute the hit. A ball located far to either side will increase rotation and side bending needed for ball contact (60,64).

The forehand and backhand ground strokes are executed with upper body movements and should produce little change in flexion and extension, and minimal rotational change should occur with ball contact. However, the movements affecting the low back are rapid alternating rotations to the right and to the left with forehand and backhand volleys; these volleys and the impact transmitted from the ball to the racquet to the body must be absorbed

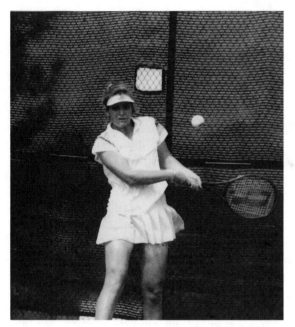

Fig. 5-10 It has been contended that the two-handed backhand can place excessive stress on the lumbar spine because the nondominant shoulder must rotate more completely with the follow-through (63). (Courtesy of the *Lady Vol Media Relations Office,* University of Tennessee, TN.)

(60). During the start of the forehand, the shoulders are perpendicular to the net; then there is a rotation away from the net of approximately 30 degrees to initiate the back swing. The stroke is finished after the upper body derotates with the follow-through, with very little transition flexion to extension (60,63,64). Although the open stance forehand involves less trunk rotation, rotational acceleration may be greater than in a close stance (63).

In the one-handed backhand, there is less trunk rotation than in the forehand during the forward swing because the hitting shoulder is already facing the net (63). However, as the arm holding the racquet crosses the body, the initial rotation is accentuated, and the resulting rotary motion increases the potential for low back injury (60,64). The two-handed backhand can place greater stress on the

lumbar spine because the nondominant shoulder must rotate more completely with the follow-through (63) (Fig. 5-10). If the athlete is reaching for a wide ball with the two-handed backhand stroke, the lumbar spine can be placed at increased biomechanical risk because the pelvis is typically fixed (65).

All strokes differ in the amount of force generated in flexion, extension, and rotation of the spine; thus, each stroke can be affected by aerobic and anaerobic fitness (64). A low center of gravity can decrease the amount of lumbar flexion necessary for ground stroke execution. Thus, muscle endurance for the lower extremities is important. Conversely, the player with a straight-legged stance must use more lumbar flexion to reach low balls; this in turn increases lumbar strain. Lumbar flexion coupled with the rotation needed to make the shot may be enough to cause significant lumbar spine trauma.

Another factor to consider is that racquet sport participants asymmetrically load the trunk and shoulders. The dominant hitting shoulder and the nondominant side of the trunk initiate powerful movements, especially during the overhead hit or serve. Furthermore, forces generated from the ball to the racquet and from the court to the feet are transmitted to the primary and stabilizing muscles and the spine. These forces all seem to play a part in the susceptibility of the lumbar spine to injury in racquet sports; an attempt to promote symmetry may be in order.

Posterior Element Injury. Overall, vertebral fractures and acute spondylolysis are unusual in racquet sports because neither the acute compressive loads causing fractures nor the excessive loading with hyperextension is a normal part of racquet sports' stroke mechanics (63). However, decreased back extension flexibility and repetitive forced hyperextension with overhead volleys and serves may lead to facet joint irritation. Repetitive compression and hyperlordotic changes affect the facets; long-term changes could lead to spinal stenosis. Facet impingement or locking can occur with trunk flexion and slight rotation, causing the facet joint to shift out of normal alignment and trigger a reflex muscle spasm (64). Facet impingement may also occur with acute hyperextension; however, a healthy disc should prevent this.

Anterior Element Injury. Torsion increases intradiscal pressure, and if rotation is carried beyond normal ROM limits, circumferential tears in the annulus can result. Because of the viscoelastic behavior of connective tissue, torque strength of a joint is stronger when the rate of axial rotation is increased. This could account for the racquet sport athlete's ability to withstand most of the joint problems associated with torsion. However, repetitive loading and unloading, as typically occurs in matches, could result in gradual deformation of the disc and distortion of its ability to dissipate the energy transmitted to the spine.

Racquet sport participants may be at increased risk of disc trauma because the annulus acts as a restraint against rotation; this is particularly true in flexed postures. Disc trauma may occur if lumbar support muscles are deconditioned or continually overloaded and fatigued. Certain strokes, in particular the overhead shot or serve, can place the disc at increased risk of annular tears due to repetitive rotational forces, especially when coupled with hyperextension (63). The combined trunk flexion-and-rotation coupling motion, which is magnified in the two-handed backhand, can also lead to discogenic problems.

Flexibility and Strength   In tennis players, both flexibility and strength are important attributes. Poor flexibility in the hamstrings will preclude hinging at the iliofemoral joint, and this in turn will place greater stress on the lumbar spine and lead to repetitive stress at end ROM. As previously mentioned, lower extremity fatigue may compromise hip and knee flexion; this could, for example, force flexion to occur in the lumbosacral area when executing ground strokes, thereby putting the spine at additional risk. Increasing the strength of the lateral abdominal musculature could theo-

retically lessen the torsion stresses placed on the spine in tennis. In tennis matches, muscle endurance seems to play an important role, for as the tennis player becomes more fatigued, body mechanics suffers, and the individual becomes more vulnerable to injury.

Injury to the shoulder complex can limit upper trunk rotation, forcing the lower trunk to generate more rotational force; this, too, increases the potential for low back strain. Flexibility exercises should focus on the trunk rotators and extensors and on upper and lower extremity muscles (64). Strength and flexibility of the extremities are important for preventing weak links in the kinetic chain that can increase the stress applied to the low back. If faulty stroke mechanics exist, having good flexibility and strength is unlikely to protect the back from repetitive stress.

Core strength development and the implementation of a lumbar stabilization program will promote awareness and control of trunk and spine position to reduce static and dynamic loads. These exercises function to limit hyperextension, improper trunk flexion, and forced trunk rotation.

Rowing

Low back pain is one of the most common complaints of rowers, and its incidence is far greater in rowers than in the general population (65–68). The conversions made to the rig and changes that comprise the modern style of rowing have been implicated in the sudden increase in injury incidences in this sport (69–71).

Rowing involves projecting one oar (sweep) or two (sculling) through the water for propulsion. Both forms place an individual facing the stern of the shell with a seat that moves fore and aft on a set of tracks. The swivel oarlocks and the gliding seat increase the mechanical advantage and propulsion of the shell (71). In a review on the evolution of rowing, Greene (69) called shell modifications a transformation from "comfort to contortion." The changes in the oar and rig have decreased the forward lean from the hips by 60% and the need to twist from the anterior axis by 50%.

FROM THE UNITED STATES ROWING ASSOCIATION

"The rowing stroke is divided into two events, the catch and finish, and into two phases, the drive and recovery. . . . The knees are fully flexed, and the shoulders and elbows are extended and the back in a forward flexed position. The movement consists of lifting the hands and tensing the back for the drive phase. During the drive phase, the shell is accelerated through the water. The leg drive, the back swing into the oars and bringing the hands into the body are the three stages that comprise the drive phase. The low back acts as a braced cantilever, serving as the linkage between the upper and lower extremities. The recovery phase begins by moving the hands away from the body and flexing the knees and then sliding the seat. This is followed by a back swing into the stern to set the body for the next catch. Elbow extension and scapular adduction promote the swing of the hands away from the body. Trunk, hip and knee flexion all promote proper positioning for the catch" (71).

General Mechanical Considerations Most injuries occur around the time of the catch (71) (Fig. 5-11A). In comparison with the older upright straight-back style of rowing, the style of accentuated forward flexion may predispose rowers to increased risk of injury (11). At the catch, there is a rapid generation of force at the oar; this force accelerates to a peak near the middle of the drive phase (71). The position of the rower at the catch is sitting bent forward up to 20 degrees or more; competitive rowers in a season may spend up to 2 h per day intermittently in this position (68,71). In relation to Nachemson's work on intradiscal pressure in different postures, the second highest pressure recorded in the disc was in a seated position with a similar forward bend (67). Furthermore, the greater the forward flexion at the catch, the greater the compressive load on the front edge of the disc and the higher the tensile forces on the posterior elements of the lumbar vertebrae (71). The increase in forward flexion at the catch decreases the efficiency of the body position for the back muscles; they must exert sufficient force to straighten the back and take on the load of the

boat. If the catch occurs too early or if the boat rocks off balance during the catch, the stresses on the muscles increase even more and add an extra burden to the low back (70).

Posterior Element Injury. Rowing itself produces predominantly flexion injuries (71). A twisting motion in sweep rowing places a stress torque on the spinal extensors and rotators; this asymmetrical movement can lead to strength imbalances. Scullers are at an advantage in comparison with sweep rowers because they keep their backs straight toward the stern at the catch, whereas sweep rowers reach at the catch and rotate their shoulders and extend the back. This increases the stresses on the facet joints and in particular on the muscles opposite the oar side (70). Most rowing injuries are usually caused by overuse or poor technique; faulty technique may be due in part to anatomic abnormalities magnified through the rowing action (72). Back pain in rowers usually involves the low back, mainly around the midpoint, but occasionally radiating out to the sides; pain is usually felt on the side away from the oar (70).

Anterior Element Injury. Intervertebral disc trauma is the most prevalent cause of LBP in rowers. Peak compressive loads on the lumbar vertebrae occur in the later part of the drive phase as the upper torso extends over the low back; at this point, the average peak compressive load for males is 6066 N and for females is 5031 N (71) (Fig. 5-11B). When normalized for body weight, the peak compressive loads for both sexes are close to the same (7 times body weight for males; 6.85 times body weight for females); loads such as these can produce disc and pars interarticularis trauma (71). The forward bending position, in which rowers spend the greatest amount of time, causes a marked increase in intradiscal pressure (26); the resulting alterations may include disc height reduction, herniation, or protrusion (68).

Flexibility and Strength Adequate flexibility and strength for trunk flexion, extension, and rotation

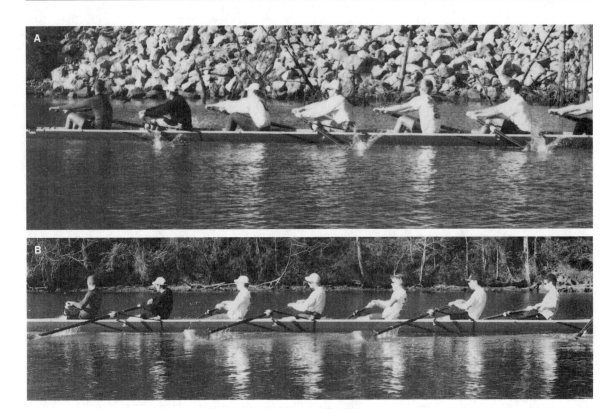

Fig. 5-11 Rowing eights. **(A)** The catch phase as the blade enters the water. **(B)** The end of the drive phase as the blade is removed from the water. The constant flexion bias in rowing places high compressive forces on the disc. (*Courtesy of Dartmouth College Rowing Team.*)

are essential. A flexibility program should be designed to increase ROM of the low back and hamstrings to extend the catch or to reach it more comfortably. Hyperflexion of the lumbar spine may be needed to achieve full rowing motion; this enables rowers to reach farther forward and increases the available ROM to generate power during the drive. However, hyperflexion is strongly related to injury and could eventually impede performance. Stretching joints that are already hypermobile should be avoided; instead, special emphasis should be on developing extensor flexibility and strength (67).

Muller et al. (73) found that elite rowers exhibited stronger isometric trunk torque in all planes when compared with those participating in sports such as tennis and swimming. Their elite rowers

also had lower extension-to-flexion ratios, superior coordination, and a smaller decrease in velocity during endurance testing. According to the United States Rowing Association (71), a balance of strength of at least 1.3 to 1 for extension to flexion is ideal.

If full power is used while reaching beyond normal limits, the potential for injury is increased. Lifting the heels may cause an overreach and decrease power; this can be avoided by keeping the heels in touch with the stretcher (70). Quitting before excessive fatigue results is also important. As fatigue develops, subtle changes in stroke and motion occur; these changes recruit muscles that are weaker and less trained.

Figure 5-11 shows a flexion bias not only in the catch phase (Fig. 5-11A) but also as the drive is completed (Fig. 5-11B). This flexion bias exists through the entire stroke and places an emphasis on the posterior ligamentous system, with the gluteus maximus and the hamstrings being the drivers for the movement. In addition to spending an inordinate amount of time in this posture (68,71), the flexion bias may be increased as rowers hang on their ligaments while relaxing immediately after a rowing work bout. This would suggest that McKenzie-type extension exercises (see Chaps. 6 and 8) may be a prophylactic measure that rowers could take immediately after practice or competition.

Track and Field

The incidence of LBP in a study on high school track and field athletes was 7.3% of all injuries, and the fifth ranked injury occurrence (74). Because a direct correlation was found between performance level and the incidence of injury, it would appear that as an athlete pushes toward excellence in a competitive event, the chance for injury increases. Because the events in track and field are so diverse, field events are presented first and then running events are presented (hurdle events are included with field events). As has been our practice throughout this chapter, we present only those events in which the research is deemed sufficient.

Field Events

Field events often involve asymmetric movements that may predispose an athlete to develop LBP and trauma. These injuries frequently involve unilateral spondylolysis with structural changes of the isthmus on the opposite (nondominant) side; cases of spondylolysis have been found in throwers, high jumpers, triple jumpers, and hurdlers (75,76). Worobiew (77) contended that most track and field injuries are a result of these underlying mechanisms. Procedure and training errors are also causes of low back problems in track and field athletes. Forced loads using a limited number of specific training methods to speed up performance and a lack of current training techniques may contribute to injury. There may also be a lack of awareness of available scientific training information in addition to incorrect interpretation or application of this information (77).

Training errors and injuries occurring in the weight room must also be taken into consideration for track and field athletes. For example, it is estimated that a shot putter typically makes 30,000 lifts of 300 to 400 pounds in a season of training; the weight lifted could accumulate to approximately 6 tons per season (78).

General Mechanical Considerations   The weakest link in the chain in field athletes is often the feet (jumpers and throwers) and the muscle corset of the trunk (throwers and jumpers). These weak links lead to overloading and improper force distribution in the lumbar spine.

Hammer Throw.   Dapena and McDonald (79) studied the angular momentum vector of the hammer throw during the turns and the contribution made to it by the thrower and hammer subsystems. Different styles or techniques among the throwers caused different degrees of pelvic tilt. Dapena and McDonald contended that the compressive stress on the spine at the low point of the hammer path in the last rotation could be reduced if the thrower countered with the hips; however, the shear stress would then be greater. Also, differences in the bending moments may be produced at different levels of the spine. Actual stresses to the spine differ across specific techniques; it is possible that the thrower who countered with the hips in early turns may have tilted the trunk backward during the late turns to decrease some type of stress to the spine. If spinal stress is the limiting factor that forces throwers to counter with the shoulders in the late turns, it may be unwise to counter with the hips without increasing the risk of injury (Fig. 5-12).

High Jump.   The potentials for low back injury in high jumpers arise from the Fosbury flop style of jumping (Fig. 5-13). This technique requires the jumper to thrust the hips forward while the upper body and legs hang downward, forcing the lumbar spine into an abnormal hyperextended curvature. Some athletes throw their heads backward, which further accentuates the arch. Furthermore, the higher the jump, the greater the arch required to clear the bar (18). Through continued repetition with this excessive hyperextension, enormous stress is placed on the neural arch (76), articular processes, and the supporting ligamentous structures (18). Rossi (75) found that five of six high jumpers in his study who used the Fosbury flop had spondylolysis (as seen on plain radiographs).

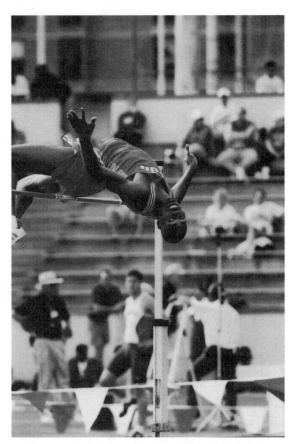

Fig. 5-13 The Fosbury flop style of high jumping can place a forceful hyperextensive stress on the spine. (Courtesy of the *Vol Sports Information Office*, University of Tennessee, TN.)

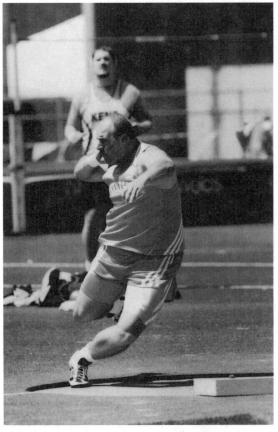

Fig. 5-12 Although the shot putter may typically place less stress to the spine than either the discus or hammer thrower, the potential stress is there, particularly in the athlete lacking in technique. (Courtesy of the *Vol Sports Information Office*, University of Tennessee, TN.)

Pole Vault. In pole vaulting, the lumbar spine is forcefully cycled from hyperextension and hyperflexion during the pole plant and the swing of the athlete on the pole; these forces can be very high, and their rapid acceleration can produce great stress on the lumbar spine, leading to spondylitic fractures (80,81). Gainor et al. (81) filmed a pole-vaulter and then plotted the position of the vertebrae anatomically. They discovered that the thoracic and lumbar vertebrae began in a neutral position but rapidly hyperextended 40 degrees during the pole plant. The spine then flexed 130 degrees in 0.65 s as the pole uncoiled and the athlete was propelled toward the bar. Angular velocities of the lumbar spine reached 348 degrees per second during both extension and flexion; torque about the spine was approximately 169 Nm during extension and 203 Nm in flexion (81). Although the torque required to initiate acute pars fractures in pole vaulters may be unknown, repeated overload could produce fatigue failure.

Running Events

The incidence of LBP and trauma among runners has been reported to range from 2 to 8% of all running injuries (82,83). Runners may be predisposed to injury because of the repetitive stress and accumulative impact loading that occur with this activity (83). Nevertheless, back injuries in runners are commonly seen with at least one other injury-related factor (e.g., asymmetry with respect to leg length, foot strike, etc.) (84,85).

Symptoms related to the spine, restricting running and other strenuous activities, occur most commonly between the ages of 30 and 50 years (84). This may relate more to the concomitants of aging rather than to any other specific causes. If so, part of this reason may be explained by changes in disc viscosity because with advanced age disc viscosity decreases and the disc loses its energy-absorbing capacity (86). Although low back complaints are infrequent in runners younger than 25 years because of the intermittent nature of symptoms, many may tend not to report their discomfort; thus, the exact incidence of back problems in runners is difficult to ascertain (84).

General Mechanical Considerations   Running differs from walking in that an airborne phase alternates with the support phase; this requires the absorption of impact. Up to 2000 N of compressive force occurs at a heel strike (87). The impact increases with velocity and the weight of the runner; therefore, shock absorption is a key to remaining injury free (85). When the compressive load exceeds the interstitial osmotic pressure of the disc, the reduction of disc height occurs (84).

Spinal shrinkage due to disc height reduction has been implicated in running. Leatt et al. (88) evaluated spinal shrinkage as an indicator of spinal loading in circuit weight training and running regimens. Spinal length was measured after all subjects performed two sets of circuit weight training, and novice runners ran a 6 K and trained runners ran a 25 K. Although spinal shrinkage was not significantly different between the weight training group and the 6-K runners, it was greater for the 25-K runners. Reversal of spinal shrinkage was observed after a night's sleep; however, no recovery occurred during a 20-min postexercise rest period. The loss of disc height from spinal loading in distance running has implications for the timely scheduling of activities that place significant loads on the spine.

Runners may be predisposed to injury because of repetitive stress and accumulated impact loading (89). In running the lower extremity is loaded to 1.2 to 2.1 times the body weight at heel strike and 2.5 times the body weight during toe-off; on average, the runner strikes the ground more than 50 to 70 times per minute for 1000 times per mile (82,90). Because of this repetitive motion, the vertebral column may be subjected to loading by gravity, changes in motion, trunk muscle activity, external forces, and external work. Intervertebral disc height could depend on not only the weight and velocity of the runner but also on the type of shoes worn, the distance run, the running surface, and the duration of running (91). Obviously, soft running surfaces and a well-cushioned shoe are important; however, shock absorption does not stop here. A heel-to-toe gait is important; this helps ankle, knee, and hip joint cushioning. Although physiologic efficiency may not always benefit, forces can be dissipated further if the runner tries to run as quietly as possible by cushioning each step up through the kinetic chain.

Running posture may also be a factor; an erect trunk will enable the lumbar spinal-pelvic unit to dissipate the forces further (85). Nachemson (26) showed how forward leaning postures increase the compression force within the intervertebral disc; this occurs because the erector spinae muscles must contract forcibly with their small force vectors to counterbalance the forward leaning posture. Running up hills can have the same effect; conversely, downhill running results in hyperextension of the lumbar spine. Because running on pitched surfaces (e.g., shoulder of a road) would result in asymmetric loading, individuals with back problems should run on surfaces as flat and soft as possible.

The trail of the hind leg in running is associated with hyperextension of the lumbar spine, which may cause lumbar pain (92). This repetitive hyperextension may be particularly accentuated in more competitive and faster runners than in their slower counterparts. Running, with its demands of repetitive ROM of the lumbar spine and in particular the increasing lordosis related to the trail leg, may be enough to overload the spine to the point of pathology (92).

Minor anatomic and biomechanical abnormalities that produce no noticeable symptoms in walking may produce injury while running (82,90). Additional causative factors include inadequate warm-up, improper stretching, uphill running, poor flexibility, changes in running style, and running on hard surfaces (93). There is an association between running and exaggerated lumbar mobility. This leads to lumbar postural changes, such as an increased lumbar lordosis with leg extension, particularly with long strides. Shorter runners may be at an even greater risk for back injury because of their longer stride patterns (93).

Ogon et al. (94) investigated the influence of medial longitudinal arch height on the shock wave that repetitively reaches the lower back during running. They hypothesized that the lower back would be subjected to less impact loading in a low-arch group than in a high-arch group during running. Their results indicated that the high-arch foot was a better shock absorber for the low back than a low-arch foot. These findings contradict other reports in the literature that seem to support that individuals with low arches are at decreased risk for low back problems (94). Further research in this area is required before general conclusions can be made.

Posterior Element Injury. It appears that posterior element injury is definitely the exception in runners unless there is a preexisting injury. Although stress fractures have been reported in the lumbar vertebral bodies and in the pars interarticularis in young distance runners, the symptoms are usually unilateral and without radiculitis (82). Moreover, runners with pars defects are often unaware of the spondylolysis or spondylolisthesis until detected during radiographic examination (84).

Anterior Element Injury. As mentioned previously, the incidence of LBP and trauma rises with increases in mileage. Interestingly, Brunet et al. (90) reported more numerous incidences of LBP and disc problems with increased mileage in women only. They concluded that, once a certain threshold is reached, the increased bone mineral content resulting from the physical activity is overcome by the hypoestrogenic effect of higher production of beta endorphins. The net effect is premenopausal osteoporosis; this may help explain the higher prevalence of back pain and disc trauma that is sometimes seen in women (90).

Flexibility and Strength Adequate flexibility in the lumbar spine and its surrounding musculature, including the hip flexors and hamstrings, are essential. Abdominal strength and back extensor strength are essential to protect the lumbar spine from trauma in track and field events. Weak abdominal muscles can lead to abnormal pelvic tilt, thereby accentuating the lumbar curve in the low back.

During periods when LBP and injury prevent an individual from performing regular running workouts, running in water is highly recommended; this is followed by a gradual progression to dry-land running. Although swimming is recommended for cardiovascular maintenance, strokes such as freestyle, breaststroke, and the butterfly may aggravate back pain; side and backstroke swimming are recommended in such situations (82). If running in water is used, efficient and proper running form must be followed. Relaxed posture is paramount to allow the trunk and arms to move synchronously with the running pace (84).

Volleyball

In a study of injuries sustained in a United States Volleyball Association National Tournament (95), the total injuries sustained were 154 in 1520 athletes during 7812 combined hours of competition. This resulted in an injury rate of 2.0 injuries per 100 h of play, with women sustaining slightly more injuries than men. Low back injury was the second most frequent injury, comprising 14.2% of all injuries. Bartolozzi et al. (96) evaluated magnetic resonance imaging (MRI) readings for the incidence of intervertebral disc abnormalities in 45 professional volleyball athletes for 3 to 7 years. A 44% incidence of disc alteration was found, including eight cases of disc degeneration; more than one lesion was discovered in eight athletes. Among the 26 athletes with LBP, 13 had positive findings with MRI; of the 19 asymptomatic athletes, 7 had noticeable disc alterations. It was also observed that, among those who were trained with exercise that produced significant overload, 16 had disc changes (61.5%). The investigators concluded that the correlation between disc alteration incidence with the type of training and overload is more important than the correlation between age and overall period of athletic activity.

High-level players average 150 1-m vertical leaps per match, and the velocity of the spike can reach speeds of 80 miles per hour (95). During the spike, the body is unsupported and the low back is rotated and hyperextended before impact, and significant potential for injury to the low back results (Fig. 5-14). Jacchia et al. (97) observed an increase in lumbar lordosis and hypermobility of the lumbar segment in volleyball athletes. These findings were associated with hypomobility of the higher segments probably related to the greater muscular hypertrophy of the shoulder girdle after the prevalent use of the upper limbs.

Diving

Groher and Heidensohn (98) investigated the incidence of LBP in divers; of the 60 active and former divers, back pain was reported in 50%. The 18 to 27 age group showed an 81.3% incidence of back pain; 17 of these athletes were selected for plain radiographs, and 14 of the 17 exhibited spinal abnormalities of the lumbar spine. The incidence

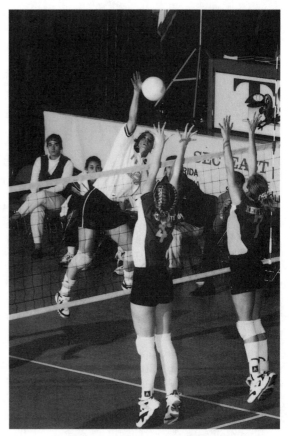

Fig. 5-14 In the volleyball spike, the body is unsupported and the low back is rotated and hyperextended before impact; this can place significant strain on the spine. (Courtesy of the *Lady Vol Media Relations Office*, University of Tennessee, TN.)

of spondylolysis or spondylolisthesis was 34% (5 of the 17 cases selected).

In an examination of lumbar spine radiographs of 1430 competitive athletes of different sports, Rossi (75) found pars interarticularis defects in 83.3% of the divers and spondylolysis in 63.33%. A more recent study by Rossi and Dragoni (76) showed only a 43.13% incidence of spondylolysis in divers.

The high incidence of LBP and spinal abnormalities in diving may be attributed in part to diving mechanics and repetition (75). Extreme rotational and hyperextension movements and the significant number of dives done in a career can be predisposing factors (76). Pain may be produced by extreme hyperflexion resulting from technique errors during water entry; furthermore, because of the inordinate number of training dives performed, only a small percentage is bound to be executed correctly (75).

Impingement syndrome of the spinous processes of the lumbar vertebrae can occur with extreme hyperextension. This position may potentially be magnified to almost 90 degrees, a position in which the spinous processes nearly touch (80). Bubble machines have also been implicated in the contribution to LBP and trauma because these machines can cause underwater forces that twist the body violently during vertical entry. In addition, techniques used to save imperfect dives, such as arching the back, may also contribute to low back trauma (80).

Lower extremity and trunk mechanics should be evaluated for low back injury prevention and treatment in divers. Proper flexibility in the lumbar spine, hamstrings, hip flexors, and calf muscles is essential. These muscles may cause abnormal mechanics in the lower extremity and place excessive stress on the lumbar spine (99).

Swimming

The incidence of LBP and trauma in swimming is common but not as prevalent as that seen in diving. It has been reported that every fifth competitive swimmer will incur chronic back pain, in particular butterfly swimmers (100) (Fig. 5-15). The primary cause of spinal injury in swimming, as might be expected, is from repetitive microtrauma (19). Goldstein et al. (49) reported that 15.8% of all swimmers had some form of spine abnormalities.

General Mechanical Considerations   Swimming training usually starts at an early age; because the spine is not yet matured, it is susceptible to trauma (101). Garges et al. (19) described a "motion cascade" in which a dysfunctional shoulder could affect the low back. These researchers identified

vulnerable areas at the junctions between the cervical/thoracic spine and thoracic/lumbar spine; these are transitional zones between more mobile and less mobile areas of the column. They also contended that back pain incidence relates to the specific swim stroke performed. Mutoh's (101) earlier findings support this contention. In that study, it was found that the percentage of abnormalities was higher in butterfly swimmers than in nonbutterfly swimmers; this swim stroke may be the most problematic because of the mechanical stresses imposed on the lumbar spine.

Wilson and Lindseth (102) followed three competitive high school swimmers treated for backache for more than a 3-year period. Back pain was reported to increase with swimming, especially the butterfly stroke. All three swimmers were diagnosed with Scheuermann's kyphosis. Scheuermann's disease is believed to be common in young swimmers, especially those who swim the butterfly stroke, whose repeated hyperflexion and hyperextension lead to trauma and degeneration of the vertebrae (80). It is uncertain whether the forceful contraction of the pectoral and abdominal musculature during the power phase of the butterfly stroke caused the vertebral abnormalities or was merely an aggravating factor. Nevertheless, the three high school swimmers experienced dramatic pain relief by eliminating the butterfly stroke and concentrating on other swim strokes (102).

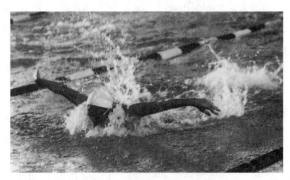

Fig. 5-15 The swimming stroke that accounts for the most low back problems in swimming is the butterfly (100). (Courtesy of the *Lady Vol Media Relations Office*, University of Tennessee, TN.)

Posterior Element Injury. The butterfly stroke and breaststroke accentuate lumbar extension that may predispose the posterior elements to injury (19). Spondylolysis and intervertebral disc narrowing was found in 22% of the butterfly competitors in Mutoh's study (101). Greater back strength was also a characteristic of these swimmers; those well trained in the butterfly stroke have stronger spine extensors than flexors because of the special breathing action and the dolphin kick. However, the strong dolphin kick with its vigorous back extension subject the lumbar spine to repeated stress. The lumbosacral angle was also greater in those who competed in the butterfly; this increased angle is an indication of increased lumbar lordosis that may be associated with LBP. It is possible that the vigorous spine extensions required in the butterfly stroke may cause the increased lumbar lordosis and possibly LBP (101).

Fowler and Regan (103) believed that LBP and spinal abnormalities have also been connected to the breaststroke; in this stroke many swimmers tend to pull with earlier elbow flexion and increased arm abduction. The elbow-up position is prolonged, propelling the upper torso above the water; this may aggravate an already lordotic curve of the low back. With this stress, a variety of low back problems may occur, including stress fractures of the pars interarticularis and frank spondylolisthesis. More often, this swim stroke aggravates a spondylolysis or possibly a mechanical LBP from facet irritation, thus limiting training (103).

Anterior Element Injury. The freestyle and the backstroke increase axial rotation and therefore increase torque forces most; these forces may render the annular fibers vulnerable. Excessive lateral lumbar flexion and rotation may be produced if proper form or technique is not adhered to (e.g., improper hand entry, decreased body rotation during the pull phase, or inadequate body roll during the recovery phase). These excessive motions increase the stresses on both the posterior and anterior elements of the lumbar spine (19).

Flexibility and Strength Pieper et al. (100) showed a high occurrence of muscular imbalance

patterns in a study involving 46 elite competitive swimmers. Their most significant finding was that the shortening of the hip flexors with corresponding weakening of the abdominal musculature causes an excessive hollow back. They emphasized the potential for these imbalances to lead to overloading of the lumbar spine and contended that the cause for the muscular imbalances was incorrect strength training rather than sport-specific loading caused by swimming (100).

Several recommended preventive strategies are designed to protect the lumbar spine from excessive stress during swimming. Improving abdominal strength increases the force of their contraction and decreases the magnitude of the anterior moment supporting the lumbar spine (80,103). Increasing low back flexibility is also important; when muscles, tendons, and ligaments are stretched regularly, their forces on the lumbar spine at the extremes of motion are decreased (80). Shortened postural musculature and any core-strength deficits must be identified and remedied; these corrections will facilitate optimal loading capacity, thereby reducing the risk for injury (100).

Low back injury and pain related to the butterfly stroke should focus on proper training and progression (80). Adolescents are not recommended to engage in back extensor muscle work because these muscles are generally well developed, and the strength imbalance between the abdominal muscles and back extensors may predispose low back injuries. Instruction of the butterfly stroke should be avoided by beginning swimmers unless they have enough strength. The training should consist of different swim strokes. Long-term training of the butterfly stroke exclusively should be avoided.

Developing eccentric lower abdominal strength is critical for swimmers to control the extension forces on the lumbar spine (19). Adequate flexibility of the back, shoulder, and hip flexors will also serve to reduce trunk extension forces. Poor breathing technique may be a source of LBP; therefore, focus should be on breathing with the chin tucked and executing the body roll through the entire trunk to reduce the extension tone of the lower back musculature. Maintaining neutral spine during the stroke, rolling, and kick-turns will reduce the forces in the lumbar spine (19).

Weight Training

Mazur et al. (104) contended that most injuries occur during the aggressive use of free weights; they reported that more than 17,000 cases of weight lifting injuries requiring emergency room visits occur annually among athletes between the ages of 10 and 19 years. The lower back has been reported as the most common site of injury during weight training among children and adolescents (105). Lack of proper instruction and supervision are factors relating to the high incidence of weight training injuries in young individuals.

Granhed and Morelli (106) evaluated the occurrence of LBP in top ranked heavy weight lifters and wrestlers 20 years after retirement from their sport. The incidence of LBP among the weight lifters was 23%; there was also a significant decrease in disc height among the weight lifters. Decreases in disc height have been shown from single sessions of weight training; this "spinal shrinkage" is due to extrusion of tissue fluid through the disc wall when the applied load exceeds the imbibition pressure of the disc and the osmotic gradients across the disc membrane (107).

Billings et al. (108) contended that many athletes will undergo more rigorous physical exercising in their training over a more prolonged period than might be required in actual competition. This, combined with the high occurrence of poor supervision, sets the stage for a dangerous situation.

General Mechanical Considerations Basford (109) contended that many low back injuries sustained during weight training occur in lumbar hyperextension, such as in an incorrectly performed bench or military press. Thus, he implicated poor lifting technique; however, he also believed that an underlying spondylolysis or spondylolisthesis could make an individual more susceptible to injury. Lifting heavy weights overhead, especially with forward flexion of the trunk, causes very high shear forces within the lumbar

vertebrae (80). The "good morning" lift can present excessive shear forces (Fig. 5-16). Rotation and combined rotation and flexion movements of the low back have also been identified as common mechanisms of injury (108).

Repetition and the cumulative effects of lifting also play a major role in injury occurrence. For example, it has been estimated that a middleweight athlete of international caliber, in 5 days of weight lifting, for 5 h per day, lifts more than 70,000 kg (75).

Posterior Element Damage. Neural arch trauma in weight lifting may occur in isolation or with disc degeneration, spondylolisthesis, or multiple defects (108). Aggrawal et al. (110) found that spondylolysis occurred only in those cases in which the individual had been weight training for more than 4 years and that pain was not necessarily associated with spondylolysis. Kotani et al. (111) also reported a correlation between years of experience and incidence of low back trauma; they also found a high occurrence of spondylolysis among experienced lifters, especially those with at least 4 years of training. The overall incidence of spondylolysis in the latter study was 30% (8 of 26); in their comparison population, the incidence was 5 to 7%. Rossi (75) and Rossi and Dragoni (76) reported the incidence of spondylolysis in weight lifters to be 36.20% and 22.68%, respectively. They pointed out that the fundamental lifting technique in the snatch and jerk involves maximal lumbar extension (Fig. 5-17). The squat and power clean can also lead to this type of stress because it also requires hyperextension of the lumbar spine (112).

Another possible injury to the low back from weight training involves apophyseal fractures in adolescents. Although rare, the effects of axial loading, especially when combined with rapid extension of the trunk, may produce this type of injury. Controlling weight lifted is therefore essential to ensure proper lifting technique in the skeletally immature athlete (113). In some cases, pure carelessness that results in extremely poor mechanics can be a precipitating factor (Fig. 5-18).

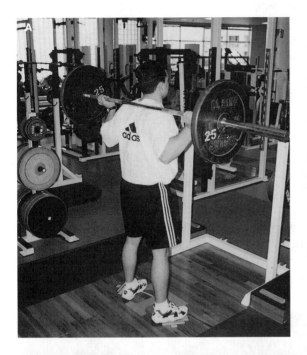
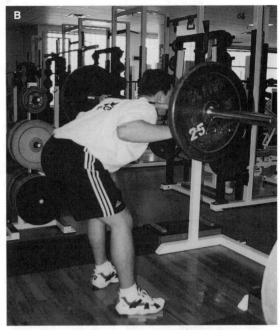
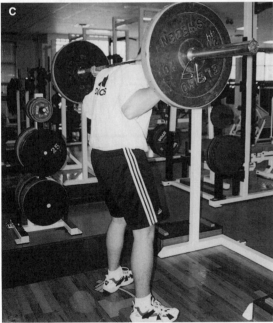
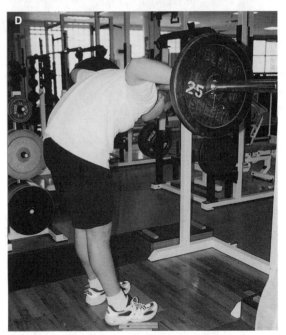

Fig. 5-16 The "good morning" lift. **(A)** and **(B)** show good mechanics; however, the greater degree of bend causes the greater shear force. **(C)** and **(D)** show poor mechanics; executing this type of lift with a heavier load could be extremely dangerous.

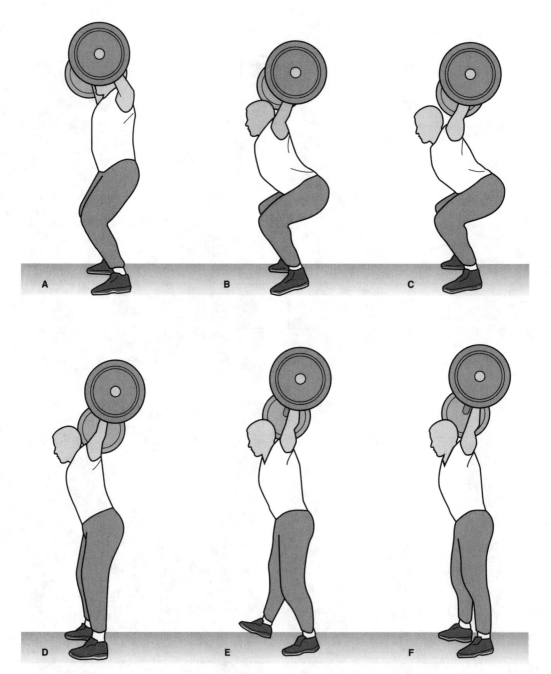

Fig. 5-17 This sequence was drawn from videotape frames (30 f/sec) of a lifter performing the snatch lift. In **(A)** (f8) the lifter has almost completed leg extension and is thrusting the weight to shoulder height. In **(B)** (f10), arm extension has been completed but there is considerable stress on the lumbar spine. In **(C)** (f11), the head is thrust forward and the weight shifts backward; this increases the turning moment and places more stress on the posterior aspects of the motion segment of the lumbar spine. In **(D)** (f13), knee extension is completed but the lifter is losing control because of the magnitude of the turning moment. In **(E)** (f15), the lifter has stepped back with the left leg and is in the process of stepping back with the right leg to reduce the turning moment. In **(F)** (f16) the lifter has recovered. (Artist drawing from video frames supplied by *Elaine Seat*, College of Engineering, University of Tennessee, TN.)

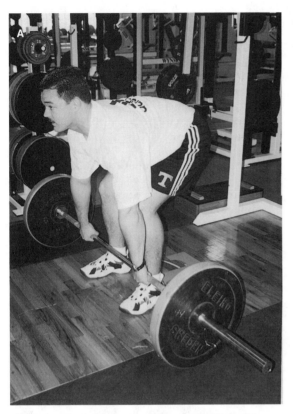
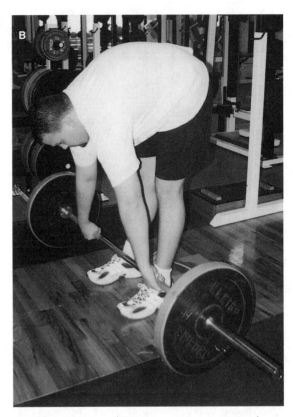

Fig. 5-18 The importance of good technique. **(A)** presents good mechanics and **(B)** presents very poor mechanics. Carelessness and/or fatigue can result in poor mechanics and increase the chance for injury.

Anterior Element Injury. One of the most common lumbar spine injuries from weight lifting is to the intervertebral disc. Evidence of degenerative disc disease is present by the first decade in males and by the second decade in females; by age 40, 80% of males involved in weight lifting have evidence of degenerative disc disease versus 65% of females involved in weight lifting (114). The association between participation in several specific sports, the use of free weights, and the use of weight-lifting equipment and herniated lumbar discs were examined in a case epidemiologic study (115). It was found that most sports are not associated with an increased risk of disc herniation and may in fact protect against such trauma.

Flexibility and Strength   Back and trunk flexibility and strength are essential in protecting the lumbar

spine against trauma, whether acute or chronic, during weight lifting. Increased muscle strength allows the motion segment to better withstand and thus reduce strain in response to overloads. In activities requiring repetitious movements of the spine, muscles with greater endurance can provide the strength needed to reduce loads for longer periods without fatigue, thereby reducing the risk of injury. Furthermore, appropriate strength may enhance the reaction time of the neuromuscular control system to suddenly applied loads, thereby protecting the spine in dynamic and static situations (115).

Proper form and technique are paramount in preventing injuries during specific exercises and when moving weights around the weight room. A stable lifting position with a good grip, the weight close to the body, and using the hip and knee joint musculature to perform the lifting are important fundamental principles of good lifting form. With regard to form, good control over the movement of the bar is essential (104).

EPILOGUE

As was indicated in the beginning of this chapter, there was no attempt to cover all sports. Although those sports selected for inclusion differ considerably in the number of participants that they attract, one thing in common is that low back injuries are prevalent in each. Although the sports are different, there are often similarities between the movement patterns and the mechanical stresses present. For example, comparable hyperextension stresses may be seen in interior line play in football and in wrestling. However, one of the common denominators that pervades all sports is weight room activity; and as previously discussed, some would contend that many low back injuries have their genesis in the weight room (4,12). Nevertheless, it is in the weight room that training activities can be developed to enable athletes to better resist the incumbent stresses in their particular sports. It is hoped that this chapter will be helpful in this endeavor.

REFERENCES

1. Kirkaldy-Willis, W.H. Three phases of the spectrum of degenerative disease, in *Managing Low Back Pain*, W.H. Kirkaldy-Willis and C.V. Burton, editors. 1992, New York: Churchill-Livingstone. p. 105–119.
2. Michelli, L.J., and R. Wood. Back pain in young athletes. Significant differences from adults in causes and patterns. *Arch Pediatr Adolesc Med* 1995, 149(1): p. 15–18.
3. Halvorsen, T.M., Nilsson, S., Nakstad, P.H. Spondylolysis and spondylolisthesis. *Tidsskr Norske Laegeforen* 1996, 116(7): p. 1999–2001.
4. Saal, J.A. Rehabilitation of football players with lumbar spine injury (part 1 of 2). *Phys Sports Med* 1988, 16(9): p. 61–68.
5. Saal, J.A. Rehabilitation of football players with lumbar spine injury (part 2 of 2). *Phys Sports Med* 1988, 16(10): p. 117–125.
6. Weir, M.R., and D.S. Smith. Stress reaction of the pars interarticularis leading to spondylolysis. A cause of adolescent low back pain. *J Adolesc Health Care* 1989, 10(6): p. 573–577.
7. Gerbina, P.G., and L.J. Micheli. Back injuries in the young athlete. *Clin Sports Med* 1995, 14(3): p. 571–590.
8. Morita, T., Ikata, T., Katoh, S., et al. Lumbar spondylolysis in children and adolescents. *J Bone Joint Surg (Br)* 1995, 77(4): p. 620–625.
9. Saal, J.A. Common American football injuries. *Sports Med* 1991, 12(2): p. 132–147.
10. Comstock, C.P., et al. Spondylolisthesis in the young athlete. *Phys Sports Med* 1994, 22(12): p. 39–46.
11. Stallard, M.C. Backache in oarsmen. *Br J Sports Med* 1980, 14(2-3): p. 105–108.
12. Barber, F.A. The lumbar spine in football, in *The Spine in Sports*, S.H. Hochschuler, editor. 1990, Philadelphia: Hanley & Belfus. p. 152–156.
13. Rovere, G.D. Low back pain in athletes. *Phys Sports Med* 1987, 15(1): p. 105–117.
14. Brady, T.A., Cahill, B.R., Bodnar, L.M. Weight training-related injuries in the high school athlete. *Am J Sports Med* 1982, 10(1): p. 1–5.
15. Nagaosa, Y., Kikuchi, S., Hasue, M., et al. Pathoanatomic mechanism of degenerative spondylolisthesis. *Spine* 1998, 23(13): p. 1447–1451.
16. Herskowitz, A., and H. Selesnick. Back injuries in basketball players. *Clin Sports Med* 1993, 12(2): p. 293–306.
17. Saal, J.A., and J.S. Saal. Sports related lumbar injuries to the adult/degenerative spine: evaluation and treatment strategies. *Sports Med Arthrosc Rev* 1997, 5: p. 216–225.
18. Miller, R.D. Spinal lordosis in the flop. *Athletic J* 1978, February: p. 100–106.
19. Garges, K.J., White, A.H., Scott, J. Acute lumbar spine problems in the competitive adult athlete. Sport specific: baseball, football, and swimming injuries. *Sports Med Arthrosc Rev* 1997, 5: p. 172–181.
20. Watkins, R.G. Chronic spine pain in the competitive adult athlete: golf, baseball, and rehabilitation. *Sports Med Arthrosc Rev* 1997, 5: p. 207–215.
21. McFarland, E.G., and M. Wasik. Epidemiology of collegiate baseball injuries. *Clin J Sports Med* 1998, 8: p. 10–13.
22. Minkoff, J., Simonson, B.G., Sherman, O.H., et al. Injuries in basketball, in *Clinical Practice*

of Sports Injury Prevention and Care, P.A.F.H. Renstrom, editor. 1994, London: Blackwell Scientific Publications. p. 303–353.

23. Hickey, G.J., Fricker, P.A., McDonald, W.A. Injuries of young elite female basketball players over a six-year period. *Clin J Sport Med* 1997, 7(4): p. 252–256.

24. Tall, R.L., and W. DeVault. Spinal injury in sport: Epidemiologic considerations. *Clin Sports Med* 1993, 12(3): p. 441–447.

25. Herskowitz, H.N., Paolucci, B.J., Abdenour, M.A. Basketball, in *The Spine in Sports*, R.G. Watkins et al., editors. 1996, St. Louis: Mosby. p. 430–435.

26. Nachemson, A.L. The lumbar spine—an orthopaedic challenge. *Spine* 1976, 1: p. 59–71.

27. Fairbanks, J.C.T., Pynsent, P.B., Van Poortvliet, J.A., et al. Influence of anthropometric factors and joint laxity in the incidence of adolescent back pain. *Spine* 1984, 9(5): p. 461–464.

28. Ferguson, R.J., McMaster, J.H., Stanitski, C.L. Low back pain in college football linemen. *J Sports Med* 1975, 2(2): p. 63–69.

29. McCarroll, J.R., Miller, J.M., Ritter, M.A. Lumbar spondylolysis and spondylolisthesis in college football players. A prospective study. *Am J Sports Med* 1986, 14(5): p. 404–406.

30. Day, A.L., Friedman, W.A., Indelicato, P.A. Observations on the treatment of lumbar disk disease in college football players. *Am J Sports Med* 1987, 15(1): p. 72–75.

31. McCarroll, J.R., Rettig, A.C., Shelbourne, K.D. Injuries in the amateur golfer. *Phys Sports Med* 1990, 18(3): p. 122–126.

32. McCarroll, J.R. The frequency of golf injuries. *Clin Sports Med* 1996, 15(1): p. 1–7.

33. Batt, M.E. A survey of golf injuries in amateur golfers. *Br J Sports Med* 1992, 26(1): p. 63–65.

34. Duda, M. Golfers use exercise to get back in the swing. *Phys Sports Med* 1989, 17(8): p. 109–113.

35. Hosea, T.M., and C.J. Gatt, Jr. Back pain in golf. *Clin Sports Med* 1996, 15(1): p. 37–53.

36. Mackey, S.T. The golf swing and facet syndrome. *Chiropract Sports Med* 1995, 9(1): p. 10–13.

37. Gracovetsky, S. *The Spinal Engine*. 1988, New York: Springer-Verlag. p. 505.

38. Gracovetsky, S. Linking the spinal engine with the legs: a theory of human gait, in *Stability and Low Back Pain*, A. Vleeming et al., editors. 1997, New York: Churchill-Livingstone.

39. Fischer, B., and R.G. Watkins. Golf, in *The Spine in Sports*, R.G. Watkins et al., editors. 1996, St. Louis: Mosby.

40. Mallare, C. Golf's contribution to low back pain. *Sports Med Update* 1996, 11(2): p. 20–25.

41. Batt, M.E. Golfing injuries. An overview. *Sports Med* 1993, 16(1): p. 64–71.

42. Hosea, T.M., Gatt, C.J., Galli, K.M., et al. Biochemical analysis of the golfer's back, in *Science and Golf: Proceedings of the First World Scientific Congress of Golf*. 1990, St. Andrews, Scotland: University of St. Andrews.

43. Adlington, G.S. Proper swing technique and biomechanics of golf. *Clin Sports Med* 1996, 15(1): p. 9–26.

44. Wallace, P., and T. Reilly. Spinal and metabolic loading during simulations of golf play. *J Sports Sci* 1993, 11(6): p. 511–515.

45. Burdorf, A., Van Der Steenhoven, G.A., Tromp-Klaren, E.G. A one-year prospective study on back pain among novice golfers. *Am J Sports Med* 1996, 24(5): p. 659–664.

46. Caine, D., Cochrane, B., Caine, C., et al. An epidemiologic investigation of injuries affecting young competitive female gymnasts. *Am J Sports Med* 1989, 17(6): p. 811–820.

47. McCall, E., Headache, G., Shields, K., et al. Injuries in women's gymnastics—the state of the art. *Am J Sports Med* 1987, 15(6): p. 558–565.

48. Snook, G.A. Injuries in women's gymnastics. A 5-year study. *Am J Sports Med* 1979, 7(4): p. 242–244.

49. Goldstein, J.D., Berger, P.E., Windler, G.E., et al. Spine injuries in gymnasts and swimmers. An epidemiologic investigation. *Am J Sports Med* 1991, 19(5): p. 463–468.

50. Kurzweil, P.R., and D.W. Jackson. Gymnastics, in *The Spine in Sports*, R.G. Watkins et al., editors. 1996, St. Louis: Mosby. p. 456–474.

51. McAuley, E., Hudash, G., Shields, K., et al. Injuries in women's gymnastics. The state of the art. *Am J Sports Med* 1987, 15(6): p. 558–565.

52. Saal, J.A. Lumbar injuries in gymnastics, in *The Spine in Sports*, S.H. Hochschuler, editor. 1990, Philadelphia: Hanley & Belfus. p. 207–213.

53. Tsai, L., and T. Wredmark. Spinal posture, sagittal mobility, and subjective rating of back problems in former female elite gymnasts. *Spine* 1993, 18(7): p. 872–875.

54. Ohlen, G., Wredmark, T., Spangfort, E. Spinal sagittal configuration and mobility related to low-back pain in the female gymnast. *Spine* 1989, 14(8): p. 847–850.

55. Walsh, W.M., Huurman, W.W., Shelton, G.L. Overuse injuries of the knee and spine in girls' gymnastics. *Orthop Clin North Am* 1985, 16(2): p. 329–350.

56. Witten, C., and W. Witten. Strength, flexibility and the low back syndrome in gymnastics. *Michigan J* 1985, Fall: p. 12–13.

57. Soderstrom, C.A., and M.T. Doxanas. Racquetball. A game with preventable injuries. *Am J Sports Med* 1982, 10(3): p. 180–183.

58. Kroner, K., Schmidt, S.A., Nielsen, A.B., et al. Badminton injuries. *Br J Sports Med* 1990, 24(3): p. 169–172.

59. Chard, M.D., and S.M. Lachmann. Racquet sports-patterns of injury presenting to a sports injury clinic. *Br J Sports Med* 1987, 21(4): p. 150–153.

60. Marks, M.R., Haas, S.S., Wiesel, S.W. Low back pain in the competitive tennis player. *Clin Sports Med* 1988, 7(2): p. 277–287.

61. Hutchinson, M.R., Laprade, R.F., Burnett, Q.M., et al. Injury surveillance at the USTA Boys' Tennis Championships: a 6-yr study. *Med Sci Sports Exerc* 1995, 27(6): p. 826–830.

62. Saraux, A., Guillodo, Y., Devauchelle, V., et al. Are tennis players at increased risk for low back pain and Sciatica? *Rev Rhumatisme* 1999, 66(3): p. 143–145.

63. Saal, J.A. Tennis, in *The Spine in Sports*, R.G. Watkins et al., editors. 1996, St. Louis: Mosby. p. 499–504.

64. Feeler, L.C. Racquet sports, in *The Spine in Sports*, S.H. Hochschuler, editor. 1990, Philadelphia: Hanley & Belfus.

65. Saal, J.A. Rowing, in *The Spine in Sports*, R.G. Watkins et al., editors. 1996, St. Louis: Mosby. p. 578–591.

66. Hainline, B. Low back injury. *Clin Sports Med* 1995, 14(1): p. 241–265.

67. Howell, D.W. Musculoskeletal profile and incidence of musculoskeletal injuries in lightweight women rowers. *Am J Sports Med* 1984, 12(4): p. 278–282.

68. Phillips, J., and D. Thomashow. Low back pain in rowers. *Am Rowing* 1986, August/September: p. 42–44.

69. Greene, E.A.W. Comfort to contortion: the last ten years of rowing. *Br J Sports Med* 1980, 14(2–3): p. 109.

70. Soghikian, G.W. Back pain. *Am Rowing* 1995, 27(2): p. 37–43.

71. United States Rowing Association. 1982 Technical supplement to *Proceedings of the 1981 USRA Symposium and Clinics.* 1981, Jacksonville, FL: United States Rowing Association.

72. Redgrave, S. Prevention/cure, in *Steven Redgrave's Complete Book of Rowing.* 1993, London, U.K.: Partridge Press.

73. Muller, G., Hille, E., Szpalski, M. Function of the trunk musculature in elite rowers. *Sportver Sportsch* 1994, 8(3): p. 134–142.

74. Watson, M.D., and P.P. DiMartino. Incidence of injuries in high school track and field athletes and its relation to performance ability. *Am J Sports Med* 1987, 15(3): p. 251–254.

75. Rossi, F. Spondylolysis, spondylolisthesis and sports. *J Sports Med Phys Fitness* 1978, 18(4): p. 317–340.

76. Rossi, F., and S. Dragoni. Lumbar spondylolysis: occurrence in competitive athletes. Updated achievements in a series of 390 cases. *J Sports Med Phys Fitness* 1990, 30(4): p. 450–452.

77. Worobiew, G. Prevention of pains in the lumbar region provoked by overuse injuries, in *Proceedings of the First International Amateur Athletic Federation Medical Congress.* 1985, Espoo, Finland: Sports Medicine in Track and Field Athletics.

78. Davies, J.E. The spine in sport-injuries, prevention and treatment. *Br J Sports Med* 1980, 14(1): p. 18–21.

79. Dapena, J., and C. McDonald. A three-dimensional analysis of angular momentum in the hammer throw. *Med Sci Sports Exerc* 1989, 21 (2): p. 206–220.

80. Alexander, M.J. Biomechanical aspects of lumbar spine injuries in athletes: a review. *Can J Appl Sport Sci* 1985, 10(1): p. 1–20.

81. Gainor, B.J., Hagen, R.J., Allen, W.C. Biomechanics of the spine in the pole vaulter as related to spondylolysis. *Am J Sports Med* 1983, 11(2): p. 53–57.

82. Brody, D.M. Running Injuries, in *The Lower Extremity and Spine in Sports Medicine*. Nicholas, J.A., Hershman, E.B., editors. 1986, St. Louis: Mosby. p. 1534–1580.

83. McBryde, A.M., Jackson, D.W., James, C.M. Injuries in runners and joggers, in *Sports Injuries: Mechanisms, Prevention, and Treatment.* Fu, F.H., editor. 1985, Baltimore: Williams & Wilkins. p. 395–416.

84. Regan, J.J. Back problems in the runner, in *Spinal Injuries in Sports*, S.H. Hochschuler, editor. 1990, Philadelphia: Hanley & Belfus. p. 346–350.

85. Uppal, G.S., et al. Running, in *The Spine in Sports*, R.G. Watkins et al., editors. 1996, St. Louis: Mosby. p. 475–479.

86. Bogduk, N. *Clinical Anatomy of the Lumbar Spine and Sacrum*, 3rd ed. 1998, London: Churchill-Livingstone. p. 261.

87. Lees, A., and P.J. McCullogh. A preliminary investigation into the shock absorbency of running shoes and shoe inserts. *J Hum Movement Stud* 1984, 10: p. 95.

88. Leatt, P., Reilly, T., Troup, J.G. Spinal loading during circuit weight-training and running. *Br J Sports Med* 1986, 20(3): p. 119–124.

89. Marti, B., Vader, J.P., Minder, C.E., et al. On the epidemiology of running injuries. The 1984 Bern Grand-Prix study. *Am J Sports Med* 1988, 16(3): p. 285–294.

90. Brunet, M.E., Cook, S.D., Brinker, M.R., et al. A survey of running injuries in 1505 competitive and recreational runners. *J Sports Med Phys Fitness* 1990, 30(3): p. 307–315.

91. O'Toole, M.L., Hiller, D.B., Smith, R.A., et al. Overuse injuries in ultraendurance triathletes. *Am J Sports Med* 1989, 17(4): p. 514–518.

92. Jackson, D.W., Wiltse, L.L., Dingeman R., et al. Stress reactions involving the pars interarticularis in young athletes. *Am J Sports Med* 1981, 9(5): p. 304–312.

93. Guten, G. Herniated lumbar disk associated with running. A review of 10 cases. *Am J Sports Med* 1981, 9(3): p. 155–159.

94. Ogon, M., Aleksiev, A.R., Pope, M.H., et al. Does arch height affect impact loading at the lower back level in running? *Foot Ankle* 1999, 20(4): p. 263–266.

95. Schafle, M.D., Requa, R.K., Patton, W.L., et al. Injuries in the 1987 national amateur volleyball tournament. *Am J Sports Med* 1990, 18(6): p. 624–631.

96. Bartolozzi, C., Caramella, D., Zampa, V., et al. [The incidence of disk changes in volleyball players. The magnetic resonance findings]. *Radiol Med (Torino)* 1991, 82(6): p. 757–760.

97. Jacchia, G.E., Butler, U.P., Innocenti, M. Low back pain in athletes: pathogenic mechanisms and therapy. *Chir Organ Movement* 1994, 79(1): p. 47–53.

98. Groher, W., and P. Heidensohn. [Backache and x-ray changes in diving]. *Z Orthop Ihre Grenzgeb* 1970, 108(1): p. 51–61.

99. Mangine, R.E., Rubine, B. Flexibility for diving. *Inside USA Diving* 1993, 1(3): p. 13–23.

100. Pieper, H.G., Schneider, A., Wolf, U. Muscular imbalances in elite swimmers and their relation to sports lesions of lumbar spine and knee joints. *Sportver Sportsch* 1989, 3: p. 29–31.

101. Mutoh, Y. Low back pain in butterfliers, in *Swimming Medicine IV*, B. Eriksson and B. Furberg, editors. 1978, Baltimore: University Park Press.

102. Wilson, F.D., and R.E. Lindseth. The adolescent "swimmer's back." *Am J Sports Med* 1982, 10(3): p. 174–176.

103. Fowler, P.J., and W.D. Regan. Swimming injuries of the knee, foot and ankle, elbow, and back. *Clin Sports Med* 1986, 5(1): p. 139–148.

104. Mazur, L.J., Yetman, R.J., Risser, W.L. Weight-training injuries. Common injuries and preventative methods. *Sports Med* 1993, 16(1): p. 57–63.

105. Risser, W.L. Weight-training injuries in children and adolescents. *Am Fam Phys* 1991. 44(6): p. 2104–2108.

106. Granhed, H., and B. Morelli. Low back pain among retired wrestlers and heavyweight lifters. *Am J Sports Med* 1988, 16(5): p. 530–533.

107. Bourne, N.D., and T. Reilly. Effect of a weightlifting belt on spinal shrinkage. *Br J Sports Med* 1991, 25(4): p. 209–212.

108. Billings, R.A., Burry, H.C., Jones, R. Low back injury in sport. Rheumatol Rehabil 1977, 16(4): p. 236–240.

109. Basford, J.R. Weightlifting, weight training and injuries. *Orthopedics* 1985, 8(8): p. 1051–1056.

110. Aggrawal, N.D., Kaur, R., Kumar, S., et al. A study of changes in the spine in weight lifters and other athletes. *Br J Sports Med* 1979, 13(2): p. 58–61.

111. Kotani, P.T., Ichikawa, N., Wakabayashi, W., et al. Studies of spondylolysis found among weight lifters. *Br J Sports Med* 1971, 6(1): p. 4–8.

112. Schafer, M.F. Low back injuries in athletes. *Sports Med Digest* 1986, 8(7): p. 1–3.

113. Browne, T.D., et al. Lumbar ring apophyseal fracture in an adolescent weight lifter. A case report. *Am J Sports Med* 1990, 18(5): p. 533–535.

114. Miller, J.A., Schwartz, A.S., Schultz, A.B. Lumbar disc degeneration correlation with age, sex and spine level in 600 autopsy specimens. *Spine* 1988, 13: p. 178.

115. Mundt, D.J., Kelsey, J.L., Golden, A.L., et al. An epidemiologic study of sports and weight lifting as possible risk factors for herniated lumbar and cervical discs. The Northeast Collaborative Group on Low Back Pain. *Am J Sports Med* 1993, 21(6): p. 854–860.

PART III

EXERCISE PRESCRIPTION

CHAPTER 6

EXERCISE (AND DIAGNOSIS) PROTOCOLS

Wendell Liemohn

Laura Horvath Gagnon

137

INTRODUCTION

Three prominent exercise protocols for the back are reviewed in this chapter. Williams's flexion program is the first protocol to be discussed. Although some of Williams's ideas (1,2) on the pathophysiology of the cause of low back pain (LBP) are no longer supported, his "flexion exercise protocol" was the dominant therapeutic exercise program for the spine for a number of years. McKenzie's approach (3) is the second protocol discussed; it is sometimes called an approach rather than an exercise program because it can be used to diagnose mechanical LBP (4,5). The third protocol to be reviewed is stabilization training; the San Francisco Spine Institute was one of its first proponents (6). The McKenzie approach and stabilization training are perhaps the two most dominant exercise programs used in low back rehabilitation.

WILLIAMS'S FLEXION EXERCISES (1,2)

This program began in the 1930s and was very widely used for the next three to four decades; moreover, some aspects of it are still followed today (7,8). However, some of Williams's contentions do not agree with those espoused in the extremely popular program began by McKenzie (3); these differences are addressed later in this chapter.

Theoretical Basis for Williams's Flexion Exercises

Williams (1) contended that posture was a prime cause of back pain, and McKenzie agreed (3). However, Williams believed that standing "up straight" was a cause of the problem, whereas McKenzie believed that standing up straight (with a concave lumbar curve) was part of the solution to the problem. Williams observed that the pelvic angle may vary from 20 to 70 degrees, and he argued that an individual's back would be better off if a correction did not make the individual assume an "upright" posture. If the spine were straight from the platform of the pelvis (e.g., a level sacrum), Williams

believed that the weight could be distributed evenly across the entire surface of each disc. Williams further argued that upright posture (e.g., cervical and lumbar vertebrae with concave and lordotic curves) with thoracic and sacral vertebrae with convex curves, required that the back edge of each disc in the concave curves and that the front edges of each disc in the convex curves support the body's weight. He thought that it was desirable to displace each disc's superincumbent weight evenly rather than biasing the load anteriorly or posteriorly.

Williams contended that the posterior portion of a disc in concave curves, such as that depicted in a normal lumbar lordosis, was vulnerable and apt to rupture when overloaded. He also believed that most individuals by age 20 had ruptured their L5-S1 discs. Although Williams may not really have been a proponent of an ape-like posture, he did believe it most desirable to reduce the cervical and lumbar concave curves in postures assumed in activities of daily living. He also stressed that sitting postures in which lordotic curves were assumed were incorrect and that assuming lumbar kyphotic curves was correct (Fig. 6-1). This opinion is diametrically opposite to McKenzie's recommendations, which are examined later in this chapter, but some of the postures Williams espoused for the spine in unloaded positions (e.g., recumbent) are still accepted.

Williams's Exercises

In the introduction to his exercise program, Williams admonishes: "Remember: Always sit, stand, walk and lie in a way that reduces the hollow in the low back to a minimum" (1)! His six exercises are delineated in Figure 6-2 and are discussed briefly in the next sections.

Trunk Flexion (see Fig. 6-2) Williams offered two variations of this exercise; the first one shown in Figure 6-2A is commonly called a sit-up. A full sit-up as depicted is frowned upon and deemed inappropriate for most individuals because of the disc compression forces created by contraction of the psoas and other hip flexors (9–11), but the criteria that Williams delineated for this exercise avert

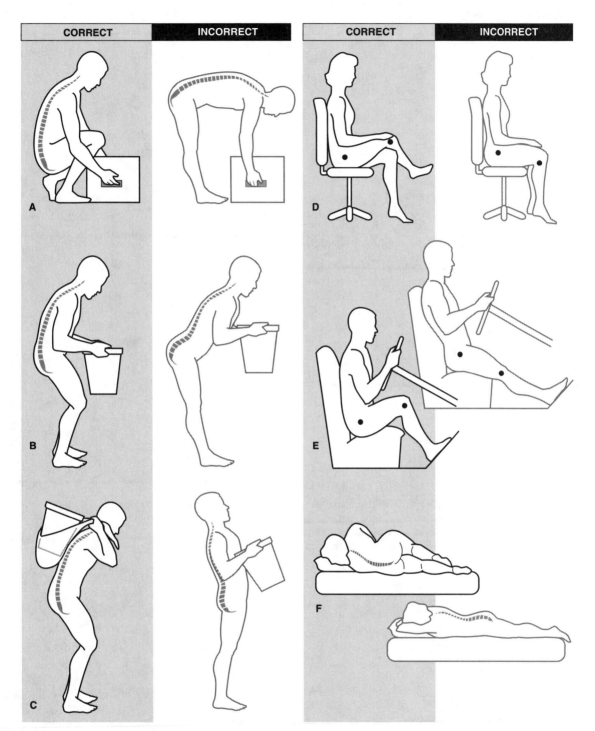

Fig. 6-1 Williams believed that the lumbar lordotic curve should be reduced as much as possible in activities of daily living; today this opinion no longer has credance. For example, although most would contend that in **(A)** Williams appropriately depicted correct and incorrect techniques, in **(D)** the posture that he identified as being incorrect is indeed correct. (Adapted with permission from Williams, P.C. *The Lumbosacral Spine.* 1965. New York: McGraw-Hill, p. 89.

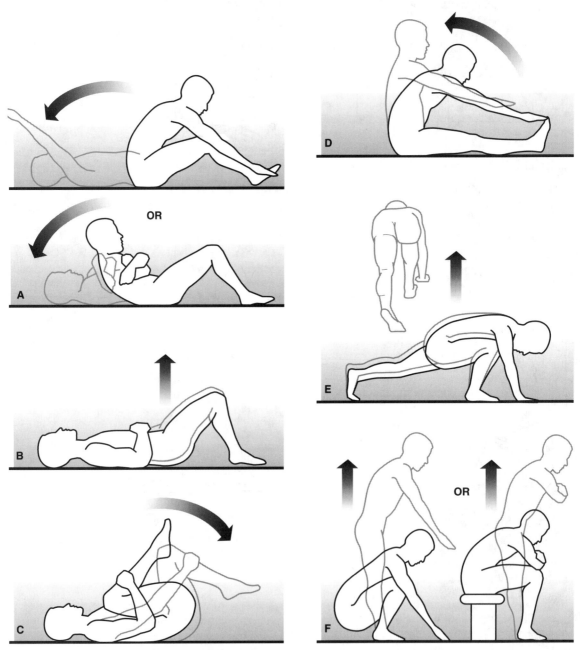

Fig. 6-2 Williams's flexion exercises. (Adapted with permission from Williams, P.C. *The Lumbosacral Spine.* 1965. New York: McGraw-Hill, p. 92.)

most of its major drawbacks. For example, his recommendations for sit-up exercise included the following points:

- Point arms toward the ceiling to reduce the chance of increasing the hollow of the back. (*This recommendation decreases the chance of extensively involving the psoas as a prime mover in the "up" phase of this exercise.*)
- Concentrate on using the abdominal muscles and sit up smoothly. (*This recommendation concerning mechanics could also tend to reduce the contribution of the psoas or other undesirable muscle substitution.*)
- Never anchor the feet or have someone hold them. (*Subsequent research backed Williams's contention that psoas activity increased with the feet supported (11,12); quite possibly he was one of the first individuals to recognize the drawbacks to exercises in which psoas activity could be detrimental to spine function.*)

Williams suggested that individuals who are unable to do the first variation do the second variation of the trunk flexion exercise shown in Figure 6-2A. Because the second variation negates the role that the psoas and other hip flexors play in trunk flexion, this exercise is more likely to be seen in exercise protocols today than is the full sit-up depicted in this figure.

Pelvic Tilt (Fig. 6-2B)   The pelvic tilt is an exercise that is still widely recommended; however, recent research cautions against its use with disc patients (13). Although Williams emphasized its role as a strengthening exercise for the gluteus maximus, all abdominal muscles and in particular the paired rectus abdominis are involved in this exercise. The pelvic tilt is also used as a lead-up to crunches or curls and the first phase in either.

Trunk Flexion (Fig. 6-2C)   This exercise is also one that is still frequently used because it provides relief to many LBP sufferers by stretching the muscles and soft tissue structures of the spine. However, although it may be a comfortable posture to some sufferers of

LBP, it may not be appropriate for some individuals with discogenic problems such as annular tears. Nevertheless, it is often recommended as an exercise in early intervention programs.

Sit and Reach (Fig. 6-2D)   This exercise is less used in the 1990s than it was previously. The reasons for its demise were discussed in Chap. 2. For example, if individuals with tight hamstrings did this exercise, the soft tissue structures of the spine may be obligated to absorb the forward bending moment of the trunk (14). Although it is viewed as an exercise that can be used to stretch the hamstrings, stretching just one leg at a time, as recommended by Cailliet, is the preferred way to perform this activity. Although the exercise depicted in Figure 6-2D is not recommended, Williams's directions to "bend the upper body slowly and smoothly forward" would avert some of its drawbacks. Williams also stated that this exercise was inappropriate for the individual with sciatica.

Iliotibial Band Stretch (Fig. 6-2E)   Williams believed that tightness in the iliotibial (I-T) band was a prime cause of increased anterior pelvic tilt (e.g., greater than 40 degrees). Although I-T band tightness is often a problem, more effective I-T band stretches than the one depicted exist.

Standing (Fig. 6-2F)   Quadriceps strengthening and learning to substitute leg action for back action are prime rationales for this exercise. Although Williams suggested that younger individuals should perform only the first variation depicted, decreasing the knee bend would be preferable because it places less stress on the structures of the knee. Otherwise, there is nothing inherently wrong with this exercise.

McKENZIE APPROACH

Because McKenzie's approach involves diagnosis and remedial exercises, calling it just a set of exercises is in error (15). More inclusive labels, such as the "McKenzie approach" or the "McKenzie method" that Donelson (4,15) uses or the "McKenzie program" that DiMagio and Mooney (16) use, are preferred.

It should be emphasized that the McKenzie approach is much more than a set of procedures that can be used by a physical therapist in working with a LBP patient. For example, Ron Donelson (an orthopedic surgeon), Research Director and Orthopedic Consultant to the McKenzie Institute International, is a strong advocate of the McKenzie approach. He believes the McKenzie assessment methods are appropriate for every LBP patient because it can be modified in accordance with the patient's level of pain and spinal motion available. Moreover, he contends that the McKenzie treatment methods based on this assessment are appropriate for most back and neck patients (personal communication 1999).

The underlying premise of the McKenzie approach is that spinal disorder and subsequent pain patterns can be categorized as mechanical or nonmechanical by use of the evaluative procedures of end range repeated movements or sustained positions. If the movement results in prolonged exacerbation of the peripheral symptoms, that particular movement should be stopped. However, if the movement results in relief of peripheral symptoms and a centralization of pain toward the body's mid-line, then the movement should be repeated (17). McKenzie's approach is one that focuses on the patient's self-awareness of the dysfunction; once the patient achieves this self-awareness, self-treatment (as appropriate) and other prophylactic measures are employed.

Background

Robin McKenzie (3), a physical therapist, was treating a patient in 1959 who had experienced a 10-day episode of low back and leg pain without resolve. McKenzie told this back patient to wait for him in an examining room. The examining room in which the patient waited had a hinged examining table that just happened to be in the up position. Rather than assume a more conventional sitting position with a back support, the patient lay prone in hyperextension (Fig. 6-3). When McKenzie returned to his patient he was astonished to see him in this posture; however, he was even more surprised when the patient told him that assuming the prone hyperextended posture resulted in a diminishment of his pain.

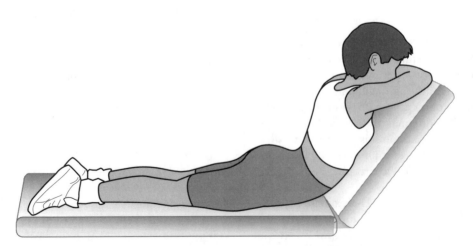

Fig. 6-3 The posture that one of McKenzie's patients inadvertently chose resulted in the development of his extension exercise protocol.

McKenzie tried this positioning with other back patients and found that their symptoms were similarly reduced in this position. After further experimentation McKenzie decided that attempting to provide tables for all patients to assume the prone hyperextended posture was impractical. Instead, he developed simple activities that could be done without a table that would create the same hyperextended posture (Fig. 6-4). Patterns emerged that led McKenzie to describe three mechanical syndromes in addition to a pattern of centralization and peripheralization of pain that could be particularly helpful in predicting outcome and choosing treatment (3,17). It is important to note that McKenzie's approach is not to diagnose the specific structure at fault but rather to make a diagnosis based on the mechanism of pain production.

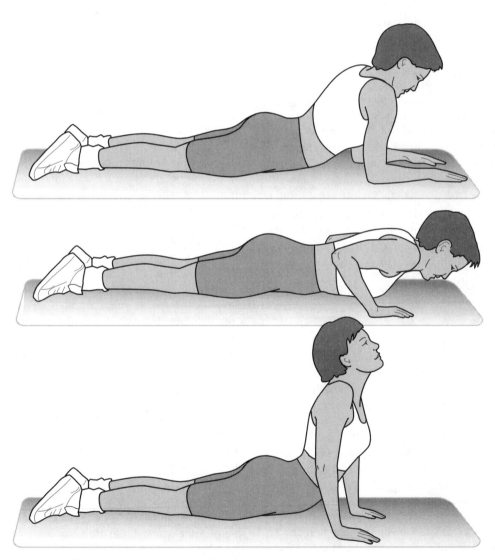

Fig. 6-4 McKenzie's extension exercise for pain that is centered.

In discussing contraindications for his technique, McKenzie (3) indicated that, if no test movement or position can be found to significantly influence the symptoms, the disorder may not be mechanical in origin. Likewise, if there is an increase in peripheral signs and symptoms with all movements, his system is likely inappropriate. Signs in these cases where there may be serious pathology include saddle anesthesia and bladder weakness (a medical emergency), anomalies of weakness and instability (fractures or spondylolisthesis), or extreme pain with twinges and transfixation on movement (3).

Theoretical Basis

McKenzie (3) outlined a pragmatic explanation for his contentions. These include predisposing and precipitating factors, causes of pain, the mechanics of the intervertebral disc in relation to McKenzie's approach, and the centralization process.

Predisposing Factors   McKenzie (3) believed that three prime predisposing lifestyle factors are the most important causes of LBP. These three factors are (a) poor sitting posture, (b) flexion frequency, and (c) loss of the ability to extend the lumbar spine. Each of these factors is presented. Subsequent research that speaks to these issues is mentioned in italic text for interested readers.

Poor Sitting Posture.   McKenzie contended that, even if sitting postures begin with an alignment that maintains the spinal curves seen in "good" erect standing posture, after a certain period there is usually a diminishment of the lordotic curves and an accentuation of the kyphotic ones. He believed that these kyphotic curves eventually place the ligamentous structures under sufficient strain to produce pain. This contention is in direct opposition to that proposed by Williams who thought that the reduction of lordotic curves was desirable (1).

Loss of Lumbar Extension Ability.   McKenzie (3) contended that most of the patients with LBP had lost the ability to extend the spine. He believed that poor postural habits could lead to adaptive shortening (possibly combined with an injury) that could lead to a reduction in the lordotic curve, thus increasing intradiscal pressures.

Flexion Frequency.   McKenzie (3) believed that in the lifestyles of Western culture the spine is constantly being flexed to its maximum but seldom extended to its maximum. He believed that this can result in a posterior migration of the nucleus against the posterior annulus; if annular tears exist, further problems are eminent.

Precipitating Factors   McKenzie cited unguarded movements and lifting as precipitating back problems. If predisposing factors as presented above have led to adaptive changes and repetitive microtrauma of the disc, even a minor stress could elicit an injury. For example, in sporting activity fatigue can lead to poor mechanics; this could set the stage for an unguarded movement. Many a patient with LBP has reported, "I just bent over to pick up something small." For athletes, lifting in the weight room could also be one such stress; the chances for injury would be magnified in the presence of either poor biomechanics or fatigue. In specific sports such as football, forces generated by someone else can quickly change postures assumed, particularly if a player is too relaxed, fatigued, or weaker than the opponent. For example, if an interior lineman is overpowered while doing a lifting-type movement in blocking, the strain incumbent in the resulting change of position could damage soft tissue structures such as annular fibers and ligaments. Although the lineman may not immediately experience pain (18), it is often the posture assumed while relaxing after the activity that eventually causes the pain (3).

There has been some disagreement with regard to the sitting postures that induce the least amount of stress on the spine; these are summarized chronologically.

- In one of a series of intradiscal pressure studies conducted by Nachemson (9), it was found that a disc flexed by 5.5 degrees has a nuclear pressure 50% greater than a disc extended by 3 degrees.
- Adams and Hutton (19) believed that the advantages of flexed posture include (a) reduced stress at the apophyseal joints, (b) less compressive stress on the posterior annulus (although they noted an increase in tensile stress), (c) improved nutrition to the disc, and (d) higher compressive strength overall.
- Hedman and Fernie (20) examined in vitro force and deformation of the lumbar spine of 12 cadavers in seated positions. The cadaver spines were subjected to sustained (30 min) loads (500 N) while flexed and extended. These are their findings. (a) The mean force at the facet joints was greater in extension (50.7 ± 32.2 N) than in flexion (5.6 ± 7.5 N); however, the mean anterior disc compressive force was greater in flexion (165 ± 133 N) than in extension (53.0 ± 46.9 N). (b) The net facet force increased only 1% over 30 min in extension, but the anterior disc force increased 32% in 30 min in flexion. (c) As a result of creep, ligament tension increased substantially in both postures over the 30 min (183% for extension and 153% for flexion).

Causes of Pain. To understand McKenzie's approach, it is important to understand his ideas about pain generators. He stated that the nociceptive system is activated either chemically or mechanically. Bogduk (21) noted that there is a wide distribution of nociceptive receptors in the periosteum, joint capsules, muscles, fascia, skin, ligaments and the outer half of the disc annulus; moreover, he also indicated that nociceptive receptors are particularly dense in the posterior longitudinal ligament. Needless to say, tension would be placed on this ligament in flexion-biased postures.

Mechanical pain occurs when force causes stress, deformation, or damage to tissue. This can occur when an end range position is prolonged or movement in any direction is excessive. Pain can remain constant while the mechanical force continues but cease when mechanical deformation is solved. Chemical pain can arise from an infective process or an inflammatory disease and may begin up to 20 days after a trauma (e.g., tissues taken beyond extensibility) (3). An important point is that chemical pain cannot be abolished by positioning; it is constant versus intermittent, and it can be perpetuated as excessive movement disrupts healing. Understanding the differences in the pain generators is essential in choosing the appropriate McKenzie exercises.

Intervertebral Disc Mechanics. Although McKenzie's model of diagnosis and treatment focuses on the type of mechanical problem rather than the exact structure, his works make extensive reference to the intervertebral disc, and understanding it is essential to choose the correct McKenzie exercises. McKenzie reported that not all discs behave the same; younger ones behave hydrostatically and absorb forces evenly, older discs are stiffer and less mobile; and middle-age discs (beginning at age 30) may begin to get fissures while still behaving hydrostatically, thereby putting the disc at risk. Treatment of derangements is based on the premise that nuclear disc material moves anteriorly with lumbar extension and posteriorly with flexion. The research of others that substantiates McKenzie's view is reviewed later in the chapter.

McKenzie's Conceptual Models of Mechanical Disorders (3)

McKenzie classified back pain of mechanical origin into three syndromes, namely postural, dysfunction, and derangement. Predictable patterns seen in the evaluative process place a patient in one of these categories, thereby directing the course of treatment.

In the McKenzie approach the evaluative procedure is essential to discerning which syndrome or combination of these syndromes the patient demonstrates. The patient's response to repeated movements or sustained positions of flexion and extension (and occasionally side glide), both loaded and unloaded, usually inform the therapist about how to classify the diagnosis and treatment. Response from the patient is reported (usually on a visual analog scale of 1 to 10) before, during, and after the application of forces (test movements). The pain or numbness responses are noted by location and marked as increased, decreased, produced, abolished, no effect, made worse, no worse, made better, or no better. The change in symptoms is noted as occurring during movement or at end range.

Postural Model   Postural pain appears by overstretching and deforming normal tissue. Patients with this syndrome are usually younger than 30, have sedentary occupations, and lack exercise. Complaints of pain are frequently in cervical, thoracic, or lumbar regions, and the pain can occur without any structural damage to the tissues under stress. For example, sitting with a slumped posture for a period can place the soft tissue structures of the lumbar spine at end range of motion (ROM); however, this pain ceases when the individual moves from a slumped sitting posture to a standing one. Before standing, structures such as mid-line ligaments, including facet joint capsules, and the annuli fibrosi may become stressed to the point that pain is perceived and persists until the displaced tissue is repositioned. If the displaced tissue is repositioned before any long-term effects such as creep or stress relaxation occur, everything "returns to normal" when the individual removes this stress by standing and hyperextending the spine or by assuming a better sitting posture (e.g., one with "a good" lordosis). Postural pain arises near the body's mid-line and does not radiate to the extremities; its characteristics differentiate it from the models to be described in the other two syndromes. Movements are normal at testing, but sustained position testing may be needed to reproduce the symptoms. Movement never induces pain from postural origin.

AN APPLICATION OF POSTURAL SYNDROME: *Once the symptoms are produced (e.g., prolonged slumped sitting), the posture is corrected, and the symptoms should disappear. The posture should be corrected; this may require the development of increased strength and endurance of select postural muscles.*

Dysfunction Model   Patients with dysfunction syndrome are frequently older than 30, underexercised, and demonstrate poor posture. The onset of symptoms is insidious. The previously noted predisposing factors of poor posture and frequent forward flexion and lack of extension allow for adaptive shortening of structures that need flexibility to perform daily activities without pain. Although minor injuries can heal quickly, the elasticity of the structure may be affected over time; this can eventually result in a reduction in ROM. The injuries incumbent in athletic activity could produce the same symptoms, but the forces imposed could cause them to occur more quickly. With each successive amount of trauma (micro to macro) to the annular fibers of the disc or to other soft tissue structures, fibrous repair would occur; however, ROM would be reduced because of scar tissue and because of the pain occurring at the diminished end ROM. Although McKenzie acknowledged that there is no sure way to determine which structures are affected at this stage of the disease process, he contended that something has contracted or fibrosed or that nerve root adherence has occurred and that this pain occurs before end ROM.

If the dysfunction model criteria are met, then the injured tissue must be remodeled. In other words, the tissue that has undergone adaptive shortening must be lengthened. Although the adaptive shortening that has occurred in the athlete may not be as great as that in the nonathlete (e.g., monitoring is less apt to be as close for the nonathlete), tissue remodeling does not occur quickly. Inextensible scar tissue developed during repair after trauma also leads to the dysfunction syndrome. McKenzie stated that the pain emanates and occurs immediately from mechanically deforming shortened soft tissues in segments that have reduced elasticity and movement. Upon assessment the pain is felt at end ROM, not during the movement. There will be a loss of function and/or movement. Pain will be referred in the dysfunction syndrome only from an adherent nerve root.

AN APPLICATION OF THE DYSFUNCTION SYNDROME: *The goal of treatment is to use exercise to stretch the shortened structures and to make postural correction. Stretching shortened structures was discussed in Chap. 2. The exercises may include flexion, extension, and side glide exercises; these should be performed daily (10 to 12 repetitions, ideally every 2 h) to the edge of pain to elongate the appropriate tissue. Once the tissue is elongated, pain should not persist. Nerve root adherence will necessitate stretching through peripheral symptoms. An adherent nerve root is treated by stretching followed by extension procedures to prevent recurrence of derangement.*

Derangement Model Patients with a derangement syndrome are usually 20 to 55 years old. They usually have a relatively sudden onset of pain and decreased function, sometimes for no apparent reason. Pain may be central or it may refer; it may be constant, and paresthesias may be present. Movements or positions alter the symptoms. McKenzie's description of this syndrome and the apparent effects of positions or movements are based on the internal dynamic disc model. When the pain changes intensity or location, the disc is changing its displacement shape or position based on the movement or position of the patient. Movement loss always occurs and may be severe, and deformities such as scoliosis or kyphosis may be seen. McKenzie reported that, with testing movements, peripheralization indicates development of the derangement and centralization reduction. Rapid and lasting changes after test movements indicate derangement. If test movements cannot reduce symptoms, the annular wall may be breached. McKenzie (3) classified posterior derangements on a basis of 1 to 6; he ranked anterior derangement as 7. For example, central or symmetric pain across L4 through L5 could meet criteria for derangement 1, whereas unilateral or asymmetrical pain across L4 through L5 and extending below the knee could meet criteria for derangement 6. The reader is referred to McKenzie's book for a more complete delineation of derangement (3).

Treatment for derangement follows four phases: reduction of derangement, maintenance of reduction, recovery of function, and prevention of recurrence or prophylaxis. Treatment exercises or mobilization technique are based on the directional preference the patient shows at mechanical evaluation. The goal is centralization and abolishment of symptoms in phase 1, as noted above. Derangement 1 is reduced by the extension principle. The treatment aim for derangements 2 through 6 is to reverse the derangement by shift correction or the extension principle to resemble derangement 1. This is centralization.

Centralization is a term coined by McKenzie (3) to describe a rapid change in the perceived location and intensity of pain from a peripheral or distal position to a more central or proximal one; this occurs in the derangement syndrome as the bulging disc reduces with exercise. A good outcome can be expected if centralization occurs.

Reduction is maintained by sitting with lumbar support, maintaining lumbar lordosis, and frequent performance of extension exercises. Function begins to recover when flexion no longer initiates onset of derangement signs. Flexion exercises or procedures are used and followed by extension. Recurrence is prevented through educating the patient to continue exercises and take precautions with prolonged bending and sitting. Treatment of derangement 7 is typically done with flexion-biased exercises or procedures and followed with extension when derangement signs are no longer present.

AN APPLICATION OF THE DERANGEMENT SYNDROME: *Assume a patient starts with unilateral back and leg pain below the knee. The patient performs 10 repetitions of standing flexion. Pain is increased distally during movement and remains worse. This may suggest to the clinician derangement behavior that further testing would confirm. Noting the symptom behavior with specific reference to effects with repeated movements is integral to evaluating and treating with the McKenzie approach. Of particular importance is to note peripheralization or centralization. McKenzie stressed the importance of repeating the movements because pain that initially decreases or abolishes with a position or movement may, when repeated, cause the condition to worsen (or the exact opposite may occur). This occurs most frequently with derangement. The reader is referred to McKenzie's book (3) or other materials such as course work through his institute for detailed descriptions of treatment of derangements.*

Research Relevant to the McKenzie Approach. When McKenzie (3) first proposed his ideas, they were somewhat controversial, in part because they were diametrically opposed to those presented in the Williams flexion exercises (1), the predominant exercise program of that era. One aspect that was difficult to demonstrate was that the nucleus pulposus would actually move anteriorly in spine extension and posteriorly in spine flexion. Clinical efficacy was also questioned; the biomechanics of nuclear movement and clinical efficacy (i.e., whether centralization or peripheralization occurs with exercise) are discussed in the next sections.

Nuclear Movement in Flexion and Extension. Schnebel et al. (22) measured the positional change of the nucleus pulposus using discography. In this study, knees-to-chest was used for flexion and a prone press-up position was used for extension. The researchers found a significant difference in the posterior position of the nucleus pulposus in normal discs between flexion and extension; the mean movement at L4–L5 and at L5–S1 was 2.2 and 2.9 mm, respectively. They concluded that extension decreased the forces on the L5 nerve root (with a herniated disc at L4–L5), whereas flexion increased the compressive and tensile forces on the nerve root.

Beattie et al. (23) investigated how the nucleus pulposus moves in lumbar flexion and extension. Subjects underwent magnetic resonance imaging while supine. Lumbar extension was considered

supine with a lumbar roll, and flexion was supine with hips and knees in flexion (~30 degrees). The anterior and posterior margins of the nucleus pulposus (NP) were measured with respect to the anterior and posterior margins of the adjacent vertebral bodies. One finding was that the nucleus pulposus of degenerated discs did not move the same as normal discs, just as McKenzie contended. A second finding from this study is that the normal nucleus pulposus did move based on lumbar vertebral movements. The distance of the posterior margin of the nucleus pulposus to the posterior margins of adjacent vertebral bodies was greater in extension than in flexion. Basically, the nucleus pulposus moved farther away from the pain-sensitive structures in the posterior spine with extension movements.

Centralization and Peripheralization. Kopp et al. (24) reported in their study of patients with a herniated NP that the use of passive extension exercises in a patient achieving normal lumbar extension is a reliable sign in determining outcome. They did not mention centralization by name, but they reported that all their patients had pain radiating below the knee. Because only 6.2% of the patients who needed surgical treatment were able to achieve extension, they concluded that the inability to achieve extension is an early predictor of the need for surgery. Of their entire population, 52% were treated successfully without surgery.

Donelson et al. (17) investigated the centralization phenomenon and concluded that 87% of patients in their study population were "centralizers" during the initial McKenzie mechanical evaluation. They concluded that the McKenzie technique of evaluation is a very accurate predictor of successful treatment outcomes and an indicator of appropriate direction of exercise.

Donelson et al. (25) reported that a nonoccurrence of centralization accurately predicts a poor treatment outcome and serves as an early predictor of the need for surgical treatment. They also noted that both the intensity and location of LBP and referred pain changed significantly as a result of end range flexion and extension testing. End range extension significantly decreased central and distal intensity and centralized referred pain for the mean of the group, in which flexion had the opposite effect. Forty percent of their group showed a directional preference for extension and improved; 7% improved with flexion. These improvements in level of pain were elicited in only one session.

Donelson et al (26) studied the validity of the dynamic internal disc model described by McKenzie (3). A dynamic spinal assessment of repeated end range movement testing, with centralization and peripheralization behavior noted, was used to predict disc level, state of annular containment, axial fissure pattern, and type of pain provocation. Diagnostic disc injection outcomes were used comparatively. Donelson et al. found that the McKenzie assessment differentiated between (a) discogenic and nondiscogenic pain and (b) competent from incompetent annuli in symptomatic discs. They also contended that this assessment was better than magnetic resonance imaging in differentiating between painful and nonpainful discs. They concluded that their research strongly supports a cause and effect relationship between the disc model and symptom response patterns of centralization and directional preferences identified during the assessment.

Conclusion. Some mistakenly view the McKenzie approach as only extension exercise. However, it is a comprehensive mechanical assessment model for diagnosis and treatment that uses extension frequently but not exclusively. A thorough understanding of the evaluative and treatment rationale is essential to a successful outcome; this point cannot be overemphasized.

DYNAMIC LUMBAR STABILIZATION

The San Francisco Spine Institute appears to be one of the first entities to promote dynamic lumbar stabilization as a therapeutic exercise for rehabilitating individuals with spine pain (27). A basic premise in lumbar stabilization training is to teach patients with LBP how to maintain functional skills that are in concert with their aims in life, whether these aims are the nominal activities of daily living or the extraordinary skills required by collegiate or professional athletes. This is achieved by learning how to dynamically stabilize diseased motion segments so that afflicted individuals can perform everyday activities satisfactorily.

Introduction to Trunk Stabilization

A few definitions must first be presented to address trunk stabilization as a form of exercise for LBP. Several terms are used interchangeably in trunk stabilization including *bracing, neutral spine,* and *muscle fusion.* Neural aspects of trunk stabilization are very important because learning stabilization requires learning new sensory motor engrams. Crucial to understanding trunk stabilization exercises is having a solid base of knowledge of what stability and instability includes biomechanically and structurally. Panjabi (28) contended that stabilization of the spine can be viewed as having three categories of support: passive, muscular, and neural. Panjabi's categories are discussed in this section. The passive system is examined with reference to the definition of stability. Muscular and neural supports are presented with reference to their inclusion in one of the two components in stability, the global or local spinal active stabilizing system.

Spinal Instability

Spinal instability has often been defined as a vertebral motion segment that exhibits excessive or abnormal quality of motion (29,30). Pope and Panjabi (31) added to this definition and suggested that "a loss of stiffness" can be used to describe spinal instability. A structure's stiffness is the ratio of the force applied and the motion that results. If a set amount of force results in a set amount of movement and the same amount of force applied to an adjacent segment results in twice the movement, the second is less stiff and therefore less stable. Subsequently, Panjabi (28,32) hypothesized beyond the traditional view of instability as movement beyond normal physiologic range and identified a neutral zone in normal range in which a decrease of control signals spinal instability. Panjabi (32) also proposed another definition for "clinical instability," namely "A significant decrease in the capacity of the stabilizing system of the spine to maintain the intervertebral neutral zones within the physiological limits which results in pain and disability" (p. 394).

Lumbar spinal instability may be triggered by an incidence of large force or trauma or by microtrauma. Microtrauma can occur in the form of sustained positions or repetitive motions. For example, it has long been accepted that combined flexion, bending, and twisting can lead to degenerative changes. With degenerative changes and a decrease in disc space, ligamentous stability may be reduced at this diseased motion segment. That level of stability will then offer less stiffness to applied loads (e.g., muscle forces and external turning moments), and an increase in segmental motion may occur. Yong-Hing and Kirkaldy-Willis (33) suggested that intersegmental motion increases in the second or intermediate stage of the degenerative process.

Spinal Stability

The biomechanics of the spine and its stability are quite complex and include the study of passive and active stabilizing systems in healthy and symptomatic backs. Saal (34) stated that spinal stabilization involves elimination of repetitive microtrauma to lumbar motion segments, thus limiting injury and allowing healing to occur. Panjabi (28) provided a model in which spinal stability is viewed as the composite of three subsystems, namely passive, active, and neural. A breakdown in any one system can constitute a spinal stabilization problem and lead to LBP. Panjabi's (28) model is presented in Figure 6-5. Each of his three systems is discussed in its relation to spinal stability.

The Passive (Ligamentous) Subsystem   The passive or ligamentous system consists of the bones, ligaments, joint capsules, and intervertebral discs. The noncontractile structures resist motion when the limit of their extensibility or stiffness is reached, but the structures do not provide substantial support in neutral joint positions. These structures adapt to stresses placed on them and behave along a stress-strain curve. When the end of the elastic range is exceeded and the plastic range is reached due to microtrauma or injury, tissue deformation is likely. This reduces the ability of the passive structure to limit motion and maintain the integrity of the spinal segment.

Movement at each vertebral segment consists of three-dimensional motions. Translation (chiefly forward or backward) and rotation at lumbar motion segments occur with flexion and extension and in lateral flexion and axial rotation in coupled motions. The facet joints limit translation and anterior sagittal rotation (35,36). The discs and longitudinal ligaments resist shear force resulting from translation; the facet joints and the disc annulus

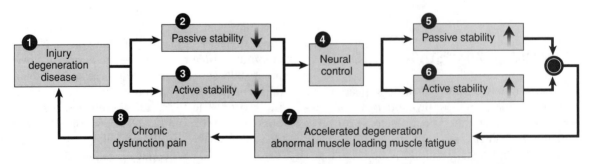

Fig. 6-5 Dysfunction of spinal stability. (Adapted from Panjabi, M.M. The stabilizing system of the spine, part I. Function, dysfunction, adaptation, and enhancement. *J Spinal Disord* 1992, 5[4]: p. 383–389.)

restrain axial rotation force (37). Dysfunction can be caused by overstretching of ligaments, tears and fissures to the annulus, and microfractures to the disc endplates. Although this passive system does not produce movement per se, it monitors nociceptive and proprioceptive receptors or, in the words of Panjabi (28), "transducer signals." Solmonow et al. (38) explained how the mechanoreceptors in the supraspinous ligament can trigger reflex contraction of the multifidus when the disc is at risk. Obviously, the health of these passive structures is integral to a functionally stable spinal unit.

The Active (Musculotendinous) Subsystem

The muscular component of spinal stability is often the weak link; conversely, it can compensate for other components in dysfunction. Gardner-Morse et al. (39) suggested that decreased muscle stiffness resulting from fatigue, degenerative changes, or injury may lead to spinal instability. The muscular system, however, has the potential to increase the stiffness of the lumbar spine and decrease inappropriate movement and improve overall spinal stability (28,39,40). The muscular system generates force that provides the active mechanical stability to the spinal segment, particularly in neutral spine.

Cholewicki et al. (41) showed that antagonistic trunk flexor-extensor coactivation (i.e., internal and external obliques, rectus abdominis, lumbar and thoracic erector spinae, and multifidus) was present in the neutral spine position in healthy individuals. This coactivation increased with increased mass added to the torso. The researchers found a variety of muscle recruitment strategies, with most subjects maintaining a constant level of internal oblique firing regardless of trunk attitude. The electromyographic (EMG) levels of coactivation in the healthy subjects overall was at a low level. This is logical because these muscles need to be able to perform daily tasks and maintain trunk stability against gravity for long periods of time; if EMG levels were constantly high, fatigue would result. Cholewicki et al. suggested that increased levels in EMG coactivation may be an objective indicator of dysfunction in the passive stabilizing system, necessitating overcompensation from the active subsystem (i.e., muscles).

Based on the level of EMG coactivation found in this study, the intensity of contraction need not be high in retraining a patient in trunk stabilization exercises.

Quint et al. (42) used cadaveric lumbar spine specimens and applied force vectors to simulate coactivation of the psoas and multifidus muscles on mobility between L4 and L5. The coactivation of these muscles was accompanied by a 20% decrease in ROM with lateral bending, thus increasing the overall stiffness of the spine. O'Sullivan et al. (43) studied the effect of spinal stabilization exercises on patients with spondylolisis and spondylolisthesis. The patients underwent 10 weeks of exercises that included emphasis on training the deep abdominal muscles (i.e., transversus abdominis and internal oblique) and the multifidus in coactivation in the performance of functional activities. The findings support a hypothesis that stability of the lumbar spine is dependent not solely on morphology of the spine but also on proper neuromuscular function. If the structure of the spine is compromised, the neuromuscular system may be trained to compensate. The muscles isolated in training in this study were the deep local muscles (see Local Stabilization System).

All skeletal muscles originating or attaching to the trunk or pelvis are involved in some fashion in stability of the spine. However, researchers have reported that some muscles more than others play pivotal roles in segmental stability. Bergmark (44) categorized the muscles of the trunk into two functional divisions. These are listed in Table 6-1.

Global Stabilization System

The global stabilizing system (see Table 6-1) includes the larger, more superficial muscles of the lumbopelvic region that have the ability to produce large torques and act on the trunk. Although they control movement of the spine, they are more involved in the transfer of external loads from the thoracic cage to the pelvis than in producing intersegmental control. They balance these loads so that the residual may be "handled" by the local smaller muscles (44). Endurance training of global muscles can increase their ability in heavy lifting and ensure that less force is trans-

Table 6-1   Categorization of Muscles Used in Trunk Stabilization

LOCAL STABILIZING SYSTEM	GLOBAL STABILIZING SYSTEM
• Intertransversarii (intersegmental) • Interspinales (intersegmental) • Multifidus • Longissimus thoracis (pars lumborum) • Iliocostalis lumborum (pars lumborum) • Quadratus lumborum (medial fibers) • Transversus abdominis • Internal oblique (fiber insertion into the lateral raphe of thoracolumbar fascia	• Longissimus thoracis (pars thoracis) • Iliocostalis lumborum (pars thoracis) • Quadratus lumborum (lateral fibers) • Rectal abdominis • External oblique • Internal oblique

Adapted from Bergmark A (*Acta Orthop Scand* 1989, 230[suppl]; p. 20–24).

ferred to the spine itself; the control of forces here is handled by the smaller local muscles (45). When O'Sullivan et al. (43) compared patients with LBP with healthy subjects as each did lifting tasks, they noted excessive global cocontraction during light weight-lifting tasks by their patients who had LBP. This suggests that excessive global contraction may be an indicator of inappropriate trunk control.

Local Stabilization System   The local stabilizing system (see Table 6-1) includes the deep muscles of the trunk and the deep portions of muscles that have their origins or insertions on lumbar vertebrae (44). These muscles have shorter lengths, are closer to the center of rotation of the spinal segment, and are therefore better suited to control motion at the segmental level (46). In addition to balancing the load not controlled by the global system, the intersegmental muscles such as the intertransversarii and the interspinales are responsible for proprioceptive feedback (37,47).

The multifidus links adjacent lumbar vertebrae and is also an efficient and important stabilizer at the local level (37). Wilke et al. (48) studied five different muscle groups and their respective contributions to stiffness at the L4–L5 motion segment and found that the lumbar multifidus contributed the most to stiffness. The segmental control of the muscle fibers of the multifidus facilitates its adjustment to applied loads (37,45).

Richardson et al. (45) contended that the transversus abdominis, one of the deep local muscles particularly emphasized in Chap. 1, is one of the

key local muscles in trunk stabilization. They stated that the transversus abdominis was the first muscle active when healthy subjects stood and performed quick upper extremity movements. This is of particular importance when teaching beginning level trunk stabilization, for the transversus abdominis contractions are the first to be emphasized as a "pulling-in" type of exercise.

The Neural Control Subsystem   In addition to monitoring the transducer signals of the passive ligamentous system, the neural control subsystem must, of course, be in command of the muscular system that is required for spinal stability. A major goal of spine stabilization activities is to develop a somewhat uniquely different control of the muscular system. This is done through the development of new engrams.

An engram can be defined as a permanent trace that a stimulus leaves in nervous tissue that describes the motor information necessary to perform a specific movement. Information that is necessary to perform this movement is stored as a unit, and once learned, it is accessed without conscious thought. Early in learning a movement, conscious control or recruitment is necessary; however, once the movement is thoroughly learned, its engram can be retrieved without conscious thought. Nevertheless, the process is not an easy one. For example, if an individual has been "turning and lifting" the same way for 20 to 30 years, that habit may be hard to break. Another reason is that not all individuals are as adroit in learning a new skill (or a new way to perform a movement) as are some other individuals. For example, some individuals can learn a new skill, such as a smooth golf swing, quickly, whereas others will need much more time before their swing even approaches smoothness.

Additional factors can affect the process. For example, the engram encoded for normal function movements may be altered because of the change in the neural system. Hodges and Richardson (49) noted a delayed onset of contraction of the transverse abdominis in patients with LBP when standing and performing quick upper extremity movements. This indicates a deficit in motor control, and they hypothesized that this resulted in inefficient muscular stability of the spine. To regain optimal spinal stabilization, a patient needs to reeducate the neural system and override the adaptive changes from either structural injury to a neural component or because of the change in afferent input due to pain. This component may be easily overlooked and merits particular attention in teaching spinal stabilization exercises.

Also, when injury occurs, the neural component may be disrupted or altered because of structural reasons (injury to a neural structure) or by change in the homeostasis of the neural feedback because of pain. An increase in afferent input increases muscle tone (spasm), leading to a change in the physiologic properties in the tissue, thus increasing pain or at least continuing the cycle. The change in muscle tone affects the ability of the muscular system to stabilize the vertebral segments adequately without overload or fatigue.

Trunk Stabilization Exercises and Bracing

Muscle fusion, bracing, and *neutral spine* are terms sometimes used interchangeably. Saal (34) defined muscle fusion as the "use of the musculature to brace the spine and protect the motion segments against repetitive microtrauma and excessively high single-occurrence loads" (p. 35). He cited the role of cocontraction of the abdominal muscles and the trunk extensors to maintain a "corseting" effect.

O'Sullivan et al. (50) used a bracing exercise as the base of their exercise protocol. They trained their patients to perform an isometric cocontraction (at low levels of maximum contraction) of the transversus abdominis and lumbar multifidus, with minimal use of the global system muscles. This was to be achieved by using the abdominal drawing in maneuver as described by Richardson and Jull (51); in Chap. 8, the maneuver is referred to as *hollowing*. They reported it was difficult to achieve because of the substitution of the rectus abdominis, external oblique, and the long back extensors. They also reported that patients had difficulty controlling breathing with this "bracing." They allowed patients to advance only when the isolated contraction could be held for 10 s 10 times. It was then incorporated into holding and dynamic tasks. They felt this was necessary to reinforce the new engram of motor control so that this stability control occurred automatically. This form of bracing in the exercise protocol produced a statistically significant reduction in pain intensity and functional disability levels at a 30-month follow-up (50).

Exercises should not recruit the lumbar stabilizers only to strengthen them but should recruit them in their most efficient functions. Small, local stabilizers need to be retrained, or educated, in the neural sense to respond when larger functional daily activities require the larger global muscles to control external forces and leave the local spinal stabilizing role to the deeper trunk musculature. Exercises including bracing need to progress to include increased load when spinal stability is performed in the simpler exercises. Compensatory usage of the global musculature (50) or release of the bracing activity in simple stability exercises point to a need for continued reeducation and training of the local stabilizers. Specific exercises are discussed in Chap. 8.

CONCLUSION

When viewing the research on spinal stabilization, many questions are answered with respect to muscular function. Many questions remain in the clinical decision of what constitutes spinal instability

(52). Some researchers, however, have shown very good results with spine stabilization exercise protocols in patients with apparent spinal stability (45,50), thereby providing a secure basis from which to prescribe trunk stabilization exercises for patients with LBP.

REFERENCES

1. Williams, P.C. *The Lumbosacral Spine.* 1965, New York: McGraw Hill.
2. Williams, P.C. *Low Back and Neck Pain-Causes and Conservative Treatment.* 1974, Springfield, IL: Charles C. Thomas. p. 82.
3. McKenzie, R. *The Lumbar Spine-Mechanical Diagnosis and Therapy.* 1981, Waikanae, New Zealand: Spinal Publications. p. 164.
4. Donelson, R. The McKenzie approach to evaluating and treating low back pain. *Orthop Rev* 1990, 8: p. 681–686.
5. Dolan, P., and M.A. Adams. The relationship between EMG activity and extensor moment generation in the erector spinae muscles during bending and lifting activities. *J Biomech* 1993, 26(4/5): p. 513–522.
6. White, A.H. Stabilization of the lumbar spine, in *Conservative Care of Low Back Pain,* A.H. White and R. Anderson, editors. 1991, Baltimore: Williams & Wilkins. p. 106–111.
7. Elnaggar, I.M., Nordin, M., Sheikhzadeh, A., et al. Effects of spinal flexion and extension exercises on low-back pain and spinal mobility in chronic mechanical low-back pain. *Spine* 1991, 16(8): p. 967–972.
8. Dettori, J.R., Bullock, S.H., Sutlive, T.G., et al. The effects of spinal flexion and extension exercises and their associated postures in patients with acute low back pain. *Spine* 1995, 20(21): p. 2303–2312.
9. Nachemson, A.L. The lumbar spine—an orthopaedic challenge. *Spine* 1976, 1: p. 59–71.
10. Axler, C.T., and S.M. McGill. Low back loads over a variety of abdominal exercises: searching for the safest abdominal challenge. *Med Sci Sports Exerc* 1997, 29(6): p. 804–811.
11. Juker, D., McGill, S., Kropf, P., et al. Quantitative intramuscular myoelectric activity of lumbar portions of psoas and the abdominal wall during a wide variety of tasks. *Med Sci Sports Exerc* 1998, 30(2): p. 301–310.
12. LaBan, M.M., Raptov, A.D., Johnson, E.W. Electromyographic study of function of iliopsoas muscle. *Arch Phys Med Rehabil* 1965, 45: p. 676–679.
13. McGill, S.M. Low back exercises: evidence for improving exercise regimens. *Phys Ther* 1998, 78(7): p. 754–765.
14. Cailliet, R. *Low Back Pain Syndrome.* 1988, Philadelphia: F.A. Davis Co.
15. Donelson, R. The McKenzie method, in *Conservative Care of Low Back Pain,* A.H. White and R. Anderson, editors 1991, Baltimore: Williams & Wilkins. p. 97–104.
16. Dimagio, A., and V. Mooney. The McKenzie program: exercise effective against back pain. *J Musculoskel Med* 1987, 4(12): p. 63–74.
17. Donelson, R., Silva, G., Murphy, K. Centralization phenomenon: its usefulness in evaluating and treating referred pain. *Spine* 1990, 15(2): p. 211–213.
18. McKenzie, R.A. *The Cervical and Thoracic Spine: Mechanical Diagnosis and Therapy.* 1990, Waikanae, New Zealand: Spinal Publications (N.Z.) Limited. p. 320.
19. Adams, M.A., and W.C. Hutton. The effect of posture on the lumbar spine. *J Bone Joint Surg* 1985, 67B(4): p. 625–629.
20. Hedman, T.P., and G.R. Fernie. Mechanical response of the lumbar spine to seated postural loads. *Spine* 1997, 22(7): p. 734–743.
21. Bogduk, N. A reappraisal of the anatomy of the human lumbar erector spinae. *J Anat* 1980, 131(3): p. 525–540.
22. Schnebel, B.E., Simmons, J.W., Chowning, J., et al. A digitizing technique for the study of movement of intradiscal dye in response to flexion and extension of the lumbar spine. *Spine* 1988, 13(2): p. 309–312.
23. Beattie, P.F., Brooks, W.M., Rothstein, J.M., et al., Effect of lordosis on the position of the nucleus pulposus in supine subjects. *Spine* 1994, 19(18): p. 2096–2102.
24. Kopp, J.R., Alexander, A.H., Turocy, R.H., et al. The use of lumbar extension in the evaluation and treatment of patients with acute herniated nucleus pulposus—a preliminary report. *Clin Orthop Rel Res* 1986, 202: p. 211–218.
25. Donelson, R., Grant, W., Kamps, C., et al. Pain response to sagittal end-range spinal motion. A prospective, randomized, multicentered trial. *Spine* 1991, 16(6S): p. S206–S212.

26. Donelson, R., Aprill, C., Medcalf, R., et al. A prospective study of centralization of lumbar and referred pain. A predictor of symptomatic discs and annular competence. *Spine* 1997, 22(10): p. 1115–1122.

27. San Francisco Spine Institute, *Workbook Dynamic Lumbar Stabilization Program.* Daly City, CA, 1989. p. 28.

28. Panjabi, M.M. The stabilizing system of the spine, part I. Function, dysfunction, adaptation, and enhancement. *J Spinal Disord* 1992, 5(4): p. 383–389.

29. Dupuis, P.R., Yong-Tiing, K., Cassidy, J.D., et al. Radiologic diagnosis of degenerative lumbar spine instability. *Spine* 1985, 10: p. 262–276.

30. Gertzbein, S.D., Seligman, J., Holtby, R., et al. Centrode patterns and segmental instability in degenerative disc disease. *Spine* 1985, 10: p. 257–261.

31. Pope, M.H., and M.M. Panjabi. Biomechanical definitions of instability. 1985, 10: p. 255–256.

32. Panjabi, M. The stabilising system of the spine, part II. Neutral zone and stability hypothesis. *J Spinal Disord* 1992, 5: p. 390–397.

33. Yong-Hing, K., and W.H. Kirkaldy-Willis. The pathophysiology of degenerative disease of the lumbar spine. *Orthop Clin North Am* 1983, 14(3): p. 491–504.

34. Saal, J.A. The new back school. Prescription: stabilization training part II. *Occup Med* 1992, 7(1): p. 33–42.

35. Twomey, L.T., and J.R. Taylor. Sagittal movements of the human lumbar vertebral column: a quantitative study of the role of the posterior vertebral elements. *Phys Med Rehabil* 1983, 64: p. 322–325.

36. Oliver, M.J., Lynn, J.W., Lynn, J.M. An interpretation of the McKenzie approach to low back pain, in *Physical Therapy of the Low Back.* L.T. Twomey, J.R. Taylor, editors. 1986, Edinburgh: Churchill Livingstone. p. 225–251.

37. Bogduk, N., and L.T. Twomey. *Clinical Anatomy of the Lumbar Spine.* 1987, Edinburgh: Churchill Livingstone. p. 166.

38. Solmonow, M., Zhou, B., Harris, M., et al. The ligamento-muscular stabilizing system of the spine. *Spine* 1998, 23(23): p. 2552–2562.

39. Gardner-Morse, M., Stokes, I.A.F., Lauble, J.P. Role of the muscles in lumbar spine stability in maximum extension efforts. *J Orthop Res* 1995, 13: p. 802–808.

40. Cholewicki, J., and S. McGill. Mechanical stability of the in vivo lumbar spine: implications for injury and chronic low back pain. *Clin Biomech* 1996, 11: p. 1–15.

41. Cholewicki, J., Panjabi, M., Khachatryan, A. Stabilizing function of trunk flexor–extensor muscles around a neutral spine posture. *Spine* 1997, 22: p. 2207–2212.

42. Quint, U., Wilke, H.J., Shiraz-Adl, A., et al. Importance of the intersegmental trunk muscles for the stability of the lumbar spine—a biomechanical study in vitro. *Spine* 1998, 23(18): p. 1937–1945.

43. O'Sullivan, P.B., Twomey, L., Allison, G.T. Dynamic stabilization of the lumbar spine. *Crit Rev Phys Rehabil Med* 1997, 9(3/4): p. 315–330.

44. Bergmark, A. Stability of the lumbar spine. A study in mechanical engineering. *Acta Orthop Scand* 1989, 230(suppl): p. 20–24.

45. Richardson, C., Jull, G., Hodges, P., et al. *Therapeutic Exercise for Spinal Stabilization in Low Back Pain-Scientific Basis and Clinical Approach.* 1999, London: Churchill Livingstone. p. 191.

46. Panjabi, M., Abumi, K., Duranceau, J., et al. Spinal stability and intersegmental muscle forces. A biomechanical model. *Spine* 1989, 14: p. 194–200.

47. Crisco, J.J., and M.M. Panjabi. The intersegmental and multisegmental muscles of the spine: a biomechanical model comparing lateral stabilising potential. *Spine* 1991, 7: p. 793–799.

48. Wilke, H.J., Wolf, S., Claes, L.E., et al. Stability increase of the lumbar spine with different muscle groups. A biomechanical in vitro study. *Spine* 1995, 20: p. 192–198.

49. Hodges, P.W., and C.A. Richardson. Inefficient muscular stabilisation of the lumbar spine associated with low back pain: a motor control evaluation of transversus abdominis. *Spine* 1996, 21: p. 2640–2650.

50. O'Sullivan, P.B., Twomey, L.T., Allison, G.T. Evaluation of specific stabilizing exercise in the treatment of chronic low back pain with radiologic diagnosis of spondylolysis or spondylolisthesis. *Spine* 1997, 22(24): p. 2959–2967.

51. Richardson, C.A., and G.A. Jull. Muscle control-pain control. What exercises would you prescribe? *Manual Ther* 1995, 1: p. 2–10.

52. Boyling, J.D., and N. Palasanga. *Grieve's Modern Manual Therapy. The Vertebral Column*, 2nd ed. 1994, Edinburgh: Churchill Livingstone.

CHAPTER 7

THE FELDENKRAIS AND ALEXANDER TECHNIQUES

Jeanne Nelson

INTRODUCTION

The combined use that the Feldenkrais and Alexander techniques have received for low back pain (LBP) patients would perhaps just be a blip on the screen when compared with the wide use that the Mckenzie and the lumbar stabilization techniques described in Chap. 6 have received. Moreover, both the Feldenkrais and Alexander techniques were developed for conditions other than LBP. However, one emphasis of the Feldenkrais technique is the development of muscle control; learning to use the trunk muscles to control pelvic positioning can be most valuable to some back patients. In stabilization training, often new sensory engrams must be learned as the patient attempts to reduce movement at a diseased motion segment; the Feldenkrais technique can be a most valuable adjunct for patients who perhaps have less coordination. The Alexander technique holds posture as one of its fundamental precepts; it has been called the "grandfather" of somatic therapies (1). The role of posture as it relates to LBP has been emphasized in Chaps. 1 and 6.

FELDENKRAIS TECHNIQUE (2)

The Feldenkrais technique, developed by Moshe Feldenkrais to rehabilitate his own knee, has been expanded to include all aspects of movement and many dysfunctions for people of all ages. The technique uses a progression of exploratory activities based on developmental movements and functional activities; it also includes abstract explorations of joint, muscle, and postural relationships. The emphasis is placed on how to move. Although the primary intent of Feldenkrais' work is not to improve strength and flexibility, often such improvement results from the training. Feldenkrais called his exercises *lessons* to emphasize the role of patients as students in learning how they currently move in addition to learning new options for performing the same motion. When individuals learn an easier way of performing a motion, they will usually incorporate the new easier pattern and discard the old

dysfunctional pattern, even though they may have used that pattern for many years (1).

As a physical therapist, I have worked with individuals with chronic LBP for 15 years. Treating such patients can be very rewarding when the pain cycle is finally broken, but too often only partial or nominal improvement is realized even after weeks of treatment. It has been estimated that 90% of individuals with acute LBP get better within 1 month despite the treatment they have received (3). Those individuals who do not improve present a challenge, not only for the medical community to treat but also for the suffering individuals to continue to function.

In individuals with chronic LBP, fluid trunk motion integrated with the extremities is usually diminished or lost due to rigid "guarding" of the trunk. Although strengthening key musculature such as that of the trunk and hip joint gives the patient more support in the low back area, torso rigidity is still often reflected in how the individual moves. Even static standing has a rigid quality as though everything would fall apart if the individual were to relax. Moreover, the patient's original complaints of pain, ache, and discomfort may persist. Why do these symptoms continue despite measurable improvements in strength?

One theory is that individuals with chronic LBP have eliminated many of their options of trunk movement and positioning over time in their attempt to become pain free. Unfortunately, pain-free (or less painful) actions or positions are not necessarily the most biomechanically advantageous and may lead to degeneration or other dysfunction elsewhere in the body. One method of addressing this dysfunction is through use of the Feldenkrais method; it can help the patient learn how to learn the movement prescribed (1).

The Genesis of the Feldenkrais Technique (2)

A flare up of an old soccer injury inspired the physicist, Feldenkrais, to follow a new direction that eventually culminated in his developing the technique. When he experienced exacerbation of an old knee injury, Feldenkrais refused to have surgery and opted instead for bed rest. The knee did not improve and traditional medicine did not have any other answers; this led Feldenkrais to search for better understanding of and control over his own body mechanics. His years of study, combined with a background in judo, led him to his own cure. After succeeding with his own difficulties, he applied his principles to total body work, which led eventually to the development of the Feldenkrais method. The Feldenkrais method consists of two parts: awareness through movement and functional integration. Each is discussed in the following sections.

Awareness Through Movement

Awareness Through Movement (ATM) consists of the practitioner verbally leading an individual through a progression of movements designed to enhance that individual's perception of motion. A method of training will power, self-control, and conscious awareness (2), ATM is very much a learning practice in that one guideline is to stop the "lesson" if mental fatigue occurs. The approach proceeds as though individuals with dysfunction have been given a blank "owner's manual" for their body, and they are asked to fill in all of their observations of the intricacies of these movements (i.e., awareness). This would be analogous to a car owner's manual that describes in great detail the electrical wiring of a car. The method is essentially educational and experiential; it is process and not goal oriented (4).

Functional Integration

Functional integration (FI) involves actual "hands on" application and differs from ATM in that it is purely manual, subconscious instruction. Feldenkrais studied the Alexander technique whose influence may be seen during the use of FI. The casual observer watching FI will witness slow, light touch applied to various aspects of the individual's body, some directly over the area of dysfunction but others much more remote. If the FI is successful,

changes will be seen immediately in breathing, posture, ability to move, and other characteristics. Feldenkrais would often leave his audiences gasping when they witnessed major improvement in function after he applied only a few minutes of FI to a patient.

Clinical Application of the Feldenkrais Technique for Chronic LBP

The Feldenkrais technique adds an extra dimension to rehabilitation of individuals with chronic LBP. As the chronicity becomes more ingrained, so do adaptive movement patterns, many of which further develop the chronicity cycle. With every painful trunk motion, the typical reaction is to restrict trunk motion even more. Sometimes bizarre motor patterns become ingrained because they are the only pain-free motor behavior that the individual knows how to use. These abnormal patterns generally cause stress (leading to possible degeneration) on crucial components of the musculoskeletal system. As more degenerative changes occur, symptoms intensify, and the cycle is perpetuated.

Pelvic Clock

The pelvic clock is a movement usually taught by asking patients to assume the supine position, with the knees bent and feet flat on the floor. Patients are instructed to picture in their minds the face of a clock lying just above their abdomen, with 12:00 pointing toward their nose, 6:00 pointing between their feet, with 3:00 and 9:00 to the right and left sides. The umbilicus is approximately in the center of the clock. Instructions are given verbally without any physical demonstration of the requested actions. The patient is asked to move the umbilicus toward 12:00 and then to the other 11 hours around the face of the clock. In other words, moving the pelvis toward 12:00 is to move the umbilicus toward the nose, moving the pelvis toward 6:00 is to move the umbilicus toward the feet, and so forth. Once patients master moving the umbilicus toward each hour of the clock, they are asked to do variations of the basic clock. These may include going clockwise or counterclockwise around the clock, changing the diameter of the clock, and moving diagonally about the clock (e.g., moving from 12:00 to 6:00, from 1:00 to 7:00, and from 2:00 to 8:00).

To heighten awareness, patients are often asked to compare the symmetry of the right and left sides of the clock, top and bottom halves, or other pairs of observations. For example, after telling patients to picture in their minds the muscles causing the motion toward 12:00, rhetorical questions such as the following might be asked to help them attain more complete awareness:

- Are the right and left side muscles working evenly or does one side initiate or cease work before the other, or does one side exhibit more force than the other?
- Are there any muscles resisting the action?
- Are muscles tensing elsewhere in the body that do not help this motion?
- What is your rib cage doing?
- Is it easier to do during inhalation or exhalation?

Patients new to the Feldenkrais technique are frequently reminded that it is the *how* of the movement that is of interest. In other words, the focus is not on the distance moved or force used to move except in the context of how those aspects affect ease of movement. The general rhetorical question to be answered is how to make a particular movement easier. Comparison is also evaluated by patients before and after the "exercise" in relation to posture. Before flexing the knees to begin the pelvic clock, patients are asked to observe how the body is resting on the mat. How much of the shoulder is contacting the mat? How much of the spine is contacting the mat? They are asked to picture in their minds the height and length of their lumbar lordosis. Do the right and left buttocks rest evenly on the mat? The technique is very flexible in that the practitioner is easily able to target critical areas and make the patient become especially aware of them.

After the "exercise" is done, patients return to their starting position to reevaluate the supine posture, noting any changes. Patients may then "test" these changes by assuming an upright posture and walking around slowly to compare the effects of gravity. Some patients appear pleased to find that upright activities now seem easier, with some reporting a sense of "walking on air."

As patients become more adept at the Feldenkrais technique, more variations of the same lesson are invented or lessons for other areas may be learned. A particular patient with whom I have worked "expanded" the pelvic clock idea. She moved the center of the clock up and down the length of the spine and then did the "clock exercise" at multiple levels of the spine. She also pictured the clock rotating about the axis of the spine, adding another dimension to the lesson. In this way, her proprioceptive/kinesthetic senses flooded the cortex with a massive amount of information regarding options for movement of the spine. She reported total amelioration of her chronic postural neck and back pain at the time of discharge from therapy.

If the reader were to perform the pelvic clock, it obviously requires activity from all of the abdominal and low back musculature in addition to adjacent musculature. Some patients who are seen in the clinic with chronic LBP have significant weakness and/or spasms in these muscles due to surgery or years of inactivity due, at least in part, to pain. They may be unable to perform a strengthening exercise such as a crunch, or they may even have trouble contracting individual abdominal muscles. The Feldenkrais pelvic clock is ideal in this situation because it allows the patient to feel those targeted muscles working.

Patients who have experienced chronic LBP for years will sometimes have long-term splinting of the musculature in this area to protect it from further painful movement. If patients are limited in their movements or their options, they are left with no choice but to reproduce the pattern of dysfunctional movements repeatedly (5). The Feldenkrais technique is very subtle to the point of merely encouraging patients to visualize motions instead of performing them immediately. This allows patients to prepare the "fearful" muscles for motion and gradually work them into the desired movement. Because the movements are performed slowly and with ease, patients understand that the attempted motions are always under control; this helps dissipate fear of new movements.

Conceptual Aspects of the Feledenkrais Technique

Most Feldenkrais work is done on the floor to reduce the effects of gravity and to induce a state of relaxation. As the dysfunctional splinting is broken down, patients discover comfortable options of movement that further break down fear and immobility that contributed to sustaining the painful syndrome. Very importantly, patients also regain responsibility for the management of their back pain (4).

By keeping movements short of tension and strain, patients' actual learning is improved significantly. Moving slowly allows the more slow-acting motor cortex to learn a new integration of movements. Conversely, moving fast evokes automatic, previously organized ways of moving so that old habits are reinforced. Ease of movement also improves learning and enhances change because it is enjoyable (2). Feldenkrais lessons not only improve perception of the function of the primary movers (such as abdominal, back, and gluteal muscles), they also enhance control of the "minor" musculature that is deeper or adjacent to the "target" area (the site of dysfunction). This has obvious relevance to the segmental stabilization discussed in Chap. 6. Thus, through the Feldenkrais technique patients can learn not only how function of the primary movers are intimately related but also how all of the different thigh, hip, and trunk musculature must work as a team.

Plotke (6) defined whole body linking as the ability to contract the upper extremities into the chest wall strongly, to stabilize the thorax through the pelvis, so that the strength and power of the lower extremities can be harnessed. If the pelvis is not stabilized sufficiently by the musculature, the transfer of power from the lower extremities does not occur. Use of the pelvic clock enables patients to be acutely aware of the pelvic musculature and how best to integrate it into their movement repertoire.

Through the Feldenkrais technique, the central nervous system is presented with many options on how to integrate a particular movement as well as many new and different movements. Because there are many ways to execute the same function, exploring alternative patterns of movement may highlight the differences in efficiency and inefficiency among patterns (7). This aspect of the Feldenkrais technique benefits patients with chronic LBP because so many of them severely limit their options of movement to control their pain and/or instability.

Many LBP patients "successfully" complete both rehabilitation and work hardening programs but continue to "distrust" their backs. Feldenkrais lessons can complete this training by leading patients through progressively more complex activities that help them learn to control these muscles and gain confidence in the intricacies of their back and discard the old inefficient movement patterns. Use of the Feldenkrais technique enhances recovery that is complete only when the patient regains balance, coordination, and confidence in performing complex movements.

Case Studies of Feldenkrais Use

Two cases are presented. One is an elderly patient and one is a teenager; however, each has relevance to understanding the Feldenkrais technique.

CASE STUDY ONE

I assisted an 84-year-old female with her rehabilitation after a series of transient ischemic attacks left her with incoordination and dyskinesia of one side of her body. She also complained of increasing chronic LBP. Her posture and mobility were typical for her age in that she had an increased kyphotic posture, "plopped" when attempting to sit, and required several repetitions of rocking to "jerk" herself up out of a chair. These two functions alone could have been the major causes of her LBP, with her sit/stand transfers adding trauma to the spine with each attempt.

The patient was initially instructed in a Feldenkrais sitting and rotation exercise that consisted of a progressive series of trunk rotation movements. Feldenkrais believed that trunk rotation is one of the first motions lost with aging (2). It is also frequently limited in individuals with chronic LBP. This lesson was expanded to teach the patient how to rise from sitting in a diagonal pattern. Basic directions such as shifting weight from one hip to the other, trunk forward bending, and trunk rotation were given; it was the patient's responsibility to learn how to synchronize the muscle recruitment pattern that was easiest.

The patient was told in what order to put the basic steps together to rise from sitting. She was also told to integrate this order into her own unique pattern as she moved from sitting to standing with the least amount of energy expenditure and pain. The patient made several attempts; successful attempts were obvious because the patient expressed her delight and surprise with regard to how easy it was to stand up when everything was "fitting together right." She also defeated her self-prophecy that "you cannot teach old dogs new tricks." Once she learned the ease of movement to stand up, she quickly learned the reverse order of movements to sit easily without her usual "plop." Over several days, not only did her chronic LBP improve but her kyphotic posture also began straightening.

CASE STUDY TWO

Back stabilization exercises were taught to a 14-year-old female diagnosed with severe spondylolisthesis in an attempt to avoid surgery to fuse the spine. The patient was having significant LBP and was being tutored at home because she was unable to tolerate sitting at school. Attempts to instruct the patient in stabilization exercises were initially unsuccessful due to the apparent total loss of proprioception in the lumbar spine. Functionally, the patient was locked into hyperextension, although she could be positioned passively to reverse the lumbar lordosis completely.

Recognizing the posture of the lumbar spine is a basic requirement of performing stabilization exercises. Some of these exercises may pull the spine into lordosis, whereas some may flatten the lordosis. It is critical for the exerciser to control the lumbar spine and maintain a neutral spine position while doing the stabilization exercises.

Because this 14-year-old was unable to control the spine enough to teach her stabilization exercises, Feldenkrais pelvic clock lessons were given. Initially they were very difficult for the patient due to her lack of proprioception and because she had been locked in hyperextension for so long. She required continual verbal feedback from her mother or the therapist to position her lumbar spine correctly. Several variations of the pelvic clock in combination with verbal feedback finally restored her proprioception to the point that she could perform some basic stabilization exercises. However, any new position (sitting, standing, bending, etc.) resulted in the patient reverting to her old habit of hyperextension. Feldenkrais lessons were necessary to change that posture and help her learn how to find the neutral spine position before reinforcing it with stabilization exercises in that position.

When last seen, this teen-age patient was pain free and could tolerate a full day of sitting at school; moreover, she could perform her stabilization exercises with minimal verbal feedback from her mother. I believe that the Feldenkrais technique was the key that unlocked this patient's hyperlordosis to allow the stabilization training, thus sparing the patient from planned spinal fusion surgery.

Research on the Feldenkrais Technique

Ruth and Kegerreis (8) examined healthy subjects to determine whether ATM lessons would result in improved neck flexion range of motion and whether the subjects would show a lower level of perceived effort in the posttest. Although their data analysis supported both hypotheses, they concluded that further investigation of Feldenkrais methods in the treatment of patients appeared warranted.

Lake (4), a physician in Australia trained in the Feldenkrais method, cited six case studies illustrating successful treatment of chronic LBP and acute LBP through the Feldenkrais method. All of the patients had previously failed to respond to a variety of traditional (including physical therapy) and alternative methods. They ranged in age from 26 to 60 years, with a variety of diagnoses including sciatica, scoliosis, degenerative disc disease, spondylolisthesis, and postoperative fusion. Symptoms had been present for a minimum of 3 months up to a maximum of 7 years. All responded favorably to the Feldenkrais method.

Advantages of the Feldenkrais Technique

The Feldenkrais method can be applied to different aspects of chronic LBP:

- Ease of use (i.e., no equipment needed)
- Patients control movement, from just imagining a movement to performing a full range and/or a complex movement
- Exploratory nature of the lessons results in learning and motivation
- It is a flexible technique that invites unique adaptations and development of individualized lessons
- It is a process, rather than a goal-oriented philosophy, potentially leading to lifetime improvement in movement
- It allows movement, the primary need of those with chronic LBP

ALEXANDER TECHNIQUE (9,10)

The Alexander technique was developed by an Australian actor, Frederick Matthias Alexander (1869–1955), who experienced progressive loss of voice while on stage. Unable to obtain relief with the assistance of physicians, voice teachers, and fellow actors, he was able to treat his "affliction" successfully after extensive self-examination and trial and error. This led to the development of his theory that "use affects functioning." He was pleased to discover

that his voice improved dramatically, as did his breathing, posture, and general quality of movement as he "finely tuned" his technique. These improvements were apparently so significant that people began asking him to help them with similar problems. Initially, the technique was developed and refined through its use with those involved in the theater, where it is still a widely used technique. Alexander worked with many famous people including George Bernard Shaw, Aldous Huxley, and John Dewey and was supported by the medical community in his approach. The principles have also purportedly improved skills in work, sport, and leisure activities in nontheatrical populations (11,12).

The Alexander Principle

In his book *Man's Supreme Inheritance* (9), Alexander stated:

conscious control is essential to man's satisfactory progress in civilization, and that the properly directed use of such control will enable the individual to stand, sit, walk, breathe, digest, and in fact live with the least possible expenditure of vital energy. This will ensure the highest standard of resistance to disease. When this desirable stage of our evolution is reached the cry of physical deterioration may no longer be heard. (p. 107)

Barlow, a teacher of the Alexander technique, defined the Alexander principle as follows (13): "There are certain ways of using your body that are better than certain other ways; that when you reject these better ways of using your body, your functioning will begin to suffer in some important respects; that it is useful to assess other people by the way they use themselves" (p. 4). In an abbreviated form, use affects function. "Use" is the manner in which we use our bodies during daily activities. It is both dynamic and static. According to Barlow, we develop so many harmful habits by age 18 that only 5% of the population is free from muscular and postural deficiencies (13).

Alexander presented the notion of "primary control" as "the certain use of the head in relation to the neck and of the neck in relation to the torso . . . constituted a 'primary control' of the mechanisms as a whole" (13, p. 16). Alexander believed that the neck is where most mechanical dysfunction begins; therefore, correction must begin with the neck to correct any other dysfunctional movement pattern. He noticed, for example, when attempting to move from sitting to standing, that there is a tendency to throw back the head while the neck is stiffened and shortened. This was a difficult pattern to change even when his students were made aware of their misuse pattern. In this area, not only does use affect function, but use may even alter physiques. For example, Alexander believed that dowager's humps were caused by this misuse; moreover, he could correct the problems of some individuals by correcting their neck posture (13). Alexander believed that the postural deformity of excessive lordosis was a consequence of the dowager hump and that only after the hump was corrected could the low back lordosis be corrected (13).

A balanced posture is critical for ideal functioning, an idea that is not exclusive to Alexander's teaching. He presented very specific points necessary for a balanced posture including cervical and lumbar vertebrae being directed up and back (instead of forward and down) to release excess muscle tension. This orientation alone would increase overall height by 1 to 2 inches. Usually he attempted to make joint surfaces open rather than contracted with his postural corrections (13); perhaps as a result of this, individuals receiving this therapy often feel taller subsequent to its application.

In addition to postural dysfunctions, Alexander believed that back pain is always accompanied and preceded by misuse. He consistently found the following three minuses: (a) a thoracic scoliosis with rotation of the lumbar spine, (b) an elevated scapula, showing that the muscular supporting work of the back is being done by the shoulders instead of the mid-back, and (c) a breathing pattern with a slight lordosis of the lumbar spine while inhaling with the front of the chest and abdomen (13).

Use of the Alexander Technique

The technique is taught in 15 or more sessions, one-on-one, for 30 to 60 mins per session. During these sessions, "students" are first shown how they misuse their bodies. Through manual adjustments, they are taught new muscle use to replace their previous, damaging movement patterns and postures. Misused muscles are gently coaxed into more efficient movement patterns by manual adjustments while maintaining proper relations between the head, neck, and torso (10). Simultaneously, the student is to project on himself a sequence of thoughts that coordinate with the instructor's manual corrections (13). These adjustments are not a form of manipulation but a method by which the student is taught to prevent previous poor habits of movement and posture and to replace them with new, more efficient patterns of use. It is not a form of hypnosis because it requires conscious attention to learn the new patterns; the new patterns must then be put into practice in functional activities such as moving from a seated to a standing position. It is not a form of relaxation therapy because the student must frequently activate previously underused muscles in new patterns of movement (13). The objective of the lessons is to encourage self-discovery, leading to improved body awareness and control; the lessons are not conditioning exercises (10).

Lessons are frequently taught in the supine position to eliminate the pull of gravity on the postural musculature; this allows the participant to focus more clearly on the interplay of muscle groups during movement and posture. The teacher may ask the student to say to himself, "neck free, head forward and out," "back lengthen and widen," "knee out of the hip," "hip free," "shoulders release and widen," in an attempt to reset the neutral resting position upon which all motion occurs (13, p. 177).

The student is cautioned to think, not perform, the orders. Alexander believed that, if the individual attempts to perform these orders, he automatically triggers a preparatory "set" in the musculature mentioned above, thus defeating the purpose of changing poor movement habits. This approach leads to heightened proprioception, with many students reporting a feeling of lightness in their bodies (13), improved flexibility, and ease of movement. Quality of movement improves such that activity becomes more flowing, without strain or jerking. Specifically, they report a freedom in the action of the eyes, less tension in the jaws and throat, and deeper breathing (10).

Alexander focused on particular areas during corrections. One was the neck, which he thought was the keystone to improvement, as noted earlier. Breathing was another critical area. He believed that many difficulties come from tendencies to keep the upper chest and abdominal musculature too tense during breathing. Ideally, breathing is a back activity; in fact, with exhalation there should be a release seen in the upper chest area (13). Alexander (10) attempted to make the student aware of breathing as it supports a particular movement and how that movement reinforces breathing. He was critical of the "military posture" because of its negative effects on breathing. Moreover, Alexander (9) contended that (a) a protruded upper chest could lead to emphysema, (b) increased lumbar lordosis could lead to back pain, and (c) a stiff neck and rigid thorax could cause heart problems, varicose veins, asthma, bronchitis, and hay fever. Furthermore, he believed that faulty breathing patterns result in displacement of the diaphragm caudally, shifting the center of gravity with a compensatory increased lordosis in the lumbar region. Austin and Ausubel (14) found a strong correlation between Alexander training and improvements in respiratory muscular strength; they contended that this improvement resulted from (a) increased strength and endurance of abdominal wall musculature, (b) decreased resting tensions of chest wall muscles, and (c) enhanced coordination of the respiratory muscles.

Research on the Alexander Technique and LBP

The literature often cites incorrect posture as having a causal relationship with LBP; moreover, very precise positioning of certain areas of the body relative to adjacent areas is sometimes stressed. Alexander believed that standing with the feet at 45 degrees to each other was critical to have the perfect base of support; however, other than that, he did not believe that there was one correct posture for everyone. Instead, he attempted to help his students achieve their most mechanically correct position, which differed from individual to individual. Alexander thought that most of the body weight should be resting on the rear of the feet and that the hips should be as posterior as possible without adversely affecting balance. Proper standing posture should allow the student to lengthen and broaden the spine; Alexander (9) felt that this could only be achieved by relaxing and lengthening the back musculature and by allowing the torso to move in any direction with the least amount of inherent strain.

Using the Alexander Technique with LBP Patients

In applying the Alexander technique to LBP, two concepts should be kept in mind. First, most people do not have the appropriate proprioception or local control of the torso to follow safe lifting instructions. Second, the way people repeatedly use and misuse their bodies determines the strain and risk of injury to their backs. Many are unaware of the back until injury or pain acutely forces their attention there. Back patients often report that they did not even know their back was there until they injured it. The Alexander technique does not focus on "fixing" the painful area but rather on how the body functions as a whole, targeting poor movement patterns wherever they may occur. Finding dysfunctional movement patterns in the neck and upper torso region that cause compensation in the lumbar region would be usual, for example (in other dysfunctional movement), leading to an injury in the lumbar region. Until the more superior dysfunction is corrected, according to Alexander's theory, the lumbar dysfunction can never be fully corrected. This would also be true if a more inferior rigidity were present.

To lift correctly an Alexander instructor would make sure that a patient's

- neck can move freely
- lower extremities can move without straining the back
- lower back can move freely
- rib cage is relaxed for unstrained breathing
- entire musculature is released so that the effort exerted in any particular movement is spread throughout the body rather than being concentrated in a particular joint
- spine maintains its natural curvature
- lengthened state is maintained to allow maximum movement
- areas, such as the shoulders, have freedom of movement that does not interfere with balance

It should be understood that the proper use of the back requires more than merely being told or shown how to use it. The individual must experience and incorporate these items into daily activities to take care of their backs (11).

SUMMARY OF THE FELDENKRAIS AND ALEXANDER TECHNIQUES

Both Feldenkrais and Alexander techniques could dovetail with other approaches for some patients, in particular those lacking in muscular control or a good sense of body awareness. The Feldenkrais technique may have more implications for working with the LBP patient than the Alexander technique because it has many implications for teaching body awareness and the muscle control that can be of value in helping the back patient learn trunk stabilization. However, the Alexander technique may be a particularly good adjunct in teaching good posture to some patients. These two techniques provide additional tools to the arsenals of those who work with chronic LPB patients.

REFERENCES

1. Miller, B. Alternative somatic therapies, in *Conservative Care of Low Back Pain*, A.H. White and R. Anderson, editors. 1991, Baltimore: Williams & Wilkins. p. 106–133.
2. Feldenkrais, M. *Awareness Through Movement.* 1977, New York: Harper & Row.
3. Moffett, J.A.K., Chase, S.M., Portek, I., et al. Controlled prospective study to evaluate the effectiveness of back school in relief of chronic low back pain. *Spine* 1986, 11: p. 120–122.
4. Lake, B. Treatment by the application of Feldenkrais principles. *Aust Fam Phys* 1985, 11: p. 1175–1178.
5. Wildman, F. Learning—the missing ink in physical therapy (A radical view of the Feldenkrais method). *Phys Ther Forum* 1988, 7: p. 1–6.
6. Plotke, R.J. The power of the center. Phys Ther Forum 1994, 9: p. 1–5.
7. Orr, R. The Feldenkrais method. On the importance and potency of small and slow movements. *Phys Ther Forum* 1990, 9(1–5).
8. Ruth, S. and S. Kegerreis. Facilitating cervical flexion using a Feldenkrais method ATM. *J Orthop Sports Phys Ther* 1992, 16: p. 25–29.
9. Alexander, F. *Man's Supreme Inheritance.* 1957, London: Re-Education Publications Limited.
10. Alexander, F. *The Resurrection of the Body.* 1969, New York: Dell Publishing Co., Inc.
11. Hall, D. Bad backs—uncovering the real problem. *Lamp* 1992, December–January: p. 24–28.
12. Maitland, J. and H. Goodliffe. The Alexander technique. *Nurs Times* 1989, 85: p. 55–57.
13. Barlow, W. *The Alexander Tecnnique.* 1973, New York: Alfred A. Knopf.
14. Austin, J.H., and P. Ausubel. Enhanced respiratory muscular function in normal adults after lessons in proprioceptive musculoskeletal education without exercises. *Chest* 1992, 102: p. 486–490.

CHAPTER 8

EXERCISE PROTOCOLS FOR LOW BACK PAIN

Julie M. Fritz

Gregory E. Hicks

INTRODUCTION

Low back pain is an extremely common disorder in our society, with lifetime prevalence rates placed as high as 80% (1). In addition, up to 20% of all sports-related injuries are reported to involve the spine (2). The rehabilitation of individuals with low back pain remains largely enigmatic to the medical community. Numerous approaches to rehabilitation have been advocated, yet, for any given individual with low back pain, the selection of a treatment method from among the many competing approaches has been said to take on the characteristics of a lottery (3), often leaving the rehabilitation specialist uncertain of the best course of action to undertake with any particular patient.

At present, there is little evidence for the effectiveness of any single method of rehabilitation. However, one fact has been established with relative certainty; bed rest and inactivity are detrimental to the recovery of individuals with low back pain (4). Bed rest has been shown to be ineffective for patients with acute or chronic low back pain, with or without leg pain (5–6). Active exercise therapy has been demonstrated to be more effective than passive forms of treatment such as modalities (e.g., ice or heat) and massage for patients with chronic low back pain (7). Given this information, the clinician should always seek to implement the most active program possible for any patient with low back pain. Reliance on passive treatments and prolonged activity restrictions should be avoided.

It may be well established that active treatment is superior to passive treatment in the rehabilitation of patients with low back pain; however the choice of a specific exercise program for an individual patient requires a more in-depth clinical understanding. The clinician must avoid the temptation to introduce patients to preexisting exercise protocols without considering the individual's unique presentation and rehabilitation goals.

The type of exercise program implemented is largely dependent on the patient's *stage*. Staging refers to the acuteness of the patient's condition and is an important consideration for setting the goals of therapy and selecting appropriate exercises for the individual. Acuteness is not based strictly on the duration of the patient's symptoms; it is also based on the severity of the patient's presentation (8). Patients who present with difficulties performing basic daily activities such as sitting, standing, or walking are considered to be in stage I (i.e., acute). Patients in stage I tend to have increased levels of pain and disability, and the goals of therapy center on reducing their symptoms and permitting those patients to move on to subsequent stages of treatment. Patients who can perform most basic daily activities but are unable to perform demanding activities such as lifting, vacuuming, and sporting activities are considered to be in stage II (i.e., subacute). Patients in stage II will generally have less severe symptoms but will tend to have had symptoms for a longer duration of time, possibly limiting their ability to work or engage in recreational activities. The goals of therapy for patients in stage II are focused on improving tolerance for work or recreational activities.

STAGE I EXERCISE PROGRAMS: CENTRALIZATION

The goals of therapy for patients in stage I are to reduce the severity of the symptoms to allow the patient to increase his or her activity level and progress to stage II. A subgroup of patients in stage I will benefit from specific exercise programs. Other therapies that may be effective for patients in stage I include mobilization or manipulation of the lumbosacral spine, spinal traction, or the temporary use of a spinal brace. The important clinical characteristic of patients in stage I likely to benefit from specific exercise routines is the presence of the centralization phenomenon. The centralization phenomenon occurs when, during active motion of the lumbar spine, the patient's symptoms are abolished or move from the periphery toward the lumbar spine. The presence of the centralization phenomenon has been found to be an important prognostic indicator and guide for prescribing exercise therapy.

Not all patients in stage I will be found to centralize with active spinal motions. Recent studies have reported that approximately 40% of patients will demonstrate the centralization phenomenon on examination (9,10). Patients in stage I who do not centralize during examination should be treated with other techniques such as lumbar traction if leg pain is present but will not centralize with any movements. Patients with suspected facet joint dysfunction will typically not demonstrate centralization and often will respond more favorably to mobilization or manipulation in stage I. Patients with spondylolisthesis or suspected segmental instability should proceed to stabilization exercises that will be described later in this chapter. If the centralization phenomenon is observed during the evaluation of the patient, the movement found to produce the centralization is used as the basis for developing a specific exercise program. The evaluation methods used to detect the centralization phenomenon will next be described, followed by the exercise routines used for the two most common movements found to produce centralization: lumbar extension and lumbar flexion.

Detecting the Centralization Phenomenon

The centralization phenomenon will be detected during the evaluation of active range of motion of the spine (Table 8-1). Active motion is first assessed with the patient standing. Before asking the patient to move, it is important to establish the baseline symptoms to judge whether centralization has occurred. The patient is then asked to side bend to the left and right, to extend backward, and flex forward. After each movement, the patient is asked

about the effect of the movement on symptoms. If symptoms are abolished or moved centrally, then centralization has occurred. If symptoms fluctuate in intensity but do not centralize, the patient is judged to be status quo. If symptoms move toward the periphery, the patient is judged to have peripheralized. Any movement producing the centralization is noted; this movement will be used as the basis for the patient's specific exercise program. Any movement causing peripheralization is also noted; this movement will be avoided in further evaluation and treatment procedures.

Movements that are judged to be status quo are tested further. This is accomplished by changing the patient's position, repeating the movement test, or sustaining the end-range test position. Spinal flexion and extension may be assessed in the seated, supine, prone, or quadruped position and while standing. The quadruped position is particularly useful for evaluation because both flexion and extension can be assessed by having the patient rock back and forth, and the position decreases the weight-bearing stresses on the spine (Fig. 8-1). The movement tests in any position can be repeated

Table 8-1 Definitions Used in the Judgment of Active Movement Testing

Centralization	Paresthesia or pain is abolished or moves from the periphery toward the lumbar spine
Peripheralization	Paresthesia or pain is produced or moves distally from the lumbar spine toward the periphery
Status quo	Pain may increase or decrease in intensity but does not move centrally or peripherally

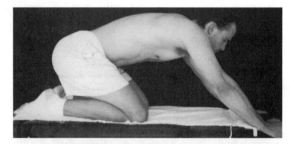

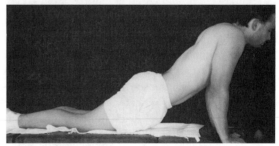

Fig. 8-1 Active movements of lumbar flexion and extension performed in the quadruped position. These movements can be used for both assessment and treatment.

5 to 10 times consecutively or can be sustained for 20 to 30 s. The patient is questioned after each test on the impact of the movement on symptoms; then the same judgments are made (i.e., did pain centralize, peripheralize, or remain status quo).

The most common movements found to centralize symptoms are extension and flexion. Extension often produces centralization in patients with signs and symptoms consistent with a lumbar disc herniation. McKenzie proposed that spinal extension "pushes" the nucleus pulposus anterior and away from the spinal nerve roots and other pain-producing structures (11). Although the magnitude and clinical relevance of nuclear movement with extension is controversial (12,13), patients who centralize with extension often respond favorably to extension exercises.

Patients who centralize with flexion tend to be somewhat older, with degenerative or stenotic spinal conditions. Spinal stenosis causes a narrowing of the spinal canals. This narrowing is exacerbated with spinal extension and relieved with spinal flexion (14). Therefore, patients with spinal stenosis will often be found to centralize with flexion movements and peripheralize with extension movements. Treatment programs based on flexion exercises are often useful for these patients.

Extension Exercise Programs

The primary goal of the initial phase of treatment is to centralize the patient's symptoms permanently and allow progression to stage II. This may be accomplished by using the extension movements found to produce centralization during the evaluation. A position that is usually comfortable for the patient and useful for beginning an extension exercise program is the quadruped one. Extension is produced by having the patient rock forward over the arms and then return to the starting position. This gentle rocking motion is repeated 10 to 20 times. The patient should not rock back into flexion at this stage of treatment. Another beginning exercise that may be useful is having the patient lie prone. Lying prone promotes extension of the lumbar spine. The prone position is sustained from 30 s up to a

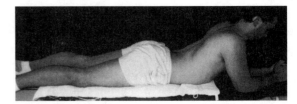

Fig. 8-2 Prone-on-elbows exercise.

few minutes. With all exercises, the response of the patient's symptoms is the key to determining their effectiveness. Exercises that help to centralize the patient's pain are continued; those that do not may be stopped.

More advanced extension exercises may include having the patient prop up on the elbows while lying prone (Fig. 8-2). This position is held for 15 to 30 s and is repeated several times. It is important that the patient be able to relax the extensor musculature in this position and keep the pelvis in contact with the support surface. Propping on elbows can be progressed to prone press-ups (Fig. 8-3); in this position the patient extends the elbows to lift the upper body while the pelvis remains in contact with the support surface. This exercise is repeated 10 to 20 times depending on the patient's upper body strength. It is important to realize that prone press-ups are a more aggressive form of extension exercise that have been shown to require substantial amounts of spinal extensor muscle activity (15). This muscle activity may not be tolerated by all patients, particularly early in the course of treatment. The response of

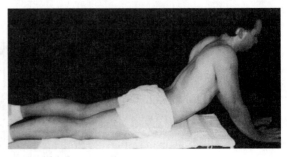

Fig. 8-3 Prone press-up exercise.

the patient's symptoms will dictate whether or not an exercise will be continued.

Motions that produce a peripheralization of symptoms should be avoided during the initial stage of treatment. The motion most often of concern is lumbar flexion. Lumbar flexion exercises, which are described in the next section, should be avoided.

Flexion Exercise Programs

Patients who are somewhat older with degenerative spinal conditions will frequently centralize their symptoms with flexion motions and thus are likely to benefit from flexion exercises in stage I treatment. In these patients the movement of lumbar extension will often cause a peripheralization of symptoms and therefore needs to be avoided early in the rehabilitation process.

Flexion exercises are easiest to perform in the supine or quadruped positions. Patients who require a flexion exercise program will frequently find the supine position with the hips and knees flexed (i.e., the "hook-lying position") to be a very comfortable one from which to exercise. From this position, the patient may bring a single knee or both knees to the chest, creating further flexion of the lumbar spine (Fig. 8-4). This position can be sustained for 20 to 30 s and repeated. Another simple flexion exercise to perform from this position is a posterior pelvic tilt. The patient is instructed to flatten the back against the support surface, thereby reducing the lumbar lordosis and increasing lumbar flexion. The posterior pelvic tilt is rightly conceived to be a

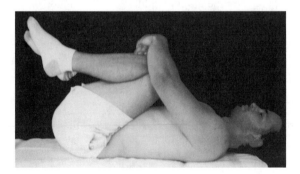

Fig. 8-4 Supine knees-to-chest flexion exercise.

lumbar flexion exercise and not an abdominal strengthening exercise; this will be discussed further in the next section. From the quadruped position the patient can move from the neutral position back onto the heels to promote lumbar flexion. This motion can be repeated as a gentle rocking movement from neutral to flexion.

Once the patient's lower extremity symptoms have been centralized to the lumbar region with either flexion or extension exercises, the rehabilitation program can be progressed to stage II. It is generally not necessary to have a patient continue to perform an extensive flexion or extension exercise program. Instead, the goal of treatment is shifted from the centralization of symptoms to allowing the patient to increase the activity level and decrease the level of disability. Important considerations in stage II of the rehabilitation process are stabilization exercises for the lumbar spine and general aerobic conditioning activities. These exercises are described in the next section.

STAGE II EXERCISE PROGRAMS: LUMBAR STABILIZATION

The lumbar spine consists of both static and dynamic components that are responsible for stability of the spine during daily activities of living. Vertebral bodies, intervertebral discs, ligaments, facet joints, and joint capsules constitute the static component of the spine. Muscles and tendons of the trunk comprise the dynamic component. According to in vitro studies, the lumbar spine, without assistance from the dynamic component, buckles under compressive loads of less than approximately 90 N, whereas the in vivo spine can withstand loads of up to 18,000 N (16). The ability of the in vivo spine to tolerate such high loads is mainly attributable to the dynamic stabilizing capacity of the trunk musculature supporting the spine in all planes of motion.

The trunk muscles support the spine in a fashion similar to guy wires supporting a ship's mast (17). If any of the trunk muscles do not perform at optimal levels, the stabilizing capacity of the spine will be compromised. Each muscle associated with the lumbar complex has a specific role in the dynamic stabilizing process needed for performance of daily activities. These muscles must work together in a coordinated fashion for optimal spinal stability. The purpose of this section is to identify the importance of specific muscles needed for stability and to identify the best methods for training these specific muscles (Table 8-2).

Transversus Abdominis

As discussed in Chap. 1, the transversus abdominis stabilizes the spine by forming a corset or rigid cylinder around the static component of the spine. Recent evidence has demonstrated that a feed-forward postural response occurs with regard to transversus abdominis contraction and limb movement (18,19). Before upper extremity motion, the transversus should contract to stabilize the spine in preparation for movement. However, in patients with low back pain, there is a delay in onset of transversus abdominis contraction. This finding suggests that people with low back pain lack the optimal

stability of the spine needed for activities requiring arm movement such as lifting or pulling.

With regard to spinal stabilization exercises, the best program will incorporate exercises that produce high levels of muscle activity and low levels of stress to the static spinal component. One of the most effective methods for training the transversus abdominis, along with the internal obliques, is the abdominal hollowing maneuver (20). This maneuver is performed by instructing the patient to draw the navel up toward the head and in toward the spine so that the stomach is flattened (Fig. 8-5). Mastery of this hollowing maneuver is important because it serves as a foundation for further exercise progression.

Many patients with back pain have a difficult time performing this seemingly simple maneuver. The key to this exercise is to isolate the deep abdominals and avoid substitution by the rectus abdominis. The following instruction method will purposely incorporate rectus activity into the early stages to ensure activation of the transversus abdominis and make the patient aware of how rectus abdominis muscle activity would present. From a supine starting position,

Table 8-2 Components of the Lumbar Stabilization Exercise Program

MUSCLE GROUP	EXERCISE PROGRESSION
Transversus abdominis	Abdominal hollowing ↓ Hollowing in hook-lying with leg movements ↓ Hollowing in hook-lying with bridging
Erector spinae and multifidus	Quadruped single arm or leg lifts ↓ Quadruped opposite arm and leg lifts ↓ Prone trunk lifts
Quadratus lumborum	Horizontal side support (knees flexed) ↓ Horizontal side support (knees extended)
Oblique abdominals	Horizontal side support (knees flexed and then extended) ↓ Curl-ups with trunk rotation ↓ Hanging leg lifts

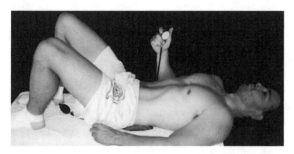

Fig. 8-5 Performance of abdominal hollowing exercise. The patient is using a pressure sensor under the lumbar spine to avoid a posterior pelvic tilt.

the patient is instructed to perform maximal cervical flexion while palpating the lower portion of the rectus abdominis muscle. While flexing the neck, the patient should feel the rectus abdominis protrude into his or her fingers. Once this occurs, the patient is instructed to draw in the abdomen away from the fingers as tightly as possible; this will produce transversus abdominis contraction. Then, while holding the abdominal contraction, the patient should lower his or her head to the start position. Once the patient is able to perform abdominal hollowing in this manner, eliminate the cervical flexion component and just focus on the drawing in of the abdomen for progressively longer periods. Self-palpation for muscle contraction by the patient just medial to the anterior superior iliac spines will often provide helpful feedback with regard to proper performance.

There are several substitution patterns that the patient must avoid while performing the hollowing maneuver (20). One of the most common strategies is to use the rectus abdominis to perform a pelvic tilt; that would appear to flatten the stomach in the same way as the hollowing procedure, but it would also cause flexion of the lumbar spine. For this reason, the patient must be taught by the use of verbal or tactile cues to maintain a neutral spine throughout the contraction. Another common substitution pattern is for the patient to hold his or her breath; this would also give the appearance of a flattened stomach. The remedy for this problem is to keep the patient talking throughout

performance of this exercise. It is also helpful to instruct the patient to count aloud as he or she holds the contraction to facilitate normal breathing.

For some patients, it is easier to learn the hollowing procedure in the quadruped position because it is more difficult to substitute the rectus abdominis in this position. As with the supine position, it is important to watch for signs of substitution such as posterior tilting of the pelvis. Another advantage of the quadruped position is that the therapist can offer tactile cues through the posterior spine to facilitate the direction of the hollowing.

Once the patient has mastered the abdominal hollowing maneuver without substitution, more challenging activities can be added to this core exercise. For example, from the supine hook-lying position, leg movements (i.e. marching or leg raises) can be incorporated while maintaining the abdominal hollowing (Fig. 8-6). Performing bridging exercises while maintaining the hollowing is also a challenge to both the transversus abdominis and the gluteus maximus muscles (Fig. 8-7). It is important to note that the addition of other challenges to the abdominal hollowing maneuver is useful only if the hollowing is consistently maintained. Without proper hollowing technique, these other components will not be useful. As the hollowing becomes more natural, it should be combined with other aspects of the stabilization program, described in the next sections. Eventually, the abdominal hollowing should be incorporated into more functional positions and postures that would challenge each individual patient in everyday activities. For example, if the patient complains of pain

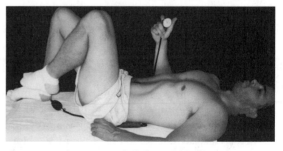

Fig. 8-6 Performance of abdominal hollowing exercise with repetitive leg movements.

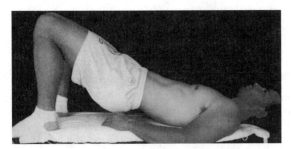

Fig. 8-7 Performance of abdominal hollowing exercise with a bridging movement. It is important to avoid hyperextension of the lumbar spine during this exercise.

while sitting, the hollowing procedure should be advocated for use in that position. The options for use of the abdominal hollowing should not be limited to the clinic. The ultimate goal of this exercise is use with all activities of daily living.

Multifidus and Erector Spinae Muscles

The extensor musculature of the lumbar spine plays an important role in stabilizing the spine and in providing the force required for bending and lifting activities. As discussed and depicted in Chap. 1, the lumbar extensor musculature can be divided into two groups. Most of the fibers of the erector spinae span the lumbar region and attach only to the thoracic spine and the pelvis; the segmental extensor portion attaches to individual lumbar vertebrae. The erector spinae fibers that span the pelvis are active in producing the extensor force needed for lifting; the segmental extensor portion and the multifidus are more concerned with the stabilization of individual lumbar segments. (The erector spinae and the multifidus can be viewed in Fig. 1-17.)

The multifidi are small intrinsic muscles that are the primary segmental stabilizers of the spine in the lumbar region (21). Current evidence demonstrates that poor endurance of multifidus and the segmental fibers of the erector spinae is a predictor of increased recurrence of low back pain (22). Moreover, the multifidi do not automatically recover full strength and endurance after the first episode of

low back pain unless specific rehabilitation is done (23). These findings emphasize the need for clinicians to focus attention on rehabilitation of the extensor musculature, with a particular focus on regaining endurance of the segmental musculature.

As noted in Chap. 1 and earlier in this chapter, the most effective exercises will produce high levels of muscle activity and low levels of spinal loading. Both the erector spinae and multifidus muscles will be trained most effectively with extension exercises; however, these types of exercise also tend to produce high levels of compression on the lumbar spine that may not be tolerated by all patients. The safest position from which to exercise these muscles is the quadruped position because it decreases the effects of gravity on the spine. For example, after assuming the quadruped position, the patient is asked to extend one leg or one arm while maintaining abdominal hollowing (Fig. 8-8). Raising the opposite arm and leg (Fig. 8-9) simultaneously offers the most efficient training of multifidus and erector spinae, with muscle activity levels in the realm of 30% of their maximal voluntary contraction (MVC), which is more than sufficient for

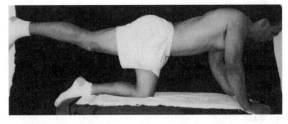

Fig. 8-8 Single leg extension exercise performed in the quadruped position.

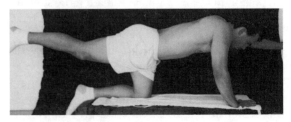

Fig. 8-9 Opposite arm and leg extension exercise performed in the quadruped position.

retraining these muscle groups (24). This exercise also produces safe levels of lumbar compressive loads. If the clinician feels that he or she needs to be more conservative with regard to spinal loading, the quadruped single leg or arm elevation is used. These exercises produce even lower lumbar compression forces and elicit multifidus activity in the range of 20% MVC. The patient should maintain abdominal hollowing while performing quadruped extension exercises to maintain the spine in a neutral position and avoiding flexion or extension.

If a greater challenge for the lumbar extensors and multifidus is desired, extension exercises in the prone position can be employed. From a prone lying position, the patient is asked to raise the trunk and legs off the support surface so that only the pelvis remains in contact. As an alternative, the patient may lie prone with the upper trunk off the edge of the support surface and the legs fixed on the surface. The patient flexes the trunk forward and then extends against gravity to return to the starting position. These exercises produce high levels of activity in the erector spinae and multifidus (40 to 60% MVC); however, the compressive loads on the lumbar spine increase substantially over the quadruped position exercises. In addition, the anterior shear forces on the lumbar spine are increased with these activities (25); therefore, these exercises should be avoided by patients with lumbar segmental instability. However, these prone extension exercises should be appropriate for athletes who are hopeful of returning to competition or for others who have demanding work activities; their spines should more easily tolerate the additional compressive and shear forces produced by these exercises.

Quadratus Lumborum

The quadratus lumborum appears to play a large role in stabilization of the spine in the frontal plane. When compression is applied to the spine in an upright position, quadratus lumborum activity most closely correlates with the increased need for stability caused by the compression (26). The horizontal side support exercise produces the highest

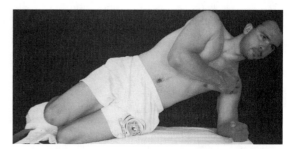

Fig. 8-10 Beginning position for the horizontal side support exercise, with the knees flexed.

muscle activity in the quadratus lumborum (54% MVC) with low compressive loads. This exercise also effectively challenges the lateral oblique abdominal muscles.

To perform the horizontal side support, the patient lies on his or her side with knees bent and upper body supported on the lower elbow (Fig. 8-10). From this position the patient is instructed to lift the body from the table with all weight borne on the knee, lower leg, and elbow. The side support is performed on both sides of the body. If a patient has unilateral low back symptoms, it may be more difficult for the patient to perform the exercise on the side of the dysfunction. This exercise can be done for a sustained isometric hold or in a more dynamic fashion with lowering and raising repetitions of the body. The patient should perform this exercise for progressively longer sustained periods of time and more repetitions. It should also be a goal to achieve symmetry between the left and right sides.

As this starting position for the horizontal side support exercise becomes less challenging, the base of support can be changed from the knees to the feet (with knees extended) during the elevation (Fig. 8-11). This makes it more difficult for the patient to raise the body against gravity, thereby providing a greater challenge to the quadratus lumborum and the oblique abdominal muscles. Another progression for the horizontal side support is the addition of the abdominal hollowing maneuver, which will more effectively train the muscles to work together.

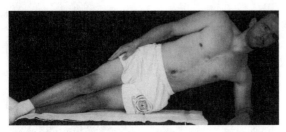

Fig. 8-11 Advanced position for the horizontal side support exercise, with the knees extended.

Oblique Abdominal Muscles

The transversus abdominis has been shown to have a unique role in stabilization of the lumbar spine, but the internal and external oblique muscles also deserve consideration during the rehabilitation of patients with low back pain. The oblique abdominal muscles form the abdominal wall, extending around the torso from anterior to posterior; as discussed in Chap. 1, the internal oblique also has an attachment on the lateral raphe (thoracolumbar fascia). The oblique abdominal muscles assist in producing rotation of the spine but also serve as important stabilizers by cocontracting with the spinal extensors during side-bending or extension movements (27). The rectus abdominis is primarily a trunk flexor and is of less importance than the lateral abdominal muscles in rehabilitating patients with low back pain.

As described in the previous section, the horizontal side support exercise has been shown to produce high levels of activity in the oblique abdominal muscle (50% MVC) with low levels of compression forces. Therefore, this exercise may be used as an effective training tool for both the quadratus lumborum and oblique abdominal muscles. Performing curl-ups with a rotation of the torso has also been found to target the oblique abdominals while imposing low compressive loads. Performing curl-ups without any trunk rotation will target mostly the rectus abdominis muscle and therefore are not useful to the rehabilitation process. A more challenging exercise for the oblique abdominals is a hanging straight leg raise. To perform this exercise the patient hangs from a bar and lifts both legs to the horizontal position (i.e., 90 degrees of hip flexion). This exercise provides very

high levels of oblique abdominal activity (nearly 100% MVC) and maintains relatively low levels of spinal compression (28).

STAGE III EXERCISE PROGRAMS: DYNAMIC STABILIZATION

Patients with low back pain have been shown to have deficits in dynamic control of the trunk. For example, individuals with low back pain have increased postural sway, increased reaction times, and decreased spinal positioning accuracy when compared with individuals without back pain (29). Progressing patients to dynamic stabilization activities after establishing a core of strength and endurance in the important muscle groups can help a patient return to full levels of activity.

Dynamic stabilization training may be performed with an unstable support surface such as a therapy ball. Exercises performed while sitting on the therapy ball may begin with simple weight shifting from

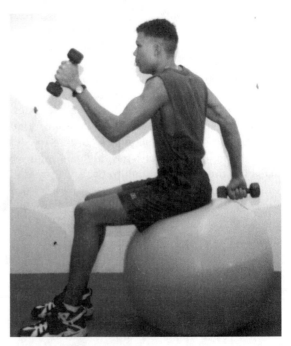

Fig. 8-12 Performance of upper extremity exercises while maintaining spine stability using a therapy ball.

side to side to encourage balance reactions from the trunk to maintain an upright position. Once the patient is able to demonstrate the ability to balance on the ball during weight-shifting activities, extremity exercises can be used, beginning with unilateral movements such as shoulder flexion, extension or abduction, hip flexion, or knee extension. This may be progressed to contralateral upper and lower extremity movements, with or without weights for resistance (Fig. 8-12). More complex and challenging movements can be performed including proprioceptive neuromuscular facilitation patterns for the upper extremity or sport-specific activities such as catching and throwing while maintaining balance and control of spinal posture. Throughout the performance of these exercises, the patient should be encouraged to maintain abdominal hollowing to promote spinal stability during the exercise.

More advanced exercises can also be performed with the therapy ball, such as bridging exercises with the legs supported on the ball. Exercises from the prone position can also be performed; one such exercise is isometric single extremity motions (Fig. 8-13). Resistance to this activity could be added with leg weights. Spinal extension exercises from a prone position could also be performed over the therapy ball by having the patient flex over the ball and then raise the upper body into a neutral position; as discussed earlier, these activities will produce high compressive and shear forces on the lumbar spine. Nevertheless, a therapy ball can be used for numerous exercises, limited only by the creativity of the clinician, provided that the patient is able to demonstrate control of the spine during all of these activities.

Dynamic exercises can also be performed in the standing position. These activities should focus on tasks that the individual patient will need to return to full activity. Dynamic activities such as catching and throwing can be added for patients involved in sporting activities. The surface may be made less stable by having the patient stand on a foam roll, trampoline, or wobble board (Fig. 8-14). Progression is then made to running and cutting activities and a gradual addition of sports-related drills. Individuals returning to activities involving lifting activities can begin with light lifting exercises performed in a limited range and progress with increased weights and increased ranges of movements. Throughout these progressions, the patient is encouraged to maintain abdominal hollowing to stabilize the spine. The clinician should closely monitor the performance of

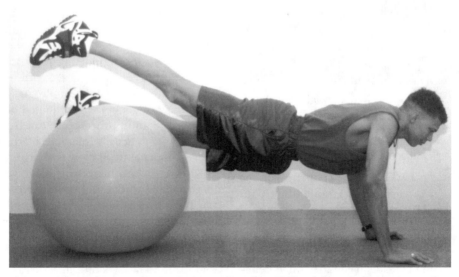

Fig. 8-13 Single leg extension exercise performed with the therapy ball. It is important to avoid hyperextension of the lumbar spine during this exercise.

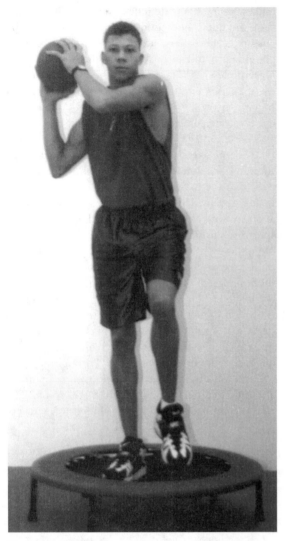

Fig. 8-14 Catching and throwing a weighted ball while balancing on a trampoline provides a challenging exercise for spinal stability.

activities for the patient's ability to control his or her spinal posture and avoid extreme positions or positions that reproduce symptoms.

Stabilization Exercise Prescription

The most important factor to consider when determining the appropriate number of repetitions of these exercises is the endurance and not the strength of the trunk muscles. Because stabilization is the main function of these muscles, sustained, submaximal efforts will be the key to effective training. Evidence suggests that low back exercises are most effective when performed on a daily basis (30). Another important factor to remember with regard to a stabilization program is persistence. Changes due to retraining of the trunk musculature will not occur quickly. It may take as long as 3 months to see desired results. It is vital that the clinician prepares the patient for the level of persistence and patience that is needed for optimal results.

STAGE III EXERCISE PROGRAMS: AEROBIC EXERCISE

Higher levels of aerobic fitness have been linked to a decreased incidence of low back injury (31); this was also discussed in Chap. 4. There is some evidence that low stress aerobic exercise may be effective in the treatment of acute and chronic low back pain (32,33). The safest forms of aerobic activity for patients with low back pain will be those that provide the benefits of an aerobic activity while placing the least amount of stress on the lumbar spine. Current evidence has demonstrated that low levels of compressive load are placed on the lumbar structures during walking (25). Because walking requires a constant, submaximal effort from the stabilizing muscles of the trunk and places very low loads on the supporting soft tissue, it serves as an ideal aerobic exercise for the appropriate patient with low back pain. Progressive walking programs can generally be initiated quite early in the rehabilitation process and can be progressed as the patient's activity tolerance increases.

Not all patients with low back pain can tolerate walking as an aerobic activity. Walking places the lumbar spine into a more extended position and therefore may cause a peripheralization of symptoms in certain patients. For example, an older patient with degenerative lumbar spinal stenosis will frequently be found to have increased symptoms in the low back and lower extremities while walking, with a near complete resolution of symptoms while sitting. As has been described in this chapter, any activity that creates a peripheralization of symptoms is to be avoided. This patient may be better suited to stationary cycling as an aerobic activity. Stationary cycling allows the patient to assume a seated position, placing the spine in more flexion and allowing the patient to exercise without peripheralization of symptoms.

Another option for aerobic activity in patients who cannot tolerate walking is the use of aquatic exercise. Having the patient walk while in a pool takes advantage of the buoyancy of the water in reducing the compressive forces of gravity. This usually permits a patient to walk for aerobic exercise without an increase in symptoms. The depth of the water will correspond to the amount of reduction in compressive force; therefore, progression can be achieved by having the patient walk in progressively more shallow water, until he or she can tolerate ambulation outside of the pool without increased symptoms. (Therapeutic aquatic activities are discussed extensively in Chap. 10.)

More recently, the use of deweighted ambulation on a treadmill has been described as an option for patients who do not tolerate regular walking because of low back pain (34). Deweighted treadmill walking uses a traction harness system to decrease the total amount of weight that the body must support during walking. The use of deweighting during ambulation has been shown to reduce the compressive forces experienced during the activity (35). When beginning an aerobic exercise program with deweighted treadmill ambulation, the clinician should use sufficient traction force to permit the patient to walk without any increase in symptoms. The amount of traction force can then be gradually reduced over the course of treatment until the patient is able to ambulate a sufficient distance without any external support.

Another popular and effective aerobic exercise is jogging or running. Running has not been associated with an increased risk for developing low back pain and has actually been found to have a lower risk of developing degenerative changes of the lumbar intervertebral discs than other activities such as soccer or weight-lifting (36). Running

has been shown to create increased compressive loads on the spine (37) and therefore is not tolerated by some patients attempting to rehabilitate from an episode of low back pain. If returning to running is a goal of a patient, caution should be exercised in resuming the activity. A gradual return should be employed. If a patient has trouble in returning, the use of deweighting and running on a treadmill may be useful tools.

Numerous other aerobic activities could be used in the rehabilitation of patients with low back pain. Regardless of the particular aerobic exercise used, the goal is to improve the patient's endurance and thereby reduce the level of disability related to low back pain. Patients should be strongly encouraged to continue with a low stress aerobic exercise program even after completion of their formal rehabilitation program. This will provide general health benefits to the individual and may help reduce the likelihood of suffering a recurrence of low back pain.

SUMMARY

Active exercise programs are a critical element in the successful rehabilitation of patients with low back pain. The selection of a specific exercise routine should be based on the presentation of the individual patient. The clinician must consider the stage of the patient's condition and the goals of treatment when selecting appropriate activities. For many patients, the initial stage of treatment will focus on exercises that produce a centralization of the symptoms. Later in the rehabilitation process, the emphasis will shift to improving the endurance of key muscles involved in stabilization of the lumbar spine and improving the overall conditioning level of the patient.

REFERENCES

1. Valkenburg, H., and H. Haanen. The epidemiology of low back pain, in *Idiopathic Low Back Pain*, A. White and S. Gordon, editors. 1982, St. Louis: CV Mosby. p. 9.

2. Cypress, B.K. Characteristics of physician visits for back symptoms: a national perspective. *Am J Pub Health* 1983, 73: p. 389.

3. Sikorski, J.M. A rationalized approach to physiotherapy for low back pain. *Spine* 1985, 10: p. 571.

4. Waddell, G., et al. Systematic reviews of bed rest and advice to stay active for acute low back pain. *Br J Gen Pract* 1997, 47: p. 647.

5. Vroomen, P., et al. Lack of effectiveness of bed rest for sciatica. *N Engl J Med* 1999, 340: p. 418.

6. Deyo, R.A., et al. How many days of bed rest for acute low back pain? *N Engl J Med* 1986, 315: p. 1064.

7. Kankaanpaa, M., et al. The efficacy of active rehabilitation in chronic low back pain. Effect on pain intensity, self-experienced disability, and lumbar fatigability. *Spine* 1999, 24: p. 1034.

8. Delitto, A., et al. A treatment-based classification approach to low back syndrome: identifying and staging patients for conservative management. *Phys Ther* 1995, 75: p. 470.

9. Werneke, M., et al. A descriptive study of the centralization phenomenon. *Spine* 1999, 24: p. 676.

10. Fritz, J.M., and S. George. The use of a classification approach to identify subgroups of patients with acute low back pain: inter-rater reliability and short-term treatment outcomes. *Spine* 2000, 25: p. 106.

11. McKenzie, R.A. *The Lumbar Spine: Mechanical Diagnosis and Therapy.* 1989, Waikanae, New Zealand: Spinal Publications Limited.

12. Beattie, P.F., et al. Effects of lordosis on the position of the nucleus pulposus in supine subjects: a study using magnetic resonance imaging. *Spine* 1994, 19: p. 2096.

13. Brault, J.S., et al. Quantification of lumbar intradiscal deformation during flexion and extension, by mathematical analysis of magnetic resonance imaging pixel intensity profiles. *Spine* 1997, 22: p. 2066.

14. Penning, L. Functional pathology of lumbar spinal stenosis. *Clin Biomech* 1992, 7: p. 3.

15. Fiebert, I., and C.D. Keller. Are "passive" extension exercises really passive? *J Orthop Sports Phys Ther* 1994, 19: p. 111.

16. Cholewicki, J., and S.M. McGill. Mechanical stability of the in vivo lumbar spine: implications for injury and chronic low back pain. *Clin Biomech* 1996, 11: p. 1.

17. Crisco, J.J., and M.M. Panjabi. The intersegmental and multisegmental muscles of the lumbar spine: a biomechanical model comparing lateral stabilizing potential. *Spine* 1991, 16: p. 793.

18. Hodges, P.W., and C.A. Richardson. Inefficient muscular stabilization of the lumbar spine associated with low back pain. *Spine* 1996, 21: p. 2640.

19. Hodges, P.W., and C.A. Richardson. Delayed postural contraction of transversus abdominis in low back pain associated with movement of the lower limb. *J Spinal Dis* 1998, 11: p. 46.

20. Richardson, C.A., and G.A. Jull. Muscle control-pain control: what exercises would you prescribe? *Manual Ther* 1995, 1: p. 2.

21. Panjabi, M.M. The stabilizing system of the spine. Part II. Neutral zone and instability hypothesis. *J Spinal Disord* 1992, 5: p. 390.

22. Sihvonen, T., et al. Movement disturbances of the lumbar spine and abnormal back muscle electromyographic findings in recurrent low back pain. *Spine* 1997, 22: p. 289.

23. Hides, J.A., et al. Multifidus muscle recovery is not automatic after resolution of acute, first-episode low back pain. *Spine* 1996, 21: p. 2763.

24. McGill, S.M. Low back exercises: evidence for improving exercise regimens. *Phys Ther* 1998, 78: p. 754.

25. Callaghan, J.P., et al. The relationship between lumbar spine load and muscle activity during extensor exercises. *Phys Ther* 1998, 78: p. 8.

26. McGill, S.M., et al. Quantitative intramuscular myoelectric activity of quadratus lumborum during a wide variety of lift tasks. *Clin Biomech* 1996, 11: p. 170.

27. Gardner-Morse, M.G., and I.A.F. Stokes. The effects of abdominal muscle coactivation on lumbar spine stability. *Spine* 1998, 23: p. 86.

28. Axler, C.T., and S.M. McGill. Low back loads over a variety of abdominal exercises: searching for the safest abdominal challenge. *Med Sci Sports Exerc* 1997, 29: p. 804.

29. Gill, K.P., and M.J. Callaghan. The measurement of lumbar proprioception in individuals with and without low back pain. *Spine* 1998, 23: p. 371.

30. Mayer, T.G., et al. Objective assessment of spine function following industrial injuries; a prospective study with comparison group and one-year follow-up. *Spine* 1985, 10: p. 482.

31. Cady, L.D., et al. Strength and fitness and subsequent back injuries in firefighters. *J Occup Med* 1979, 21: p. 269.

32. van Tulder, M.W., et al. Conservative treatment of acute and chronic nonspecific low back pain. A systematic review of randomized controlled trials of the most common interventions. *Spine* 1997, 22: p. 2128.

33. Bigos, S., et al. *Acute Low Back Problems in Adults.* AHCPR Publication 95-0642. 1994, Rockville, MD: Agency for Health Care Policy and Research, Public Health Service, US Department of Health and Human Services.

34. Fritz, J.M., et al. A nonsurgical approach for patients with lumbar spinal stenosis. *Phys Ther* 1997, 77: p. 962.

35. Flynn, T.W., et al. Plantar pressure reduction in an incremental weight-bearing system. *Phys Ther* 1997, 77: p. 410.

36. Videman, T., et al. The long-term effects of physical loading and exercise lifestyles on back-related symptoms, disability and spinal pathology among men. *Spine*, 1995, 20: p. 700.

37. White, T.L., and T.R. Malone. Effects of running on intervertebral disc height. *J Orthop Sports Phys Ther* 1990, 12: p. 139.

CHAPTER 9

HISTORY AND PRINCIPLES OF AQUATIC THERAPY

Bruce E. Becker

INTRODUCTION

The history of aquatic therapy is very rich because it has been in use for more than two millennia. The physical and physiologic principles that are the foundation of aquatic therapy are presented in this chapter. They are important because they provide the reader with an explanation of the important scientific precepts on which aquatic therapy is based.

HISTORY OF AQUATIC THERAPY

Rehabilitation in the aquatic environment predates recorded medical history. The ancient Greeks and Romans documented the widespread use of water immersion for medicinal purposes for a variety of ills including arthritis. Observations were made that immersion in thermal mineral waters resulted in shrinking of peripheral edema, reduction of joint pain, and improvement in joint mobility. Hydrotherapy combined with heat is among the oldest rehabilitative treatments for arthritis (1), and passive and active treatments in the aquatic environment still play a unique role in the rehabilitation of acute and chronic musculoskeletal problems. Contemporary aquatic rehabilitation represents the evolution of classic medical traditions in combining the use of healing water pools with 20th century advances in the understanding of disease and immersion physiology.

Early Uses of Aquatic Therapy

Since the beginning of recorded history, the sick and suffering have resorted to springs, baths, and pools for their soothing and healing waters. Taking the waters, soaking in baths and pools, and resting at places called spas played an important social and spiritual role in the river valley civilizations of Mesopotamia, Egypt, India, and China. Ritual bathing pools were widely used for individual, religious, and social renewal and healing and appeared in ancient Greek, Hebrew, Roman, Christian, and Islamic cultures. Whereas the Greeks considered bathing as an additional function to the gymnasium, the Romans viewed the bathing process and pools as central to social activities that might include exercise in a gymnasium. The Roman physician Galen is said to have had his office in the Baths of Hadrian.

During the European Middle Ages, grand healing pools developed around thermal springs, including Baden-Baden in Germany, Bath in England, and Spa in Belgium. By the 19th century, Bad Ragaz in Switzerland developed into a major health resort spa, where today the aquatic rehabilitative procedure known as the "Bad Ragaz method" is taught and practiced. Similar aquatic histories and traditions are found at other European spas that have served European medicine for centuries, and many are even today a component of standard traditional health care practice.

The Rise of American Medical Hydrology

Postwar American culture focused on the powers of science and technology. Few physicians remembered how earlier civilized cultures used and revered the regenerative powers of healing waters. During the early 1950s, the spread of poliomyelitis affected nearly 58,000 Americans each year. The National Foundation for Infantile Paralysis supported the corrective swimming pools and hydrogymnastics therapies of physician Charles Lowman and the therapeutic use of pools and tanks for the treatment of poliomyelitis. The development of the Salk vaccine and the subsequent demise of poliomyelitis in the late 1950s reduced the medical community's perception of the need for complex aquatic therapy regimens, and pools became far less important to hospital practice. Advances in aquatic practice made immediately before and during the war years began to lose prominence as pools went into disrepair, therapists lost interest in the old techniques, and reimbursement mechanisms made alternate forms of therapy more profitable.

The late 1960s and early 1970s were golden times in American basic science research. Research funds became plentiful as the United States attempted to move man into space. It was in this frame that much aquatic physiology was studied. The human body in water has parallels with the human body in space: both conditions cause the body to respond as though it were weightless, both result in similar cardiovascular effects, and both present common concerns regarding the manipulation of tools. Thus, as researchers prepared to send humans into space, they needed information on how the body might respond in this new technologically controlled environment. Ironically, many answers were found in a simulation of humans' first environment: thermoneutral total body immersion. Much of this research laid the foundation for today's medical rationale for aquatic rehabilitation.

PHYSICAL PRINCIPLES OF AQUATIC THERAPY

Matter on earth at normal temperatures commonly exists in three states: solid, liquid, and gas. A solid maintains a consistent shape and size that typically does not change without significant force. Liquids, in contrast, readily alter shape but typically retain volume despite force. Gases are the least fixed, lacking both stable shape and size. Both liquids and gases can flow, and because flow properties are more related to density than to any other factor, both are called fluids. Although water is therapeutically used in all its forms, this chapter deals with water only in its liquid form. Nearly all of the biologic effects of immersion are related to the fundamental principles of hydrodynamics. An understanding of these principles makes the medical application process far more rational.

Density and Specific Gravity (2)

Density is defined as mass per unit volume and is represented by the Greek letter ρ (rho). The relationship of density to mass and volume is characterized by the formula:

$$\rho = m/V$$

where m is the mass of a substance whose volume is V. Density is measured in the international system

by kilograms per meter cubed and occasionally as grams per centimeter cubed. A density given as grams per centimeter cubed must be divided by 1000 to convert to kilograms per cubic meter. Density is a temperature-dependent variable, although this is much less true for solids and liquids than for gases. Water reaches maximum density at 4°C and is unusual in this characteristic because liquids typically become more dense as they freeze, but this rather unique property of water is important. If water were a typical liquid, as it froze into ice it would sink into the mass of still liquid water, thus allowing lakes to freeze from the bottom, killing off most of the biomass within.

In addition to density, substances are defined by their *specific gravity*, the ratio of the density of that substance to the density of water. By definition, water has a specific gravity equal to one at 4°C. Because this number is a ratio, it has no units of measurement. Although the human body is composed mostly of water, the body's density is slightly less than water and averages a specific gravity of 0.974, with males having a higher average density than females. Lean body mass, which includes bones, muscle, connective tissue, and organs, has a typical density near 1.10. In contrast, fat mass, which includes both essential body fat plus fat in excess of essential needs, has a density of about 0.90 (3). Consequently, the immersed human body displaces a volume of water weighing slightly more than the body, lifting the body upward by a force equal to the volume of the water displaced, as will be described.

Hydrostatic Pressure

Pressure is defined as force per unit area, where the force expressed by convention as F is understood to act perpendicularly to the surface area A. This relationship is:

$$P = F/A.$$

The standard international unit of pressure is called a pascal (Pa) and is measured in Newtons per meter squared. Other common measurement units are dynes per centimeter squared, kilograms per meter squared, millimeters of mercury per foot, and pounds per square inch (also known as ψ).

Fluids have been experimentally found to exert pressure in all directions, as the swimmer and diver are well aware. At a theoretical point immersed in a vessel of water, the pressure exerted on that point is equal from all directions. Obviously, if unequal pressure were exerted, the point would move until the pressures on it were equalized.

Pressure in a liquid increases with depth and is directly related to the density of the fluid. If we consider a theoretical point immersed to a distance h below the surface, the force exerted on the point is due to the weight of the column of fluid above it. Pressure is directly proportional to both the liquid density and the immersion depth in cases where the fluid is incompressible, as water is at the depths used in therapeutic environments. The pressure of the Earth's atmosphere is an important contributor to the total force from immersion. Water exerts a pressure of 22.4 mmHg/ft of water depth, which translates to 1 mmHg/1.36 cm (0.54 inches) H_2O depth. Thus, a body immersed to a depth of 48 inches is subjected to a force equal to 88.9 mmHg, which is slightly greater than diastolic blood pressure. This is the force that aids the resolution of edema in an injured body part.

Buoyancy

Immersed objects have less apparent weight in water than on land because a force opposite to gravity acts on these objects. This force is called *buoyancy* and equals an upward force generated by the volume of water displaced. The force arises from the fact that pressure in a fluid increases with depth. Thus, buoyant force is equal to the weight of the fluid displaced. This principle, discovered by Archimedes (ca. 287–212 BC) is the reason why we float, why water can be used as a laboratory for mimicking weightlessness, and why it can be used to advantage in managing medical problems requiring weight off-loading. The principle applies equally to floating objects. A human with specific gravity of 0.97 will reach floating equilibrium when 97% of his or her volume is submerged.

Buoyancy's upward force is an important consideration in the therapeutic aquatic environment. The center of gravity is a point at which all force moments are in equilibrium. For a human being standing in the "anatomic" position, this point is slightly posterior to the mid-sagittal plane and at the level of the second sacral vertebra because the human body is nonuniform with respect to density. For example, the lungs obviously are less dense than the lower limbs. The center of gravity is really the physical aggregate of the centers of gravity of all the body parts, whereas the center of buoyancy is defined as the center of all buoyancy force moments. Consequently, the human center of buoyancy is in the mid-chest. When both centers are aligned in a vertical plane, only vertical vector forces are apparent, which may produce a compressive or distractive force on the body. When these points are not aligned vertically, rotational force results. The product of a force and a distance over which the force acts is called a *moment*; it may also be called *torque*. Although the terms are technically equivalent, torque is often used with reference to circular motion. Torque in this context is the horizontal displacement of centers and the vector magnitude difference between the upward force on the center of buoyancy and the downward force on the center of gravity. This torque force may help the floating human to maintain an upright head-out posture or, when buoyancy devices are used, to float face down or face up. These same forces will affect a limb and become a vector continuum as the limb moves through water.

Joint Effects

As the body gradually immerses, water is displaced, creating the force of buoyancy. This offloads the immersed joints progressively. With neck immersion, only about 15 pounds of compressive force (the approximate weight of the head) is exerted on the spine, hips, and knees. A person immersed to the symphysis pubis has effectively displaced water equivalent to about 40% of body weight, and when further immersed to the umbilicus, approximately 50% of body weight. Xiphoid immersion produces 60% or more off-loading, depending on whether the arms are over the head or next to the trunk. A body suspended or floating in water essentially counterbalances the downward effects of gravity by the upward force of buoyancy. This effect may be of great therapeutic use in the management of many spine and musculoskeletal problems. For example, a fractured pelvis may not become mechanically stable under full body loading for many weeks. However, with water immersion, gravitational forces may be partly or completely offset so that only muscle torque forces are present on the fracture site(s), allowing "active-assisted" range of motion activities, gentle strength building, and even gait training. The same principles may substantially off-load an injured intervertebral disc.

Time-Dependent Properties

Water at motion becomes a very complex physical substance. In fact, despite centuries of study, many aspects of fluid motion are still incompletely understood. Nevertheless, the major principles of flow are valid and apply to general activities.

Flow Motion   Water may have several characteristics in motion. When water moves smoothly inside a vessel, with all layers moving at the same speed, the water is said to be in *laminar* or *streamline flow*. In this type of movement, all molecules are moving parallel to each other, and paths do not cross. Typically, laminar flow rates are slow, as when water moves rapidly, and even minor oscillations create uneven flow that knocks parallel paths out of alignment. When this occurs, another type of pattern emerges, called *turbulent flow*. Within the mass of water, flow patterns arise that run dramatically out of parallel and may even set up paths running in opposite directions. These paths are called *eddy currents* and appear like whirlpools in response to obstacles in the flow path or to irregularities in the surface of flow-directing vessels. Examples of the latter are the eddy holes that occur in fast-moving streams behind boulders and eddy currents that form in

the blood stream behind irregularities in arterial walls due to cholesterol plaques. Turbulent flow absorbs energy at a much greater rate than streamline flow, and the rate of energy absorption is a function of the internal friction within the fluid. This internal friction is called *viscosity*. The major determinants of water motion are viscosity, turbulence, and speed.

Viscosity and Drag   When an object moves relative to a fluid, it is subjected to the resistive effects of the fluid. This force is called *drag force* and is due to fluid viscosity and turbulence, if any is present. With faster movement, the drag force begins to increase at the rate of the square of the velocity. Streamlining reduces the frontal aspect of an object and reduces the force necessary to move through the fluid, but turbulence is still produced behind the object and is known as a *wake*. At low speeds the force increases with the square of the velocity; however, as the speed increases, there is an abrupt increase in drag force. This force is due to turbulence produced not only behind the moving object but also in the layer of fluid passing over the object, known as the *boundary layer*. The greatest surface area drag in a person swimming is the head, although the negative pressure following the swimmer causes the greatest force resisting forward movement. There is turbulence produced by the moving body's surface area, and a drag force is produced by the turbulence behind.

Viscosity, with all its attendant physical properties, is a quality that makes water a useful strengthening medium. Viscous resistance to movement of a limb through water increases as more force is exerted against it. However, that resistance drops to zero almost immediately with cessation of force because the inertial mass of the limb is small compared with the inert mass of the surrounding water. Viscosity effectively counteracts inert momentum. Thus, when a rehabilitating person feels pain and stops movement, the force drops precipitously and water viscosity damps movement almost instantaneously. This allows great control of strengthening activities within the "envelope" of patient comfort.

Thermodynamics of Water

Water is used therapeutically in all its forms: solid, liquid, and gas. A major reason for its usefulness lies in the physics of aquatic thermodynamics.

Specific Heat   All substances on Earth possess energy stored as heat. This energy is measured in a quantity called a *calorie* (cal). A calorie is defined as the heat required to raise the temperature of 1 g of water by 1°C, from 14.5 to 15.5°C. Sometimes the energy required to raise temperature is defined in kilocalories, the amount required to raise 1 kg of water 1°C, and this unit by convention is termed a *Calorie* (Cal). This is the unit in which food energy content is measured. A mass of water possesses a definable, measurable amount of stored energy in the form of heat. By Centimeter Gram Second (CGS) system definition, water has a specific heat capacity equal to one. Air, in contrast, has a significantly lower specific heat capacity (i.e., 0.001). Thus, water retains heat 1000 times more than an equivalent volume of air.

Thermal Energy Transfer   The therapeutic utility of water is greatly dependent on both its ability to retain heat and its ability to transfer heat energy. Exchange of energy in the form of heat occurs in three ways: conduction, convection, and radiation. Conduction may be thought of as occurring through molecular collisions that take place over a small distance in the absence of movement. Convection requires the mass movement of large numbers of molecules over a large distance. Liquids and gases are generally poor conductors but good convectors. Radiation transfers heat through the transmission of electromagnetic waves. Conduction and convection require contact between the exchanging energy sources; radiation does not. Substances differ widely in their ability to conduct heat. Water is an efficient conductor of heat and transfers heat 25 times faster than air.

The human body produces considerable heat through the conversion of food calories into other energy forms, but only about one-fifth of this converted energy is used to do work. The remaining four-fifths is converted into thermal energy. Core temperature would rise about 3°C per hour during light activity if it were not for the body's ability to dissipate heat. This dissipation process occurs through all heat transfer mechanisms but by far the most important is convection, which occurs through the flow of warm blood from the core to the skin and lungs, where contact with the cooler air occurs. Because energy must be dissipated further, the body uses another mechanism that allows energy loss through the latent heat of evaporation of sweat and respiratory loss, further cooling the skin. This mechanism is remarkably efficient, as the evaporative loss of 2.5 mL of water cools the body 0.94°C (2°F). Heat transfer increases as a function of velocity so that a swimmer will lose more heat when swimming rapidly through cold water than a person standing still in the same water. Fortunately for the swimmer, heat is produced through exercise. This thermal conductive property and the high specific heat of water make the use of water in rehabilitation very versatile because it retains heat or cold while delivering it easily to the immersed body part.

PHYSIOLOGIC PRINCIPLES OF AQUATIC THERAPY

Immersion in the aquatic environment has profound biologic effects that essentially involve all biologic systems. There are both immediate and delayed physiologic effects that allow water to be used with therapeutic efficacy in a great variety of rehabilitative problems. Aquatic rehabilitation is beneficial in the management of patients with diverse musculoskeletal and neurologic problems, cardiopulmonary pathology, and various other medical concerns. Not only may this broad range of problems be treated, but the margin of therapeutic safety is wider than almost any other treatment milieu. Thus, knowledge of these biologic effects is important to the skilled rehabilitative clinician.

Circulatory System Mechanics

The column of blood contained within the arterial system is under pressure generated by the left ventricle during systolic contraction; at rest, this is typically less than 130 mmHg. It remains under pressure during diastole (the period of ventricular relaxation) because of the closure of the aortic valve, and the elastic properties of the arterial system sustain the pressure at 60 to 70 mmHg on average in the normotensive adult. The diastolic pressure is largely determined by the autonomic nervous system through its control of the smooth muscle within the vessel walls of the peripheral vascular tree.

Pressure in the venous side of circulation is much lower than pressure on the arterial side of the system. Venous pressures differ, depending on the part of the body and its vertical relationship to the heart. Venous pressures are controlled in part by a system of valves that prevent back flow. These one-way valves act to divide the large vertical column of venous blood into many short columns with little vertical height. They also create much lower hydrostatic pressure gradients inside the vein and shorten the effective fluid column so that the maximum venous pressure is 30 mmHg peripherally. Venous pressure decreases steadily so that the blood reaching the right atrium has a negative pressure of 2 to 4 mmHg. The role of these valves in maintaining a low-pressure system is critical; if they fail, venous varicosities develop because of insufficient vessel wall strength to support the increased fluid column.

This low-pressure venous gradient system is the driving force returning blood to the heart. Consequently, venous return is very sensitive to external pressure changes, including compression from surrounding muscles and, more importantly in this chapter, external water pressure when the body is immersed. The immersed individual is subjected to external water pressure in a gradient; because the water pressure exceeds venous pressure, blood is forced upward through this one-way system, first into the thighs, into the abdominal cavity vessels, and then into the great vessels of the chest cavity and into the heart. External water pressure is proportional to immersion depth. For example, right atrial pressure is −2 to 4 mmHg in an individual standing on land; however, this pressure rises to +14 to 17 mmHg when the individual is standing in water up to the neck (4,5). Pulmo-

nary blood flow consequently increases with increased central blood volume and pressure.

The healthy cardiac response to increased volume (stretch) is an increased force of contraction, a phenomenon known as Starling's law (6). Stroke volume increases because of this increased stretch. Normal resting stroke volume is about 71 cc per beat, and the additional 25 cc from immersion equals about 100 cc, which is close to the exercise maximum for a sedentary deconditioned individual on land (7). Mean stroke volume increases 35% on average with immersion to the neck; there is both an increase in end diastolic volume and a decrease in end systolic volume (8). These changes are compared to preimmersion status in Fig. 9-1.

Stroke Volume Stroke volume is one of the major determinants of the rise in cardiac output seen with training because heart rate response ranges are relatively fixed (9). In an untrained individual, subtracting age from a pulse rate of 220 beats per minute approximates maximum heart rate. The upper limit in an untrained indi-

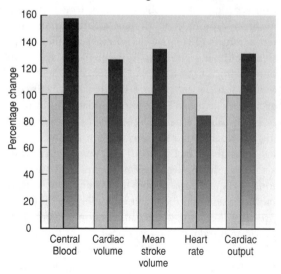

Fig. 9-1 Comparative changes in cardiologic function.

vidual differs only 10 to 15% less from that of a trained one (9). As heart rate increases beyond an optimal point, cardiac output begins to decrease due to shortening of diastole, which reduces time for ventricular filling (6). Maximum stroke volume is reached at 40 to 50% of maximum oxygen consumption, which equals a heart rate of 110 to 120 beats per minute on land. This is generally accepted as the rate at which aerobic training begins to occur (9).

As cardiac filling and stroke volume increase with increase in immersion depth from symphysis to xiphoid, the heart rate typically drops (8). This drop is variable, with the amount of decrease dependent on water temperature; typically, at average pool temperatures, the rate lowers by 12 to 15% (10). There is a significant relationship between water temperature and heart rate. For example, at 25°C, heart rate drops approximately 12 to 15 beats per minute (11); at thermoneutral temperatures, the drop in rate is less than 15%. In warm water, the rate generally rises significantly, which contributes to the major rise in cardiac output at high temperatures (10,12).

Immersion Depth   During immersion to the neck, systemic vascular resistance decreases by 30% (4). Decreased sympathetic vasoconstriction contributes to this drop, with peripheral venous tone diminishing from around 17 to 12 mmHg at thermoneutral temperatures (13). Total peripheral resistance drops steadily during the first hour of immersion and persists for a time thereafter. This fall is related to temperature, with higher temperatures producing greater decreases. This lowers end diastolic pressures. Systolic pressures always increase with increasing workloads but appear to be approximately 20% less in water than on land (14). Venous pressures also drop during immersion because less vascular tone is required to support the system. Much study has been done on the effect of immersion on blood pressure. Very short-term immersion (10 min) in thermoneutral temperatures has been found to very slightly increase both systolic and diastolic temperatures, perhaps as part of the "cool water" accommodation process (8).

In an important study for aquatic rehabilitation, Corruzi et al. (15) found that longer immersion produced significant decreases in mean arterial pressure, with group I hypertensive patients showing an even greater drop (−18 to −20 mmHg) than normotensive patients and group II patients showing a lesser drop (−5 to −14 mmHg) (15). No studies have demonstrated consistent sustained increases in systolic pressure with prolonged immersion, although several have found no significant decrease. Based on a substantial body of research, the therapeutic pool appears to be both a safe and potentially therapeutic environment for both normotensive and hypertensive patients.

Cardiovascular Fitness   Water-based exercise has often been said to be less effective than land-based exercise for improving cardiovascular fitness. However, during exercise, maximal myocardial oxygen consumption efficiency (peak heart muscle efficiency) occurs with a stroke volume increase because a heart rate rise is a less efficient means of increasing output (6,9,12). Stated another way, the most efficient way for the heart to deliver more blood is to increase stroke volume; it would be inefficient to attempt to make up the difference by an increase in heart rate. Energy is wasted at the onset of myocardial contraction, when the heart is contracting but moving no volume, and at the endpoint of contraction, when the heart is moving little volume and the myocardium is maximally contracted. The optimal length-to-tension relationship develops with increased stroke volume. Thus, as cardiovascular conditioning occurs, cardiac output increases are achieved with smaller increases in heart rate but greater stroke volumes. This is the reason that conditioned athletes are able to maintain lower resting pulses while maintaining similar cardiac outputs when compared with matched deconditioned individuals. Older individuals also increase stroke volume more rapidly than younger individuals do at equivalent cardiac workloads.

Cardiac output is the product of stroke volume times pulse rate per unit time. Cardiac index is the ratio of cardiac output to body surface area, thus compensating for size and sex differences. Because the ultimate purpose of the heart as an organ is to pump blood, its ultimate measure of performance is the amount of blood pumped per unit of time.

Submersion Effects   Submersion to the neck increases cardiac output greater than 30% (8). Output increases by about 1500 ml/min, of which 50% is directed to increased muscle blood flow (4). Normal cardiac output is approximately 5 L/min in a resting individual. Maximum output in a conditioned athlete is about 40 L/min; this is equivalent to 205 ml/beat times, or 195 beats per minute. Maximum output at exercise for a sedentary individual on land is approximately 20 L/min, equivalent to 105 ml/beat, or beats per minute (9). Because immersion to the neck produces a cardiac stroke volume about 100 ml/beat, a resting pulse of 86 beats per minute produces a cardiac output of 8.6 L/min and is already producing cardiac exercise. The increase in cardiac output appears to be somewhat age dependent because younger subjects show greater increases (up 59%) than older subjects (up only 22%) (7). The increase is highly temperature dependent as it changes directly with temperature increases from 30% at 33°C to 121% at 39°C (10).

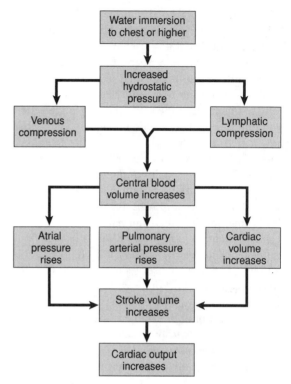

Fig. 9-2 Immersion-induced cardiovascular cascade.

Cardiac Output   Recent research has shown that conditioned athletes demonstrate an even greater increase in cardiac output than untrained control subjects during immersed exercise and that this increase is sustained for longer periods than in the control group (16). Therefore, the myth that water exercise is not aerobically efficient is faulty, for it can be an ideal cardiovascular conditioning medium. The total cascade of cardiovascular responses is summarized in Fig. 9-2.

Gleim and Nicholas (17) found that maximum oxygen consumption (VO_2) was three times greater as a given (53 m/min) speed in water than on land. Thus, looking at the reverse effect of this fact, during water walking and running, only one-half to one-third the speed was required to achieve the same metabolic intensity as on land (10). It is

important to note that the relationship of heart rate to VO_2 parallels the relationship seen in land-based exercise, although water heart rate averages 10 beats per minute less, for reasons discussed earlier (8). Consequently, metabolic intensity in water may be predicted as on land from monitoring heart rate.

Pulmonary System

The pulmonary system is profoundly affected by immersion of the body to the neck. Part of the effect is due to shifting of blood into the chest cavity, and part is due to compression of the chest wall itself by the water. The combined effect is to alter pulmonary function, increase the work of breathing, and change respiratory dynamics.

A brief overview of pulmonary physiology is helpful to understanding the changes involved. When an individual is at rest and breathing comfortably, the normal excursion of air during inspiration and expiration is called *tidal volume*. At the endpoint of a nonforced expiration, there is still a volume of air left in the lungs that can be expelled with increased effort. This volume is called the *expiratory reserve volume* (ERV). This may be experienced by simply exhaling normally and then exhaling forcibly to the maximum amount. Even when this last volume has been expelled, there is air left in the lungs that cannot be voluntarily expelled. This remainder is called the *residual volume* (RV). The combination of ERV and RV is called the *functional residual capacity* (FRC). It is felt that this volume of residual air serves a buffering role for blood oxygen and carbon dioxide saturation levels, preventing extreme fluctuation.

At the end of comfortable inspiration, there is room for more air to be inhaled and this is called the *inspiratory reserve volume* (IRV). As one exercises and increases the need for more oxygen, tidal volume increases, reducing both ERV and IRV. The combination of both inspiratory and expiratory reserve volumes plus tidal volume is called *vital capacity* (VC) and represents a laboratory measurement of the maximum amount of air that can be inhaled and subsequently exhaled. These relationships are graphically demonstrated in Fig. 9-3. Vital capacity differs widely with stature, sex, and individual differences. A low VC per body mass reduces the amount of oxygen potentially available for metabolism, whereas a large VC-to-body mass ratio increases aerobic potential.

Functional residual capacity reduces to about half of the normal value with immersion to the xiphoid [18]. Most of this loss is due to reduction in ERV, which decreases three-fourths at this level of immersion [19]. The change in this volume may readily be perceived at poolside: while sitting on the edge of the pool, exhale normally and then expel the rest of the reserve volume forcibly. Enter the water to neck level and perform the same experiment; the difference is very perceptible. Little air remains to exhale at the endpoint of

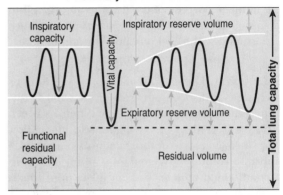

Pulmonary function divisions

Fig. 9-3 Pulmonary function terminology.

relaxed exhalation. Expiratory reserve volume is reduced to 11% of VC [20]. There is some loss of RV, which drops by 15% [21]. Vital capacity decreases about 6 to 9% when comparing neck submersion with xiphoid submersion; about half of this VC reduction is due to increased thoracic blood volume and half is due to hydrostatic forces counteracting the inspiratory musculature [20,21]. Pressure on the rib cage shrinks the rib cage circumference by approximately 10% during submersion [20]. Vital capacity does appear to fluctuate somewhat with temperature, decreasing with cooler water immersion (25°C) and increasing slightly in warm water immersion (40°C) [22]. Figure 9-4 shows the changes in pulmonary function during immersion.

The ability of the alveolar membrane to exchange gases is called *diffusion capacity*. Diffusion capacity of the lungs is reduced slightly as the lung beds become distended with blood shifted from the extremities and abdomen. This causes airway resistance to the movement of air to double, resulting from reduced lung volume [20,21]. Expiratory flow rates are reduced, increasing the time to move air into and out from the lungs. Chest wall compliance is reduced due to the pressure of water on the chest wall, increasing pleural pressure from -1 to $+1$ mmHg [4].

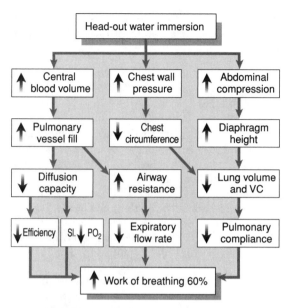

Fig. 9-4 Immersion-induced changes in pulmonary function.

The combined effect of all these changes is to increase the total work of breathing. The total work of breathing for a tidal volume of 1 L increases by 60% during submersion to neck, 75% of which is attributable to increase in elastic work (redistribution of blood from the thorax) and the rest to dynamic work (hydrostatic force on the thorax) (21).

For an athlete used to land-based conditioning exercises, a program of water-based exercises can result in a significant workload challenge to the respiratory apparatus. This challenge can raise the efficiency of the respiratory system if the time spent in water conditioning is sufficient to achieve a training effect for the respiratory apparatus.

Renal and Endocrine Systems

Aquatic immersion has many effects on renal blood flow, on the renal regulatory systems, and on the endocrine systems. These effects have been extensively studied in both the American and international literatures (15,23). Epstein (20), one of the most skilled and prolific researchers in study-

ing immersion effects on the human, published an exhaustive summary of these effects in 1992. The flow of blood to the kidneys increases immediately with immersion. This causes an increase in creatinine clearance, a measure of renal efficiency, initially with immersion.

Overall, immersion-induced central volume expansion causes increased urinary output accompanied by significant sodium and potassium excretion, beginning almost immediately with immersion, steadily increasing through several hours of immersion, and gently tapering off over subsequent hours. These time-dependent changes in urinary excretion are shown in Fig. 9-5.

The combined effect of the renal responses, the autonomic responses, and the cardiovascular responses on blood pressure has been quite intensively studied, with different results. During sustained immersion in water of neutral temperature, blood pressure does not appear to change greatly. During immersion in water of neutral temperature, patients with essential hypertension often show lowered blood pressure (20). The combination of these renal and sympathetic nervous system effects typically is to lower blood pressure in the immersed hypertensive individual during sustained immersion and to create a period of lowered pressure for a time thereafter (15).

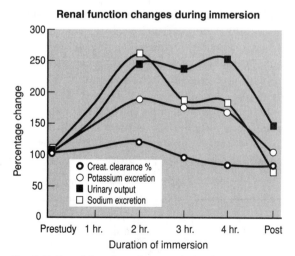

Fig. 9-5 Renal function changes during immersion.

Accompanying the renal hormone effects are changes in the autonomic nervous system neurotransmitters, collectively called *catecholamines*, which act to regulate vascular resistance, cardiac rate, and force. The most important of these are epinephrine, norepinephrine, and dopamine. Catecholamine levels begin changing immediately with immersion (24,25).

Musculoskeletal System

Water immersion also causes significant effects on the musculoskeletal system. The effects are caused by both the compression caused by immersion and the reflex regulation of blood vessel tone. It has been concluded that during immersion it is likely that most, if not all, of the increased cardiac output is redistributed to skin and muscle rather than to the splanchnic beds (20). To resist blood pooling during dry conditions, sympathetic vasoconstriction tightens the resistance vessels of skeletal muscle. Immersion pressure removes the biologic need for vasoconstriction, thus increasing muscle blood flow. Resting muscle blood flow has been found to increase from a dry baseline of 1.8 ml/min per 100 g of tissue to 4.1 ml/min per 100 g of tissue with neck immersion (21). In the same study, xenon clearance in the tibialis anterior during immersion to heart level was found to increase 130% above dry land clearance, essentially an identical rise to the cardiac output during immersion. Hydrostatic forces add an additional circulatory drive. Because 0.5-inch water depth equals 1 mmHg, immersion to only 36 inches of depth causes a pressure head exceeding average diastolic pressure and acts to drive out edema, muscle lactate, and other metabolic end products. Thus, blood flow and consequent oxygen delivery to muscle are significantly increased during immersion, as is the removal of muscle metabolic waste products.

CONCLUSION

This chapter presented the history of aquatic therapy and the physical and physiologic principles that are cogent to this medium. In Chap. 10, these principles are applied to aquatic exercise therapy.

REFERENCES

1. Harrison, R.A. Hydrotherapy in rheumatic conditions, in *Physiotherapy in Rheumatology*, S.A. Hyde, editor. 1980, Oxford: Blackwell Scientific Publications.
2. Giancoli, D.C. *Physics, Principles with Applications*, 2nd ed. 1985, Englewood Cliffs, NJ: Prentice Hall.
3. Bloomfield, J., et al. *Textbook of Science and Medicine in Sport.* 1992, Champaign, IL: Human Kinetics.
4. Arborelius, M., et al. Hemodynamic changes in man during immersion with the head above water. *Aerosp Med* 1972, 43(3): p. 593–599.
5. Risch, W.D., et al. The effect of graded immersion on heart volume, central venous pressure, pulmonary blood distribution and heart rate in man. *Pflügers Arch* 1978, 374: p. 117.
6. Hurst, J.W., editor. *The Heart*, 6th ed. 1986, New York: McGraw-Hill. p. 51.
7. Tajima, F., et al. Renal and endocrine responses in the elderly during head-out immersion. *Am J Physiol* 1988, 254 (*Regul Integr Comp Physiol* 23): p. R977–R983.
8. Haffor, A.A., et al. Effects of water immersion on cardiac output of lean and fat male subjects at rest and during exercise. *Aviat Space Environ Med* 1991, 62: p. 125.
9. McArdle, W.D., et al. *Exercise Physiology, Energy, Nutrition and Human Performance*, 3rd ed. 1991, Malvern, PA: Lea & Febiger. p. 435–436.
10. Weston, C.F.M., et al. Haemodynamic changes in man during immersion in water at different temperatures. *Clin Sci (Lond)* 1987, 73: p. 613–616.
11. Evans, B.W., et al. Metabolic and circulatory responses to walking and jogging in water. *Res Q* 1978, 49(4): p. 442–449.
12. Dressendorfer, R.H., et al. Effects of head-out water immersion on cardiorespiratory responses to maximal cycling exercise. *Undersea Biomed Res* 1976, 3(3): p. 183.

13. Epstein, M. Cardiovascular and renal effects of head-out water immersion in man. *Circ Res* 1976, 39(5): p. 620–628.

14. Bishop, P.A., et al. Physiological responses to treadmill and water running. *Phys Sports Med* 1989, 17(2): p. 87–94.

15. Coruzzi, P.A.A., et al. Low pressure receptor activity and exaggerated naturiesis in essential hypertension. *Nephron* 1985, 40: p. 309–315.

16. Claybaugh, J.R., et al. Fluid conservation in athletic responses to water intake, supine posture, and immersion. *J Appl Physiol* 1986, 61: p. 7–15.

17. Gleim, G.W., and J.A. Nicholas. Metabolic costs and heart rate responses to treadmill walking in water at different depths and temperatures. *Am J Sports Med* 1989, 17(2): p. 248–252.

18. Agostoni, E., et al. Respiratory mechanics during submersion and negative pressure breathing. *J Appl Physiol* 1966, 21(1): p. 253.

19. Hong, S.K., et al. Mechanics of respiration during submersion in water. *J Appl Physiol* 1969, 27(4): p. 535–536.

20. Epstein, M. Renal effects of head out immersion in humans: a 15-year update. *Physiol Rev* 1992, 72(3): p. 563–621.

21. Balldin, U.I., et al. Changes in the elimination of [133]Xenon from the anterior tibial muscle in man induced by immersion in water and by shifts in body position. *Aerosp Med* 1971, 42(5): p. 489.

22. Choukroun, M.L., and P. Varene. Adjustments in oxygen transport during head-out immersion in water at various temperatures. *J Appl Phys* 1990, 68(4): p. 1475–1480.

23. Borg, G.A.V. Psychophysical bases of perceived exertion. *Med Sci Sports Exerc* 1992, 14(5): p. 377–381.

24. Grossman, E., et al. Effects of water immersion on sympathoadrenal and dopa-dopamine systems in humans. *Am J Physiol* 1992, 262 (*Regul Integr Comp Physiol* 31): p R993–R999.

25. Krishna, D., and J. Sowers. Catecholamine responses to central volume expansion produced by head-out water immersion and saline infusion. *J Clin Endocrinol Metab* 1983, 56(5): p. 998.

CHAPTER 10

AQUATIC EXERCISE THERAPY

Bruce E. Becker

INTRODUCTION

Aquatic exercise therapy has made long strides in the last 10 years of the 20th century. This is exemplified by the fact that many therapy centers now use pools; moreover, pool therapy is also used by trainers and therapists employed by universities and professional athletic teams to rehabilitate athletes. Moreover, shortly after underwater treadmills became popular for lower extremity rehabilitation in athletes, the underwater treadmill was installed in at least one veterinary medicine teaching hospital.

This chapter discusses the use of aquatics in exercise therapy, with an emphasis on exercises for the spine. However, because spine pain and arthritis are both forms of joint disease, there is some overlap and commingling of exercise activities.

BASIC EXERCISE CONSIDERATIONS

There are several factors that are basic to providing aquatic exercise therapy regardless of patient symptomatology or site of dysfunction. Some patients may present symptoms for more than one dysfunction, such as an arthritic knee and low back pain. One of the advantages of aquatic therapy is that certain activities may be appropriate for more than one site or dysfunction.

Conditioning Effects

Controversy has existed regarding the utility of a program of water-based exercise in maintaining fitness in athletes who must be sheltered from gravity effects during injury recovery. For maintenance of cardiorespiratory condition in highly fit individuals, water running has the same effect as dry-land running on maintenance of maximum oxygen consumption (VO_2 max) when training intensities and frequencies are matched (1). Similarly, when aquatic exercise is compared with land-based equivalent exercise in effect on VO_2 max gains in unfit individuals, (a) aquatic exercise is seen to achieve equivalent results and (b) when water temperature is low, the gains achieved are accompanied by lower heart rate (2). Lactate thresholds are more closely correlated with training performance than with heart rate or VO_2. Blood lactate has been found to shift to the left in relation to oxygen uptake in both submaximal and maximal water running when compared with dry-land running on a treadmill (3). Thus, water-based exercise programs may be used effectively to sustain or increase aerobic conditioning in athletes needing joint off-loading such as with spine pain, when in injury recovery, or when in an intensive training program in which joint or bone microtrauma could occur.

A key question frequently asked is whether aquatic exercise programs have sufficient specificity to provide a reasonable training venue for athletes in this situation. Hamer and Morton (4) addressed this specific question and found that aquatic-based running programs did achieve significant reductions in submaximal heart rates and improved performance on graded exercise tests when compared with nonexercising control subjects.

Relative Perceived Exertion (RPE) Scales

For more than 30 years it has been recognized that the subjective experience of effort is closely related to measurable parameters of the workload. Through the years, beginning with the groundbreaking work of Borg (5) and confirmed by many other researchers, this relation has been carefully studied. It is now well known that the inner perception of effort closely correlates with VO_2, blood and muscle lactate, heart rate, and other objective measurements. Coefficients of correlation with heart rates have ranged from 0.80 to 0.90, and high levels have also been shown with all other measures of exertion. It is significant that RPE scores correlate closely with blood lactate levels (6). The human being has an accurate internal tachometer of exercise intensity, which can be effectively used in the training process.

Borg's rating scale allows an individual to relate his or her effort level to a specific scale point that can facilitate training consistency and measurement (7). This scale used values ranging from 6 to 20. It was intended to represent pulse rate increases, with average resting pulse rates at 60 that increased to 200 at maximum effort; thus, a scale measurement was approximately equal to 10 heart beats. This scale has been modified in a number of ways by many researchers. It has been found that the metabolic costs of aqua running are slightly less than treadmill running for equal RPE scores (8). A more recent variant of the Borg scale was developed specifically for water running exercise programs by Wilder and Brennan (9); they derived a 5-point scale, with 1 equaling light work and 5 equaling very hard work. They found it very helpful in high-level training and in general rehabilitation.

Open Versus Closed Kinetic Chain Issues

Aquatic exercise programs may be designed to change the amount of gravity loading by using buoyancy as a counterforce; in this way, joint movement through water can be loaded or off-loaded. A joint that is moving against a fixed resistance, such as the ground, forms what is termed a *closed kinetic chain*. Rehabilitative programs for specific joints may be more effective as either closed or open kinetic chain programs. When extensive structural reconstruction of a normally gravity-loaded joint has been performed, many rehabilitationists feel that closed chain exercises are preferable.

Shallow water vertical exercises generally approximate closed chain exercise, but with reduced joint loading because of the buoyancy counterforce. Deep water exercises are comparable to an open chain system; horizontal exercises such as swimming are also viewed as being open chain. However, paddles and other resistive equipment tend to close the kinetic chain. Aquatic programs offer the ability to check the force of movement instantaneously because of the viscous properties of water.

The effects of buoyancy and water resistance make possible high levels of energy expenditure with relatively little movement and strain on lower extremity joints (10). Off-loading occurs as a func-

tion of immersion depth, as was extensively discussed in Chap. 9. The amount of weight off-loading occurring through progressive immersion is shown in Figure 10-1. The spine is especially well protected during aquatic exercise programs; it permits early rehabilitation at a point when land-based exercise is uncomfortable or unwise.

In walking the force exerted against the floor by the feet is counteracted by the ground. This force is termed *ground reaction force* and may easily be measured through a force plate. In chest-deep

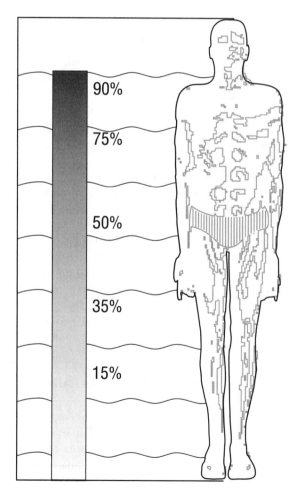

Fig. 10-1 Body weight off-loading during static standing.

water walking the forces generated are (a) substantially reduced in magnitude by more than 50%, (b) generated more slowly, and (c) transmitted over a longer time interval than in land walking (11). Clinically, this means that joint compression is less and impact strain is diminished. Because smaller forces are transmitted throughout the kinetic chain, ankles and knees are spared stress, as are the hip joints and the lumbar spine. However, as speed increases, the force development rate increases, so that when joint stress is to be avoided, the therapist should caution against overly rapid movement.

Weight Control Issues

Water exercise seems to have a fat-sparing quality because similar exercise intensities and durations do not produce similar body fat decreases (12,13). One need only compare the bodies of elite distance swimmers with those of elite track distance athletes to corroborate this research.

Implications for Overweight Patients   Aquatic exercise programs may be highly beneficial in the restoration of fitness in obese patients because of the protective effects they offer against heavy joint loading. The ability to achieve an aerobic exercise level for sufficient time to produce a conditioning effect may be difficult in this population on dry land, and a program initiating in water, transitioning to land as tolerance builds, may be the most effective method of achieving both conditioning and weight loss.

AQUATIC EXERCISE FOR SPINE PAIN

Because the common denominator in spine pain and arthritis is joint disease, there will at times be a commingling of material relevant to both of these conditions in this chapter. There are often more similarities than differences in providing exercise therapy for the adult with either spine pain or arthritis.

Spine Pain Management

An accurate diagnosis of patients' spinal injuries helps determine further therapeutic exercise treatment and should include observation of their initial responses to land-based or aquatic stabilization programs. An aquatic exercise regimen can eliminate dry-land risks, establish a supportive training environment, provide a new therapeutic activity, decrease the risk of peripheral joint injury, and often permit a quick return to prior activity. Important therapeutic considerations should include the inability to tolerate axial or gravitational loads and the need for increased support in the presence of a strength or proprioceptive deficit (14). Recent evidence indicates that there is protective value in exercise that does not involve impact loading of the skeleton but relies on joint loading forces to build strength. Joint loading exercises such as resistance training, rowing, and cycling all are capable of facilitating bone mineral retention (15). Thus, it is reasonable to infer that aquatic exercise can be included in joint loading nonimpact exercise programs. However, no published studies explicitly assessing the effect of aquatic exercise on bone mineral status have been found.

Continuing the rehabilitative course in a water-supported environment is appropriate if a dry-land environment exacerbates symptoms or if adherence to a progressive program will be improved in the water. Transition from a wet to a dry-land environment should occur if patients are doing well in the water but must return to land to meet functional training needs efficiently and attain their ultimate competitive goals (16,17).

General Stabilization Considerations

The aquatic rehabilitation programs that will be reviewed are based on the work of Cole et al. (18) in adapting dry-land spine rehabilitation techniques to the aquatic environment. Dynamic lumbar, thoracic, and cervical stabilization techniques have been previously described in Chapters 6 and 8 and have achieved wide acceptance for land-based programs. Dynamic land-based stabilization training is a therapeutic exercise program that (a) helps patients regain dynamic control of segmental spine forces, (b) eliminates repetitive injury to motion segments and encourages their healing, and (c) may alter the degenerative process. The underlying premise is that motion segments and supporting soft tissues react to minimize applied stresses and reduce risk of injury. Aquatic stabilization exercises and swimming programs incorporate these elements but incorporate the unique properties of water to reduce the risk of spine injury. Aquatic stabilization programs can help develop patients' flexibility, strength, and body mechanics, so that a smooth transition to aquatic-stabilization swimming programs or other spine stabilized activities may occur. Such programs can help first-time swimmers or patients who previously swam (19,20).

Progressive elimination of gravitational forces through buoyancy allows patients to train with decreased yet variable axial loads and shear forces. Water increases the safety margin of patient postural error by decreasing the compressive and shear forces on the spine. Velocity can be controlled by water resistance, viscosity, buoyancy, and training devices. Buoyancy increases the range of training positions. It has been contended that pain attenuation takes place in the water because of the "sensory overload" generated by hydrostatic pressure, temperature, and turbulence (21).

Aquatic Spine Stabilization Techniques

The spine stabilization principles discussed in Chaps. 6 and 8 also apply to aquatic programs; however, there are a number of exercises that can be performed on land that cannot easily be reproduced in water and vice versa. Aquatic programs can be designed for patients who cannot train on land or for those whose land training has reached a plateau. Eagleston first described aquatic stabilization in 1989 (22).

Cole et al. (19,23) described eight core aquatic stabilization exercises with four levels of difficulty to provide graded training of stabilization skills.

Programs must be customized to meet each patient's unique spine pathology, related to their musculoskeletal dysfunction, and their comfort within the aquatic environment.

JOINT REPLACEMENT PATIENTS: *Individuals who have had joint replacements require particular care during positioning in the water. The joint prostheses can change the center of buoyancy and may cause patients to sink because of their high specific gravity (24).*

When a program is mastered, patients are transitioned to a more advanced one. If patients wish to incorporate a swimming program, a series of transitional aquatic stabilization exercises are initiated. When these exercises are mastered, injured patients can soon advance to spine-safe swimming or other high-level aquatic training activities (25). It is very important to establish a spine stabilized swimming style that minimizes the risk of further spine injury and helps maximize swimming performance (18,26).

Spine Stabilized Swimming Programs

Once a patient's stabilization skills have progressed to the point where swimming is possible, a thorough analysis of stroke technique and its effect on spine motion is critical. The following overview is based on the work of Cole et al. (18) and focuses on lumbar spine injury, and it indicates the role that the cervical spine plays in the mechanics of lumbar aquatic motion. Analysis of stroke mechanics, such as gait analysis, should be done in an ordered, sequential manner so that all deficits and their relationships are carefully and fully scrutinized. Typically, the analysis begins at the head and progresses distally.

Prone Swimming   During prone swimming the patient's head should be in the mid-line. Breathing should occur by turning the whole body as a unit; the head should not lift or strain into cervical spine extension or rotation. Body roll contributes to proper breathing mechanics and is essential to minimize dysfunctional cervical positioning and subsequent pain. The cervical spine should be kept in the neutral position in the sagittal plane because excessive extension causes the legs and torso to drop in the water, and excessive flexion can cause difficulty in breathing (19,27).

The upper body arm position is evaluated by stroke phase. The freestyle stroke consists of three phases, namely the (a) entry phase, including hand entry and hand submersion ("ride"), (b) pull phase incorporating insweep, outsweep, and finish components, and (c) recovery phase, including the exit and arm swing forward. Swimming programs require that close attention be paid to proper swim stroke biomechanics and to the effect that abnormal mechanics may have on the spine. This attention ensures the most rapid rehabilitation of painful spinal disorders. There are several stroke defects that can cause poor lumbar mechanics in the freestyle (Table 10-1):

- If the arm abducts beyond 180 degrees, lateral lumbar flexion and rotation are produced.
- During the pull phase decreased body rotation can cause lateral lumbar flexion and rotation that stress the lumbar motion segments, in particular the annular fibers of the disc.

Table 10-1   Common Freestyle Stroke Defects and Consequences

PRIMARY PERIPHERAL JOINT STROKE DEFECT	SECONDARY EFFECT	SPINE REACTION
Head high	Lower body sinks	Increased cervical extension Increased lumbar extension
Head low	Upper body sinks	Increased lumbar flexion
Crane breathing	Lower body sinks Contralateral shoulder sinks	Increased cervical and suboccipital extension Increased cervical rotation Increased lumbar lateral flexion and rotation
Cross-over hand entry	Lateral body movement	Increased lumbar lateral flexion and rotation
Wide hand entry	Contralateral shoulder roll	Increased cervical rotation Increased lumbar lateral flexion and rotation
Inefficient pull power	Upper body sinks Difficulty breathing	Increased cervical rotation Increased cervical extension Increased lumbar extension Increased lumbar lateral flexion and rotation
Increased hip flexion	Decreased kick propulsion Lower body sinks	Increased cervical extension Increased lumbar extension Increased lumbar lateral flexion and rotation
Cross-over kick	Decreased kick propulsion Increased hip roll Lower body sinks	Increased cervical extension Increased lumbar extension Increased compensatory lumbar lateral flexion and rotation
Increased knee flexion	Decreased kick propulsion Lower body sinks	Increased cervical extension Increased lumbar extension
Increased ankle dorsiflexion	Decreased kick propulsion Increased hip roll Lower body sinks	Increased cervical extension Increased lumbar extension Increased compensatory lumbar lateral flexion and rotation

SOURCE: Aquatechnics Consulting Group, Inc., Aptos, CA.

- Inadequate strength in the triceps during the finish phase often results in low arm recovery, which in turn generates secondary lateral flexion and rotation through the lumbar spine.
- During recovery inadequate body roll can cause the neck to crane, which results in a struggle for air and accompanying lateral flexion and rotation through the lumbar spine.

Specialized Equipment

Although not essential, certain pieces of equipment can be used advantageously in aquatic exercise programs. A few will now be discussed.

Flotation Devices   A broad range of flotation devices have been developed for aquatic rehabilitation. For central trunk flotation, neoprene vests and foam waist belts are the most commonly used. The Bad Ragaz technique uses foam rings that are placed around the arms and legs or under the head. Kick boards, leg floats, vinyl foam flexible buoys, and combinations of these are all important pieces of the aquatic rehabilitation armamentarium, if a broad base of patients is to be treated.

Resistive Devices   As strengthening proceeds, the natural resistance of the water may be augmented through devices to increase the surface area of the moving part. Finned dumbbells, finned boots, kick boards, and flotation devices may all be used to add resistance to movement.

Performance Measurement Tools   Water is a more challenging environment for the therapist wishing to quantify performance. Waterproof heart rate monitors are useful and relatively inexpensive. Quantifying time, resistance, and movement freedom can add attributes to the treatment program that are essential for accountability, patient perception of accomplishment, and physician feedback. Standardized exercise log sheets can be useful. These sheets are completed during the treatment session and are used to monitor the patient at subsequent visits and at outpatient medical visits. If properly created, they may be used as a clinic progress note, providing support for reimbursement processes.

ARTHRITIC PATIENT

Even though this section centers on the arthritic patient, some of the activities will be most appropriate for some patients with low back pain. The therapist must decide, based on knowledge of the patient and extenuating circumstances, which activities are in the patient's best interest.

Pathology of Arthritis

Rheumatic diseases affect the joints, muscles, and connective tissues of the body and appear to be a result of a complex of interacting mechanical, biologic, biochemical, and enzymatic feedback loops (28). The word *arthritis* literally means "joint inflammation" (29). The precise mechanisms causing these structures to be attacked are not completely understood. They seem to be triggered by factors such as a preceding infectious process, a sudden autoimmune response, and in some cases a response to joint stress. There is considerable individual variation in symptom magnitude, joint involvement, and disease duration. A symptom complex of joint swelling, pain, stiffness, inflammation, and limitation of range of motion is typically produced, irrespective of cause (30).

The two most common forms of arthritis are osteoarthritis and rheumatoid arthritis. Osteoarthritis is a degenerative joint disease in which one or many joints undergo degenerative changes, including loss of articular cartilage, with the subsequent formation of osteophytes. Rheumatoid arthritis is an autoimmune disease that produces acute inflammatory and progressive joint damage. In the case of osteoarthritis, age is the most significant risk factor but, as with many other forms of arthritis, may result from an anatomic or a metabolic predisposition. More commonly, the pathogenesis is simply unknown (31). There are thought to be more than 100 types of arthritis; other examples include ankylosing spondylitis, fibromyalgia, lupus, and juvenile rheumatoid arthritis (32). Most of these are chronic conditions for which there is no definitive cure, but rather a series of medical management options.

Left untreated, the arthritic condition may be progressive and can cause significant impairment and disability. For the great majority of arthritides, medical management can be very helpful in controlling symptom magnitude and disease progression and in reducing disability. The typical approach is to (a) control the underlying disease and reduce symptoms, (b) preserve and maintain function through activity modulation and adaptation, and (c) prevent disability through activity regulation, joint protection, and activities of daily living and lifestyle adjustment.

Demographics of Arthritis

Arthritis is the number one cause of disability and the most common clinical complaint in the United States (33). Recent estimates are that, by the year 2020, 59.4 million Americans, or 18.2% of the country's population, will have some form of arthritis; the current prevalence is 15% (34). The same studies show that nearly 3% of the population is functionally limited by their arthritis. More alarmingly, Guccione (35) stated that 60 million adults in the United States were thought to have some form of osteoarthritis, an estimate much higher than the American Arthritis Foundation has suggested. As the general population ages, this number will continue to rise. Overall, women are more commonly afflicted than men; 23 million of the 40 million who suffer it today are women (30). Arthritis can strike all ages and is almost universal by age 70. Despite advanced technology and current research efforts, arthritis still accounts for 427 million days of lost work annually and is the leading cause of industrial absenteeism in the United States (33).

Disease Effects

The rheumatic diseases share common signs and symptoms including pain, general stiffness, joint inflammation, swelling, and diminished range of motion (36). The primary impairments associated with arthritis are found mainly in the alterations of normal structures and functions of bones, muscles, and joints of the musculoskeletal system. Deformities and loss of function in arthritis are caused by changes in articular and periarticular tissues that are directly or indirectly related to the disease process. Early tissue changes cause pain and stiffness that interfere with movement before there is actual loss of function (37). Muscles and joints tend to become stiff, tense, and weak; tense muscles press on nerve endings, making movements painful and difficult. Persistent pain causes restricted joint motion and inhibition of muscle contraction that results in further loss of joint mobility and disuse atrophy of adjacent muscle groups. This leads to a weakening of the muscles essential to joint protection and to a vicious cycle of lack of activity and loss of function. Inactivity causes substantial weakness and loss of tissue from all elements of the musculoskeletal system. Deficits such as poor endurance and fatigue associated with aerobic deconditioning are viewed as reversible functional losses for the arthritic patient. The weakness associated with arthritis may have multiple origins. Joint effusion has been shown to decrease active strength across the joint (38). Strength may be reduced because of decreased biomechanical integrity, with consequent reflex inhibition of the joint effector muscles; pain-induced inactivity will lead to deconditioning and atrophy (39).

The medical management of arthritis may involve medications such as corticosteroids that create muscle atrophy, even on low dose regimens (40). The arthritic process may involve muscle directly and produce inflammatory myopathy and diminished strength (41). Other causes have also been noted to cause muscle weakness, including nerve involvement, muscle fiber type alteration, and cellular metabolic process changes.

Figure 10-2 shows the vicious cycle that an active arthritic process can develop. These changes include loss of bone, muscle, and connective tissue, a reduction in joint range of motion, muscle strength, endurance, and a marked decline in fitness (42).

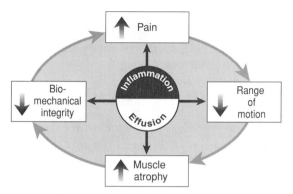

Fig. 10-2 The vicious cycle of joint inflammation.

Exercise and Arthritis

It has often been stated that exercise and rest are the cornerstones of the overall medical management of arthritic diseases. The belief that exercise is an essential part of the management of patients with arthritis dates at least to Roman times. It is not established whether exercise may or may not change the progression of the underlying rheumatic process.

Rheumatoid patients in general have overall muscle strength that is 60% below that of age-matched control subjects and have lower than expected aerobic capacity and physical performance; however, these patients do tolerate carefully structured strengthening and endurance programs and may experience gains in physical performance levels in as brief a time as 6 weeks (43). Long-term exercise regimens over many years in rheumatoid arthritis patients have been proven to be well tolerated, with resultant improvement in functional and other outcome measures (44).

Because patients with arthritis have been shown to have diminished endurance, these individuals should participate in some form of aerobic exercise to enhance their overall fitness. Studies have demonstrated the benefits of aerobic exercise for many conditions including fibromyalgia pain (45), rheumatoid arthritis (46,47), lupus (48), and osteoarthritis (49). Hampson et al. found that arthritic patients participating in exercise programs are more likely to manage their osteoarthritis with low impact exercise than with medications (50).

Because of the properties of the aquatic environment, incorporation of aquatic exercise and/or swimming (forms of low impact exercise) provides an advantageous alternative to manage arthritic symptoms. This contention has been substantiated in two studies of patient groups with nonacute rheumatoid and osteoarthritis participating in water exercise regimes. In a Danish study, Danneskold-Samsoe et al. found markedly increased isometric and isokinetic muscle strength of the quadriceps in rheumatoid subjects after only moderate training in the pool (51). Other gains in-cluded an increase in aerobic capacity, freedom of movement, and a higher degree of self-help in activities of daily living. Bunning and Materson (49) found that pool therapy was both efficacious and achieved high compliance for those with osteoarthritis; they concluded that aquatic exercise should be the cornerstone of treatment for severe arthritis. Patients who participated in the study exhibited significant improvements in aerobic capacity, walk time, and physical activity levels. Furthermore, it was felt that the use of group exercise allowed for increased socialization that counteracted the isolation felt by many arthritic patients. The overall benefits of aquatic exercise programs to the arthritic can include reduction of joint swelling and a decrease in joint stiffness and muscle soreness; this can enhance the opportunities for active motion, improve or maintain range of motion, increase muscle strength, improve coordination, increase endurance, and improve the ability to perform daily tasks.

There are many reasons aquatic therapy programs in a heated pool are an effective application of exercise for the arthritic. Water's unique properties of heat, buoyancy, resistance, and hydrostatic pressure provide a medium where passive and voluntary exercise can be performed with minimal stress. Immersion and exercise in water of therapeutic temperatures (92 to 96°F) facilitates relaxation, lengthening, and strengthening of the muscles, ligaments, and tendons. The following list shows the beneficial effects of heat on arthritic conditions:

1. increased collagen extensibility in tendons (52)
2. decreased joint stiffness (53)
3. pain relief (54)
4. pain threshold elevation (55)
5. muscle spasm relief (56)
6. increased circulation (57)
7. increased diuresis and cell metabolism (58)

Buoyancy offsets body weight and supports painful and weakened structures. When submerged to neck level, body weight is about a tenth of that on land. This can enable individuals with weakness to move comfortably. Those with atrophied muscles can experience complete freedom of movement due to achieved "weightlessness." When a gradation of weight-bearing activities is desired, exercise can begin in deep water where there is no weight bearing on the lower extremities and buoyancy unloads the compressive forces on the spine. For gradual increases in weight bearing, activities can be moved to progressively more shallow water. Patients recovering from lower extremity joint replacement surgery, such as total hip replacement and total knee replacement, benefit tremendously from this approach. Passive range of motion to prevent joint deformities and contractures is much easier to conduct in the aquatic environment. Buoyancy can be structured to assist, support, or resist motions of the extremities or trunk, and ambient body weight is reduced. Furthermore, the viscosity of the water acts as resistance to movement. As turbulence and speed of movement increases, so does the resistance. Lightly resistive aquatic equipment can be used by the arthritic to develop muscle strength and endurance.

Hydrostatic pressure assists in edema reduction. Edema can stretch intraarticular joint structures and produce pressure in the joint capsule. The pressure of periarticular edema is one of the factors that trigger pain with joint movement; this is a key in the initial loss of range of motion and in the development of joint stiffness in the arthritic patient. The benefits available through whirlpool therapy are increased with the larger therapeutic pool, which permits:

1. treatment of multiple joint problems simultaneously

2. deeper immersion in the vertical position
3. heat transference through total body immersion
4. a much broader range of therapeutic exercise
5. swimming for conditioning
6. ambulation training
7. popular spa techniques such as the Bad Ragaz ring method
8. cost-effective group treatments versus more costly one-on-one therapy treatments

Exercise Program

The aquatic environment presents a cost effective and versatile option for occupational and physical therapists to progress and expedite the goals of rehabilitation for a disease as pervasive as arthritis. Medically supervised water therapy interventions are available to the arthritic individual. The primary goals of treatment are the same for most of the rheumatic diseases:

1. mobilization of joints
2. strengthening of muscles
3. conditioning
4. reeducation of function
5. patient education for pacing, joint protection, and disease management
6. instruction in self-directed exercise regimens

Aquatic therapy techniques are not simply adaptations of conventional dry-land therapeutic exercise programs. The aquatic environment allows a different approach for achievement of the above goals for a variety of arthritic conditions. Properties of water that appear to assist rehabilitative goals at each stage of the arthritic process include buoyancy, ability to store heat, pain-reducing properties, and viscous damping properties. The approach is determined by whether the condition is acute, subacute, or chronic, inflammatory or noninflammatory, unifocal or multifocal, in addition to other considerations specific to an individual's diagnosis.

Acute Management   Traditional medical management for acute episodes or flare-ups consisted of rest, immobilization, and medication for pain. However, there has been some evidence that acute rheumatoid patients, who undergo partial weight-bearing water exercise, can decrease joint pain and inflammatory activity (59). This perhaps is due to endorphin release and in part to edema reduction. This suggests that in the acute stages, gentle range of motion, strengthening, and endurance goals can be pursued in the therapeutic pool in addition to the passive benefits of pain relief, muscle relaxation, and decreased joint stresses. Noninvolved joints may be exercised, and joints in a less acute phase may show therapeutic benefit.

In acute flares some modifications of aquatic therapy technique are recommended. These include reducing repetitions to between three and five and positioning to prevent buoyancy (or active patient motions) from forcing the joints into painful ranges of motion. Important in the acute phase of treatment are patient education and cuing for adherence to joint protection principles in the use of equipment, handrails, and grab bars. Because movement is easier in water due to joint off-loading and pain minimization, there can be a tendency to overdo; pacing should be used and sessions kept short to prevent overfatiguing the patient. The patient should be counseled that, if they incur pain persisting for a period of hours or into the next day after treatment, exercise ranges and repetitions should be decreased. In the case of severe cervical joint involvement, a patient may wear a plastizote collar during activity to protect the neck. Use of a mask and snorkel is recommended in prone horizontal activities and swimming to prevent pain, cervical joint hypermobility, or even subluxation. When temperature elevation of more than 1°C is present, admission into the therapeutic pool is generally ill advised.

Subacute Management Treatment programs can include one-on-one techniques with the therapist and more general exercises and activities designed to improve functional capacity. These include passive mobilization and relaxation, buoyancy assisted, supported, or resisted exercise, strength training, conditioning and functional posture, balance, and mobility training. Patients may be positioned in the seated, standing, horizontal supine, or prone flotation set-up positions, or suspended in deep water. Treatment may be carried out on a one-to-one basis or in groups.

Mobilization of Joints Mobilizing joints and stretching muscles, ligaments, and tendons is a common goal for many treatment protocols (60). Range of motion exercises can help maintain joint movement, relieve stiffness, promote synovial fluid production and quality, and restore flexibility. The buoyancy and warmth of the water promote general relaxation and specific relaxation of those muscle groups around painful joints (61). Once in this optimal state, exercise can progress from passive range of motion performed by the therapist to active assistive range of motion, active patient exercise, and then resistive exercise.

Passive Techniques. Mobilization of joints with contractures must involve stretching connective tissue; however, care must be taken not to overstretch periarticular structures that may cause local "flare-ups" (42). It is essential that the therapist control joint mobilization techniques and limit range and activity in a specific joint. The therapist should elicit feedback from the patient about the effects of the previous treatment. After a session of joint mobilization, one can expect the joint to be a little sore for a few hours; however, this should subside within 24 h. A stiff and painful joint must be protected by isolating therapeutic movement through adequate fixation (62). This may mean positioning the patient in a pool chair, on a bench or a water plinth, or working with a patient in a flotation set-up with stabilization being provided by the therapist, such as in the Bad Ragaz ring method. Ranging, joint mobilization, and joint oscillations can then be performed with accuracy. The Halliwick techniques such as rocking, swaying, and snaking may also be incorporated into passive treatment sessions to promote patient relaxation, elongation, and spine traction; this can decrease muscle guarding and splinting before exercise.

Active Assisted Exercise.   In active assisted exercise the individual can move the limb actively but may need some type of aid in moving it through its full range of motion. Treatment programs should begin with one-on-one techniques, with the therapist positioning the patient for utilization of buoyancy and assisting the limb through controlled available joint range of motion. Bad Ragaz ring exercises use proximally controlled handholds and are excellent for this purpose.

Active Exercise.   In active exercise the patient can move the body or body part through the water with control throughout the available joint range of motion. Exercises and activities based on improving functional patterns of motion can be performed independently in specific positioning set-ups or in groups in the shallow end of the pool. The aquatic environment is an optimal one for improving coordination of precise functional motions, with supervision and cuing on the proper use of body mechanics and joint protection. The therapist can see the patient's spinal alignment and movement patterns in functional tasks and the density and viscosity of the water slow movement for observation and analysis. Normal biomechanical alignment may be difficult in the face of spine or joint pain and produce postural deviations. The therapist can provide skilled corrections and modifications of active exercise. From poolside, careful attention to true body position is essential because the refractive properties of the water may create distortion that masks actual body posture. This is especially important in spine stabilization exercises. Calisthenic-type exercises, water walking, deep water exercises, and swimming are modes for active exercise performance.

Resistive Exercise.   Because the body has buoyancy in water, movement is easier because of weight off-loading. Movement, however, becomes more difficult against the resistance presented by the viscosity of the water. This resistance differs depending on such factors as the speed of movement, the surface area of the moving body or body part or equipment additions, and the ambient turbulence of the water. As discussed in Chap. 9, the resistance noted with increasing speed of movement is not linear but rather complex and logarithmic. However, the viscous damping properties of water make the resistance drop almost instantaneously with cessation of effort.

Water offers the arthritic patient the opportunity for protected, subtle, and measurable increases in resistive exercise to increase muscle strength and muscular endurance. When submerged to the neck, the effects of gravity on the joints with impaired integrity are negligible. Muscles can be strengthened through isometric exercises by holding a stable position (a) against the resistance of the water, (b) against turbulence created by the therapist, or (c) while being pushed through the water by the therapist (the last one is an activity of the Bad Ragaz ring method). Isokinetic resistive exercise can be performed by the patient moving the body or limb through water resistance for muscle strengthening. Because the water is a three-dimensional medium, active exercise in any direction is resistive.

There is a wide variety of aquatic exercise equipment available to grade and progress the resistive properties of water. Light weight training of 3 to 10 repetitions to specific muscle groups is indicated to minimize the debilitating effects of many arthritic conditions and for the development and maintenance of lean muscle mass. Graded isokinetic water activities provide a protective medium to accomplish this aim. It is important to slow the speed of movement through the range of motion whenever equipment is added to prevent injury.

The Bad Ragaz ring method and conventional water also prove effective in the treatment of patient weakness (62). Conventional water exercise may use flotation rings that act as added resistance when the patient performs a motion against the force of buoyancy. This method may generate considerable resistance to the muscles, depending on the buoyant object. The exercise effort may be graded by using progressively buoyant objects, through increasing the number of repetitions done in decreasing amounts of time, and through greater arcs of movement. Table 10-2 shows an example of a grid that may be used to quantify progress.

It is quite important to attempt to quantify exercise movement with joint pathology because the patient needs protection against an overload; this requires knowledge of past loads successfully managed. Thus, strength gains are achieved and joint tolerances are monitored. The faster the motion is away from buoyancy or the more air is in the flotation rings, the greater the resistance is to movement. In the Bad Ragaz ring method, the therapist acts as a fixator around which the patient works isometrically, supported by floats in supine, prone, or side-lying positions, while moving in straight or diagonal closed chains of movement. Thus, the arms, trunk, and legs can be strengthened by using a system of resistance progression readily graded by the aquatic therapist trained in this method. When working with patients who have abnormal joint physiology, care must be taken to break the momentum of initiated movements from proceeding too far by the therapist stepping forward into the direction of the joint movement when the movement approaches end ranges.

Aerobic Conditioning

Control of joint loading is paramount to the prevention and slowing of the progression of many arthritic diseases (28). Water provides a safe, versatile, and protective medium for deconditioned individuals to initiate or enhance their cardiovascular capacity. A wide variety of aerobic exercise modes can be conducted in water of different depths. Deep water exercise, in which the patient can be suspended with a flotation belt, saddle, or vest in the vertical position at the water's surface, permits a wide range of non-weight bearing underwater exercise that can be aerobically formatted. Water running, scissor kicks, cross-country skiing movements, abduction/adduction kicks with and without lower extremity water resistance equipment (e.g., fins, Hydrotoner boots) are examples of such workouts. Aerobic conditioning of very high intensity can be accomplished even while protecting injured joints.

Shallow water also offers a range of aerobic workout opportunities such as water walking, water aerobics in which calisthenics are performed in simple straight planes of motion incorporating good body mechanics, and exercising with light resistive aquatic equipment. With adaptations made for adherence to proper postural alignment and joint protection techniques, swimming is yet another aquatic aerobic option. Aquatic aerobic circuits can be designed for specific diagnoses to include functional motions such as squatting to standing, trunk flexion and extension, and ambulation.

Reeducation of Function

Improvement and maintenance of joint flexibility, muscle strength, and cardiovascular conditioning can improve physical capacity that translates into improved function. Restoration of the muscle's

Table 10-2 Clinical Progression

DATE	BUOYANCY OBJECT	NUMBER OF REPETITIONS	ELAPSED TIME (SEC)	MOVEMENT ARC DEGREES
10/1/98	Small barbells	20 extensions	1:20	90–150
10/8/98	Larger barbells	10 extensions	1:15	90–140
10/15/98	Gallon jug	15 extensions	0:55	90–170

normal pattern of movement with freedom from pain is the functional outcome measure by which to judge whether treatment interventions have been effective.

Patient Education

Group exercise classes are cost effective, offer psychological and peer support, and emphasize important patient educational goals. Pacing, joint protection skills, proper body mechanics, pain management, and self-empowering knowledge of exercise theory may all effectively be taught in groups with the end goal of long-term maintenance and independent exercise program adherence (63). Groups such as this may facilitate exercise adherence and decrease health care system utilization with its associated costs.

Certification in the content base is available for interested therapists; training materials are available through the Arthritis Foundation (64). There are 68 range of motion and strengthening exercises and an optional endurance building component. Swimming skills are unnecessary. The certification process is sufficient so that a medical practitioner may generally feel comfortable referring a patient to the program; my experience has been that patient adherence is high, therapeutic value is significant, and cost to the patient is low. The Arthritis Foundation has developed two other programs, PACE (People with Arthritis Can Exercise) and Joint Efforts; PACE is a community-based group program and Joint Efforts is a gentle exercise program for sedentary older adults. Water walking, deep water exercise, and swimming are aerobic modes from which individuals can select for conditioning.

Once discharged from water therapy and rehabilitation programs, those with arthritis should follow some type of functional maintenance program. Recognizing the importance of water exercise for those who suffer from arthritis, the American Arthritis Foundation in cooperation with the YMCA has developed a nationwide program, The Arthritis Aquatics Program. This carefully structured recreational program has incorporated the basic tenets of arthritic precautions so that safe, effective, low cost, and medically sound water exercise programs are available to those who suffer from arthritis.

CONCLUSIONS

The physical properties of water create an ideal environment for the rehabilitation of the spine pain patient, as has been known and practiced since the beginnings of recorded medical therapeutics. Watching the relief upon a patient's face as he or she slips into warm water allows no other conclusion. For the arthritic patient, these physical properties address nearly all the causes of symptoms and allow the patient an opportunity to reduce pain, increase spine flexibility and strength, and preserve and build functional capacity while in a comfortable relaxing medium. The therapeutic options range from simple warm water immersion to passive and active underwater exercise techniques, to skilled hydrotherapeutic interventions by an aquatic therapist in one-on-one or in group treatments, progressing into recreational usage of water for exercise maintenance. The therapeutic margin of safety is exceedingly high, permitting self-directed exercise programs and low cost disease management.

The decline in utilization of the aquatic environment has been to the disadvantage of patients. In a time of scrutiny of health care expenditures, it becomes critical to find safe and inexpensive treatment modalities for common problems. We must find methods that are suitable for self-management regimes, ideally across a large variety of clinical concerns, and that may be easily learned by the patient. These methods should have the added advantages of high patient compliance and consistency. The aquatic environment offers a significant step forward toward these goals. Aquatic therapy is a scientifically grounded and useful approach to a very broad range of rehabilitative problems from acute to chronic; patients find it helpful and pleasurable. Although specific aqua-therapeutic approaches are plentiful, many problems lend themselves to creative aquatic-based solutions. Successful rehabilitation may occur with a high safety margin, with low cost especially when community pools are used, and may use professional extender personnel for group programs, further decreasing cost and increasing adherence (63).

REFERENCES

1. Gatti, C.J., et al. Effect of water-training in the maintenance of cardiorespiratory endurance of athletes. *Br J Sports Med* 1979, 13: p. 162.

2. Avellini, B.A., et al. Cardio-respiratory physical training in water and on land. *Eur J Appl Physiol* 1983, 50: p. 255–263.

3. Svedenhag, J., and J. Seger. Running on land and in water: comparative exercise physiology. *Med Sci Sports Exerc* 1992, 24(10): p. 1158.

4. Hamer, T.W., and A.R. Morton. Water-running: training effects and specificity of aerobic, anaerobic and muscular parameters following an eight-week interval training programme. *Aust J Sci Med Sport* 1990, 22(1): p. 13–22.

5. Borg, G.A.V. Psychophysical bases of perceived exertion. *Med Sci Sports Exerc* 1992, 14(5): p. 377–381.

6. Glass, R.A. Comparative biomechanical and physiological responses of suspended deep water running to hard surface running. Unpublished thesis. 1987, Auburn, AL: Auburn University, PE (3039f).

7. Borg, G.A.V. Perceived exertion as an indicator of somatic stress. *Scand J Rehabil Med* 1970, 2: p. 92–98.

8. Bishop, P.A., et al. Physiological responses to treadmill and water running. *Phys Sports Med* 1989, 17(2): p. 87–94.

9. Wilder, R., and D. Brennan. Physiological responses to deep water running in athletes. *Sports Med* 1993, 16(6): p. 374–380.

10. Harrison, R.A., et al. Loading of the lower limb when walking partially immersed. *Physiotherapy* 1992, 78(3): p. 165–166.

11. Nakazawa, K., et al. Ground reaction forces during walking in water, in *Medicine and Science in Aquatic Sports/10th FINA World Sport Medicine Congress, Medicine and Sport Science, Vol. 39*, M. Miyashita et al., editors. 1994, Basel: S Karger AG. p. 28–35.

12. Gwinup, G. Weight loss without dietary restriction: efficacy of different forms of aerobic exercise. *Am J Sports Med* 1987, 15: p. 275–279.

13. Kieres, J., and S. Plowman. Effects of swimming and land exercises on body composition of college students. *J Sports Med Phys Fitness* 1991, 31: p. 192–193.

14. Minor, M.A., et al. Efficacy of physical conditioning exercise in patients with rheumatoid arthritis and osteoarthritis. *Arthrit Rheum* 1989, 32: p. 1396–1405.

15. Kohrt, W.M., et al. Effects of exercise involving predominantly either joint-reaction or ground-reaction forces on bone mineral density in older women. *J Bone Mineral Res* 1997, 12(8): p. 1253–1261.

16. Cole, A.J., et al. Swimming, in *The Spine in Sports*, R.G. Watkins, editor. 1996, St. Louis: CV Mosby. p. 362–385.

17. LeFort, S.M., and T.E. Hannah. Return to work following an aquafitness and muscle strengthening program for the low back injured. *Arch Phys Med Rehabil* 1994, 75: p. 1247–1255.

18. Cole, A.J., et al. Swimming, in *Spine Care*, A.H. White, editor. 1995, St. Louis: CV Mosby. p. 727–745.

19. Cole, A.J., et al. Getting backs in the swim. *Rehabil Mgmt* 1992, 5: p. 62–71.

20. Cole, A.J., and S.A. Herring. The role of the physiatrist in the management of lumbar spine pain, in *The Handbook of Pain Management*, 2nd ed, D.C. Tollison, editor. 1994, Baltimore: Williams & Wilkins. p. 85–95.

21. Constant, F., et al. Effectiveness of spa therapy in chronic low back pain: a randomized clinical trial. *J Rheumatol* 1995, 22: p. 1315–1320.

22. Eagleston, R. Aquatic stabilization programs. Presented at the Conference on Aggressive Nonsurgical Rehabilitation and Lumbar Spine and Sports Injuries. San Francisco Spine Institute, March 23, 1989.

23. Cole, A., et al. Aquatic therapy of spine pain, in *Comprehensive Aquatic Therapy*, B. Becker and A. Cole, editors. 1997, Newton, MA: Butterworth-Heinemann.

24. Brewster, N.T., and C.R. Howie. That sinking feeling. *Br Med J* 1992, 305: p. 1579–1580.

25. Wilder, R.P., et al. A standard measure for exercise prescription for aqua running. *Am J Sports Med* 1993, 21: p. 45–48.

26. Cole, A.J., et al. Swimming, in *The Spine in Sports*, R.G. Watkins, editor. 1996, St. Louis: CV Mosby. p. 362–385.

27. Maglisco, E. *Swimming Even Faster*. 1993, Sunnyvale: Mayfield Publishing.

28. Reed, K.L. *Quick Reference to Occupational Therapy*. 1991, Maryland: Aspen Publishers, Rockville, MD.

29. Mosby-Year Book, Inc. *Mosby's Medical, Nursing, and Allied Health Dictionary*, 4th ed. Philadelphia: Mosby-Year Book, 1994.

30. Freeman, M.A.R. Operative surgery in rheumatic diseases, in *Clinical Rheumatology*, M. Mason and H.L.F. Curry, editors. 1970, Philadelphia : J.B. Lippincott.

31. Robinson, D. Osteoarthritis, in *Scientific American Medicine*, M.E. Rubenstein and D.D. Federman, editors. 1994, New York: Scientific American. p. 1–10.

32. Verbrugge, L.M., and D.L. Patrick. Seven chronic conditions and their impact on U.S. adults' activity levels and use of medical services. *Am J Public Health* 1995, 85(2): p. 173–182.

33. Marmer, L. Preparing for the arthritis epidemic. *O.T. Advance* 1995, 11(4).

34. Center for Disease Control. *CDC, Morbidity & Mortality World Report* June 24, 1994.

35. Guccione, A.A. Arthritis and the process of disablement. *Phys Ther* 1994, 74: p. 408–413.

36. Caspers, J., and E. Ostle. Osteoarthritis and rheumatoid arthritis, in *Occupational Therapy with the Elderly*, M. Helm, editor. 1987, New York: Churchill Livingstone. p. 31–42.

37. Instill, J. Reconstructive surgery and rehabilitation of the knee, in *Arthritis and Related Disorders*, W.M. Kelly et al., editors. 1981, Philadelphia: W.B. Saunders.

38. deAndre, J.R., et al. Joint distension and reflex muscle inhibition in the knee. *J Bone Joint Surg (Am)* 1965, 47: p. 313–322.

39. Herbison, G.J., et al. Muscle atrophy in rheumatoid arthritis. *J Rheumatol* 1987, 14(suppl 15): p. 78.

40. Danneskold-Samsoe, B., and G. Grimby. The relationship between leg muscle strength and physical capacity in patients with rheumatoid

arthritis with reference to the influence of corticosteroids. *Clin Rheumatol* 1986, 5: p. 468.

41. Hicks, J.E. Exercise in patients with inflammatory arthritis and connective tissue disease. *Rheum Dis Clin North Am* 1990, 16: p. 845–870.

42. Swezey, R.L. Rehabilitation aspects in arthritis, in *Arthritis and Related Disorders*, 9th ed, D.J. McCarty, editor. 1979, Philadelphia : Lea and Febiger.

43. Beals, C. A case for aerobic conditioning exercise in rheumatoid arthritis (abstract). *Clin Res* 1981, 29: p. 780A.

44. Nordemar, R. Physical training in rheumatoid arthritis: a controlled long-term study. II. Functional capacity and general attitudes. *Scand J Rheumatol* 1981, 10 : p. 25–30.

45. McCain, G. Non-medical treatment in primary myalgia. *Rheum Dis Clin North Am* 1989, 15: p. 73–90.

46. Ekdahl, C., et al. Dynamic versus static training in patients with rheumatoid arthritis. *Scand J Rheumatol* 1990, 19: p. 17–26.

47. Perlman, S.G., et al. Synergistic effects of exercise and problem solving education for rheumatoid arthritis patients. *Arthrit Rheum* 1987, 30(suppl): p. S13.

48. Robb-Nicholson, C., et al. Effects of aerobic conditioning in lupus fatigue: a pilot study. *Br J Rheumatol* 1989, 28 : p. 500–505.

49. Bunning, R.D., and R.S. Materson. A rational program of exercise for patients with osteoarthritis. *Semin Arthrit Rheum* 1991, 21(3, suppl 2): p. 33–43.

50. Hampson, S.E., et al. Self management of osteoarthritis. *Arthrit Care Res* 1993, 6(1): p. 17–22.

51. Danneskold-Samsoe, B., et al. The effects of water exercise therapy given to patients with rheumatoid arthritis. *Scand Rehabil Med* 1987, 19: p. 31–35.

52. Gersten, J.W. Effects of ultrasound on tendon extensibility. *Am J Phys Med* 1955, 34: p. 362–369.

53. Bucklund, L., and P. Tiselius. Objective measurement of joint stiffness in rheumatoid arthritis. *Acta Rheum Scand* 1967, 13: p. 275–288.

54. Harris, E., Jr., and P.A. McCroskery. The influence of temperature and fibril stability on degradation of cartilage collagen by rheumatoid synovial collagenase. *N Engl J Med* 1974, 290: p. 1–6.

55. Benson, T.B., and E.P. Copp. The effects of therapeutic forms of heat and ice on the pain threshold of the normal shoulder. *Rheumatol Rehabil* 1974, 13: p. 101–104.

56. Don Figny, R., and K. Sheldon. Simultaneous use of heat and cold in the treatment of muscle spasm. *Arch Phys Med Rehabil* 1962, 43: p. 235–237.

57. Harris, P.R. Iontophoresis: clinical research in musculoskeletal inflammatory conditions. *J Orthop Sports Phys Ther* 1982, 4: p. 109–112.

58. Epstein, M. Renal effects of head out immersion in humans: a 15-year update. *Physiol Rev* 1992, 72(3): p. 563–621.

59. Scott, D.L. Rest or exercise in inflammatory arthritis. *Br J Hosp Med* 1992, 48(8): p. 445.

60. Melvin, J.L. Rheumatic *Disease: Occupational Therapy and Rehabilitation.* 1980, Philadelphia: F.A.Davis.

61. Pennington, F.C. Water exercise can provide relief for people with arthritis. *Dealer News* 1990, p. 19.

62. Harrison, R.A. Hydrotherapy in arthritis. *Practitioner* 1972, 208: p. 132–135.

63. Becker, B.E. Motivating adherence in the rehabilitation setting. *Back Musculoskel Med* 1991, 1(3): p. 37–48.

64. The National Arthritis Foundation, 1330 W. Peachtree, Atlanta GA 30309. Information regarding the nearest Arthritis Aquatic program may be located through the Arthritis Info-line at 1-800-283-7800.

CHAPTER 11

CONSIDERATIONS FOR THE DEVELOPMENT OF BACK EXTENSOR MUSCLE STRENGTH

James E. Graves

John M. Mayer

INTRODUCTION

Soft tissue weakness is often mentioned as a primary risk factor for low back pain (LBP) (1). As a result, the lumbar extensor musculature is considered by some to be the weak link in the kinetic chain that makes many individuals susceptible to LBP. This is not surprising when one considers the general kinesiology of the extensor muscles of the lower back.

The lumbar extensor musculature consists of two muscle groups: the erector spinae and the multifidus (2). Together, the erector spinae and multifidus muscles of the low back are often referred to as the *lumbar paraspinal muscles*. The erector spinae group, which lies lateral to the multifidus, is divided into the iliocostalis lumborum and longissimus thoracis muscles (3). These muscles are separated from each other by the lumbar intramuscular aponeurosis, with the longissimus lying medially (4). The longissimus and iliocostalis are comprised of several multisegmental fascicles (5) that allow for sagittal rotation (extension) and posterior translation when the muscles are contracted bilaterally. The fascicular arrangement of the multifidus muscle suggests that it acts primarily as a sagittal rotator (extension without posterior translation). Lateral flexion and axial rotation are possible for both the multifidus and erector spinae musculature during unilateral contraction (2,6). Because of these anatomic and biomechanical properties, it has been suggested that the lumbar extensor musculature is particularly adapted to maintain posture (7) and stabilize the spine and trunk (7,8). Whether these muscles are well suited for load bearing is a debatable issue.

MORPHOLOGY OF THE LUMBAR MUSCULATURE

Fiber type of the lumbar extensors is well documented from samples resected from patients during lumbar disc surgery and from "healthy" cadavers. For many years it has been reported that the type II (fast twitch) fibers of the erector spinae

and multifidus muscles in back pain patients are smaller than usual (9–12). Thus, the term *selective type II fiber atrophy* has been used in the literature to describe the back muscles of chronic back pain patients (9–12). This characterization has been based on the comparison of type II fibers of the back extensors with those of other skeletal muscle groups and by comparing the size of the type II fibers of the back with the type I (slow twitch) fibers of the back. Zhu et al. (10) reported a mean type IIa fiber cross-sectional area that was smaller than the type IIa fibers of a typical extremity skeletal muscle. Mattila et al. (9) found that the type II muscle fibers were significantly smaller than the type I fibers in the multifidus muscle of patients with lumbar disc herniation.

Mattila et al. (9) also analyzed the multifidus muscle fibers of "healthy" cadavers and patients with disc lesions and found no significant differences in type II fiber cross-sectional area, percentage of type II fibers, and percentage of area occupied by the type II fibers. Other investigators have reported relatively small type II fibers in "healthy" cadavers, raising the possibility that small type II fibers in the back extensor musculature are not necessarily indicative of pathology (13,14). Because generalizations made from cadaveric muscles are limited and back muscle biopsies from normal living populations have been avoided, normative data for lumbar muscle fiber characteristics have not been established.

Recently, Mannion et al. (15) evaluated the fiber type characteristics of the erector spinae muscles in a living, healthy population. They obtained muscle biopsies from the erector spinae musculature at L3 from 31 healthy and physically active men and women. The investigators stated in this report that the relatively small size of the type II fibers of the erector spinae (when compared with other skeletal muscle groups) may be attributed to a sedentary lifestyle. More importantly, they suggested that the small type II fibers should not be considered abnormal or pathognomonic for low back disorders (15). However, one cannot ignore the fact that functional capacity (strength) is correlated with muscle fiber size. Therefore, these findings (15) may only indicate that most of us are walking around with weak backs. Such weakness may help to explain the high incidence of LBP.

A follow-up study by Mannion et al. (16) examined the fiber type characteristics of the erector spinae and multifidus muscles in 21 patients with LBP and 21 healthy control subjects who were matched for age, sex, and body mass. The mean size of any given fiber type was not different between the patients and control subjects. However, the lumbar muscles of the patients had a higher proportion of type IIb fibers than did those of the control subjects. Therefore, the relative area of the muscle occupied by type IIb fibers was higher in the patients than in the control subjects. This finding is in agreement with research on other skeletal muscle groups, indicating that the percentage of type IIb fibers is associated with injury and inactivity (17). Mannion et al. (16) concluded that the lumbar extensor muscles of LBP patients display a more glycolytic profile than do healthy control subjects, which makes them less resistant to fatigue. If "selective type II atrophy" is associated with the lumbar musculature of LBP patients (as previously described), one would expect the relative area occupied by type I fibers to be greater in LBP patients than in healthy control subjects. However, the findings of Mannion et al. (16) do not support this expectation and appear to indicate the contrary. Of course, we do not know the fiber type characteristics of the LBP patients before their LBP.

PHYSIOLOGIC CONSIDERATIONS: FUNCTIONAL CAPACITY

The functional capacity of skeletal muscle is usually quantified by measures of muscular strength and endurance. *Muscular strength* refers to the ability to generate force during a single muscle action. *Muscular endurance* is the ability to resist fatigue during repeated muscle actions (18).

The relationship between morphologic and physiologic characteristics of the lumbar musculature and low back extension strength has been explored extensively with isometric strength testing procedures. The mean fiber size of the erector spinae muscles is positively correlated ($r = 0.60$, $p = 0.05$) with isometric trunk extension strength (19,20). It has been estimated that the absolute strength of the erector spinae is approximately 48 N/cm^2, based on cross-sectional area and morphologic analyses (21). Mean values for isometric trunk extension strength while standing have been reported to be between 675 and 1034 N for males and between 410 and 823 N for females (20). Furthermore, males are stronger than females even after total body mass and lean body mass are taken into consideration (20). This is consistent with sex comparisons of the relative strength of other muscle groups located in the upper body and is likely due to the fact that men as opposed to women contain a greater proportion of lean mass in the upper body (22). Patients with LBP have been shown to have lower trunk extension strength values than healthy individuals (23–28). However, the force generated during maximum voluntary contraction of the trunk extensors has failed to be a predictive factor for future incidences of LBP (29).

Morphologic and histochemical characteristics of the lumbar extensor musculature are also related to isometric trunk extension endurance (resistance to fatigue). The relative area of the erector spinae muscle occupied by type I fibers has a significant positive correlation to static endurance (isometric holding) time ($p = 0.05$) (30). The lumbar extensor muscles also have higher endurance times at various levels of submaximal forces than do other skeletal muscles (20). In addition, women as opposed to men have approximately 33% greater endurance times during a prone isometric test (30–33). Lower endurance values for patients with LBP have been reported (31,33,34), and, unlike maximum voluntary contraction, endurance values have been predictive of future incidences of LBP (31,33). Therefore, the prescription of resistance exercise for the prevention and rehabilitation of LBP should probably focus on the development of muscular endurance (lower load, higher repetitions) as opposed to muscular strength (higher load, lower repetitions).

PHYSIOLOGIC CONSIDERATIONS: EXERCISE TRAINING

A common belief within the exercise and rehabilitation communities is that conditioning the trunk flexors (abdominal musculature) should be the highest priority for exercise training protocols designed to relieve back pain. This belief arises from the theory that strengthening the abdominal muscles will increase intraabdominal pressure and also maintain a favorable balance between the strength of the abdominal muscles and the back extensors. Increasing intraabdominal pressure diminishes compressive forces on the spine and reduces the load on the intervertebral discs and posterior spinal structures (35). However, studies have shown that intraabdominal pressure does not increase during contraction of the abdominals (36). Furthermore, it is not increased after an abdominal strength-training program (36). Thus, focusing on abdominal strength and excluding the rest of the trunk musculature is probably not an effective strategy for the prevention and rehabilitation of LBP. As discussed in Chap. 1, the lateral abdominals are important for trunk stabilization during a variety of activities. Therefore, although strengthening the trunk flexors may not be the highest priority, these important muscles should not be overlooked.

Current evidence suggests that it is weakness in the lumbar musculature (possibly resulting from disuse) and not weak abdominals that is closely linked to LBP. Weak and highly fatigable trunk extensor muscles have been consistently reported in LBP populations (4,6,8,26,37–39). Low back pain sufferers also have a decreased ratio of trunk extensor to trunk flexor strength compared with asymptomatic individuals (40,41). Furthermore, morphologic changes, such as atrophy of the lumbar multifidus and erector spinae muscles, have been reported in patients with acute and chronic LBP (42). Morphologic changes to the lumbar extensors often persist long after the remission of symptoms from the first episode of back pain, leaving the individual at risk for future pathology (43). In vitro studies, for example, have shown that mul-tifidus dysfunction results in intersegmental instability and excessive vertebral rotation (8) and may lead to facet capsulitis, arthrosis of the facet joint, annular tears, disc herniation, and spondylosis (6).

It is for these reasons that spinal rehabilitation programs often attempt to incorporate back extensor muscle conditioning exercises. Progressive resistance training regimens involving the low back extensor muscles have been successful with respect to increased cross-sectional area of the lumbar extensors (43,44), decreased fatty infiltration of the lumbar extensors (27), increased strength (24,28, 44–47), increased endurance (48,49), decreased pain (24,28,49,50), improved psychosocial function (28), decreased rates of future spinal surgery (51), and reduction in lost work time (28,46,47) reported after training in chronic LBP patients. Recently, the United States Agency for Health Care Policy and Research concluded that back extensor muscle conditioning exercises are helpful in the management of LBP (52).

Although the lumbar extensors appear to be the weak link in the development of LBP (as opposed to the trunk flexors), it is our firm belief that conditioning of all of the major muscle groups is important for the development of overall functional capacity and the health benefits associated with physical activity. Therefore, although the lumbar extensors should be targeted for the prevention and rehabilitation of LBP, a well-rounded exercise program that incorporates a variety of progressive resistance exercises should be practiced by everyone.

Potential for Change

Progressive resistance exercise training with pelvic stabilization on a lumbar dynamometer effectively develops functional capacity in both healthy and LBP patient populations. Pollock et al. (53) found that 10 weeks of dynamic progressive resistance training was capable of increasing isometric lumbar extension strength from 42 to 102%. Surprisingly, the subjects in that study trained just once a week and with a low training volume (one set, 8 to 12 repetitions to volitional exhaustion). A follow-up study indicated that a training frequency of one time per week was as effective as training two and three times per week in developing isometric lumbar extension strength (54). Furthermore, after achieving strength gains from this relatively low training frequency, reduced training frequencies as low as one time every 4 weeks allow maintenance of the lumbar extension strength gains (55) for up to 3 months.

The lumbar extensor muscles exhibit morphologic changes (hypertrophy) that exceed those found in other muscle groups after a low volume of training. A 5 to 8% increase in cross-sectional area of the erector spinae musculature has been visualized after a 12-week resistance training program of one exercise session per week (56,57), whereas a 15% increase in cross-sectional area has been noted after training at a frequency of three times per week (56). The greater increases in cross-sectional area associated with more frequent training raises interesting and important questions about the prescription of lumbar extension exercise for the prevention of LBP. Low volume (one set), low frequency (one time per week) training is likely associated with significant neural (learning) adaptations (56). If improving the structural integrity of the vulnerable area through morphologic adaptation is important, more frequent training may be advantageous, even though functional measures (isometric strength) are identical between low frequency and more frequent training.

The relatively large strength gains (versus gains reported after training with other skeletal muscle groups) (58) associated with a low volume of exercise have been attributed to a low initial trained state of the low back extensor muscles (53). Because there is little pelvic stabilization during normal activities of daily living, the lumbar muscles rarely experience an overload stimulus sufficient to elicit strength gains (54). Thus, the powerful gluteus maximus and hamstring muscles, instead of the smaller lumbar paraspinals, may be responsible for the majority of torque generation during compound trunk extension. The postulation of a low initial trained state of the lumbar extensors is supported by histochemical data that

have shown smaller type II fibers in the lumbar extensor muscles as opposed to other skeletal muscles (13,15,16,30).

Pelvic Stabilization

It has been suggested that isolating the lumbar area through pelvic stabilization eliminates the contribution of the gluteal and hamstring muscle groups during exercise training, thereby allowing the lumbar extensor muscles to receive the stimulus necessary for strength gains (53). To test this hypothesis, the effect of pelvic stabilization during resistance training on lumbar extension strength was investigated by several researchers. In a 12-week training study by Graves et al. (59), exercise training with pelvic stabilization (PSTAB) on a lumbar extension dynamometer (MedX, Ocala, FL) was compared with exercise training without pelvic stabilization (NOSTAB) on other machines (Cybex, Ronkonkoma, NY; or Nautilus, Dallas, TX). All training groups exhibited significant increases in dynamic exercise load, but only PSTAB showed an increase in isometric lumbar extension strength. The researchers concluded that pelvic stabilization is required during training to strengthen the lumbar extensor muscles. However, they stated that there may have been specificity of testing and training issues related to the testing machine in the study because the PSTAB group exercised on the lumbar extension dynamometer used to obtain criterion measures, whereas the NOSTAB groups did not (59).

To minimize these exercise specificity issues, Mayer et al. (60) completed a study that allowed both the PSTAB and NOSTAB groups to train on the same lumbar extension dynamometer that was used for the isometric strength tests. In this study, isometric strength tests were performed by 33 healthy subjects with and without the pelvis stabilized on the dynamometer before training. Interestingly, lumbar extension torque values were similar for the stabilized and unstabilized tests at five of the seven angles of lumbar flexion tested. The unstabilized test produced higher torque values than the stabilized test only at the two most extended angles in the range of motion (0 and 12 degrees). After 12 weeks of progressive resistance exercise, both the PSTAB and NOSTAB groups increased lumbar extension isometric torque output during the test with the pelvis stabilized. However, only the NOSTAB group increased torque output in the unstabilized test. The investigators concluded that pelvic stabilization during testing of lumbar muscle function may not be as important as once thought. In addition, they stated that training with pelvic stabilization on the dynamometer is not necessary to increase lumbar extension strength and that training without pelvic stabilization on the dynamometer is more versatile. Training without stabilization may be more closely correlated with performance of normal activities (unstabilized).

In support of the study by Mayer et al. (60), Parkkola et al. (61) reported that training on a low back machine (Nautilus, Inc, Independence, VA), which makes little to no attempt to stabilize the pelvis, was successful in increasing back extension strength and the cross-sectional area of the lumbar extensor muscles. In addition, Lee et al. (62) reported that exercise on a Roman chair (Fig. 11-1) or lumbar dynamometer (Fig. 11-2) was successful in increasing back extension static endurance times on the Roman chair and isometric torque values on the dynamometer after 4 weeks of training by healthy, sedentary subjects and by female volleyball players.

Fujita et al. (63) compared 12 weeks of exercise training on a dynamometer with straight-leg dead lifts and Roman chair exercise. Outcomes were assessed using all exercise techniques and included a seven-angle isometric lumbar extension torque test on a dynamometer, a five repetition maximum (5-RM) test on a Roman chair, and a dead lift. After training, all groups showed significant improvement in the 5-RM test on the Roman chair and the dead lift ($p < 0.05$). The dynamometer group improved significantly at all angles of lumbar flexion during the seven-angle isometric torque test ($p < 0.05$). The dead lift group increased at 0, 12, 60, and 72 degrees of lumbar flexion. The Roman chair group did not increase their isometric torque output at any angle of lumbar flexion measured on the dynamometer ($p > 0.05$). The investigators con-

cluded that the Roman chair is not effective for increasing lumbar extension strength when testing is performed on a dynamometer. Mayer et al. (60) also reported no gain in isometric torque production on a dynamometer after 12 weeks of training with a Roman chair. The findings of these studies contradict the finding by Lee et al. (62) that Roman chair training can develop lumbar extension torque output on the dynamometer. The lack of improvement with Roman chair training in two of the three studies discussed above suggests that there may be significant specificity of testing and training effects associated with measures of functional capacity obtained when using a lumbar dynamometer.

These studies indicate that the need for pelvic stabilization during lumbar extension testing and

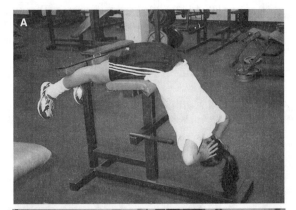

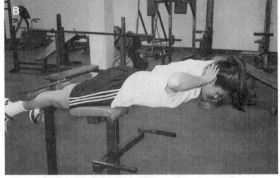

Fig. 11-1 The conventional Roman chair as used for back extension. Subject is shown in the flexed **(A)** and extended **(B)** positions in the range-of-motion.

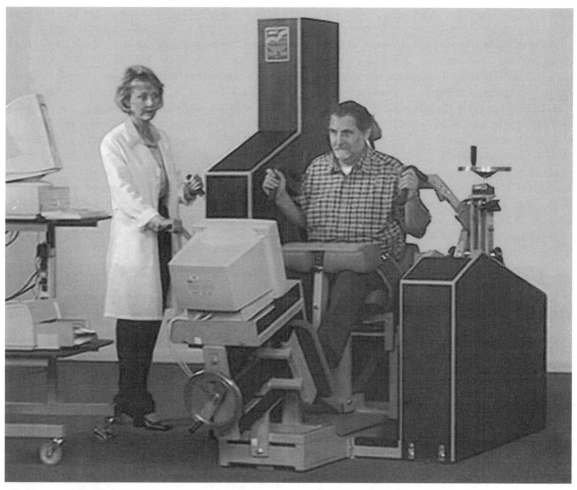

Fig. 11-2 The MEDX dynamometer. An advantage of this dynamometer is that it permits an accurate measurement of the strength of the paraspinal muscles because the contribution of the hip extensors is minimized. (*Courtesy of Med X*, Ocala, FL).

training is inconclusive and perhaps not as important as once thought. Intuitively, stabilization is essential for the isolation of specific muscle groups during progressive resistance exercise training. It is important to recognize, however, that individual muscles rarely work in isolation in the real world. The trade-off between the need to isolate a muscle to achieve maximum training benefit and the ability of a muscle to work in concert with other muscle groups to produce patterned movements will be debated for some time.

The feasibility of widespread clinical or home use of lumbar extension dynamometers has been limited by the expense and lack of portability of these machines, despite their clinical efficacy (64). Furthermore, the high cost of dynamometric methods (65–68) and the unusual posture often required for testing has put into question the true benefits of the various sophisticated dynamometric devices. In addition, the seated upright posture, which is necessary for the performance of lumbar extension exercise on some dynamometers, is associated with increased compressive forces on the spine and lumbar discs (69) and may be detrimental for some patients with LBP. However, at present, there are no known low cost, low tech alternatives to safely and effectively measure the functional capacity of the lumbar extensor musculature.

Stationary Roman chair machines, such as 45- and 90-degree benches, are unable to provide a level of resistance that is appropriate for clinical back pain populations. The lightest load for resistance on a Roman chair depends on upper body mass, which is frequently greater than the patient's initial functional capacity. In addition, the loading characteristics attributed to upper body mass through the range of trunk extension have not been determined (64).

PHYSIOLOGIC CONSIDERATIONS: ELECTROMYOGRAPHY

Electromyography (EMG) has been used extensively to quantify skeletal muscle activity associated with resistance exercise. Moritani and De Vries (70) evaluated surface integrated EMG activity (iEMG) of the elbow flexor muscles during isometric exercise and found a linear relationship between iEMG and isometric torque production, with a highly significant correlation ($r = 0.99$, $p < 0.05$). A similar relationship has been observed for the lumbar extensors (71).

Electromyography of the Lumbar Musculature

Whereas the strength and endurance characteristics of back pain sufferers are fairly well understood, the activation patterns of the lumbar muscle groups are less clear. Comparisons of surface EMG activity of the lumbar paraspinals during exercise and at rest between patients with LBP and healthy control subjects have produced conflicting results. Studies have found increased activity (72), decreased activity (73), and no difference in activity (3,71) of the lumbar paraspinal muscles in LBP patients and healthy control subjects. A disappearance of the

flexion-relaxation phenomena in patients with LBP (74–76) suggests increased lumbar muscle activity. However, chronic LBP patients studied with magnetic resonance image have displayed significantly lower signal intensity increases on T2-weighted magnetic resonance images of the lumbar extensors after Roman chair exercise than have healthy subjects (77), suggesting decreased activity. The situation is further complicated by other EMG activity studies that have observed bilateral asymmetry of lumbar muscle activity in some patients (78).

Historically, lumbar muscle function has been commonly evaluated by surface or needle EMG. Technical limitations associated with surface EMG, such as lack of reliability (79), inability to provide an indication of specific muscle patterns (80), variability in signals from electrode type and placement (81), variability associated with subcutaneous tissue (82), confounding of the myoelectric signal by cross talk between muscles (83), and the invasiveness of needle EMG, limit the ability to make definitive conclusions about muscle function from EMG. Despite these limitations, EMG has remained the procedure of choice to evaluate low back muscle activity during exercise and lifting tasks, and many researchers consider surface EMG representative of the "neural drive" to a given area. The following paragraphs highlight the research that has described the EMG activity of the lumbar musculature during exercise.

Tan et al. (84) evaluated the effects of trunk position on surface EMG activation of the lumbar musculature during isometric contractions while standing and found that the erector spinae muscles are significantly more active in the flexed postures. This finding is consistent with research using the lumbar extension dynamometer, which has shown that isometric torque output is linear and descends from 72 to 0 degrees of lumbar flexion (53). While standing with the trunk fully flexed, the lumbar paraspinal muscles exhibit a reduction in EMG activity. This phenomenon is commonly referred to as the *flexion-relaxation response* (76) and has been attributed to the elastic properties of the muscles and posterior vertebral connective tissues (75). In addition, the passive torque production commonly seen during full trunk flexion when the lumbar muscles are electrically silent has been explained by these elastic properties (85).

Udermann et al. (86) evaluated the influence of pelvic restraint during back extension exercise on EMG activation of the hamstring, gluteal, and lumbar extensor muscles with a lumbar extension dynamometer. In this study, 12 men completed two dynamic lumbar extension exercises of 12 repetitions, with a load equaling 80% of body weight. One exercise was performed with the pelvic stabilization mechanisms intact and one was performed with the stabilization mechanisms removed. No difference in EMG activity was observed between the restrained and unrestrained conditions in any of the muscle groups ($p > 0.05$). This finding supports the conclusion of Mayer et al. (60) that pelvic stabilization during training is not required for the recruitment of the lumbar musculature or for increases in lumbar extension strength.

Lee et al. (62) found that surface EMG mean power frequency patterns of muscle fatigue on a Roman chair isometric endurance test decreased after 4 weeks of resistance training on both a lumbar dynamometer and Roman chair (16.8% versus 15.2%, respectively). The investigators used these data to suggest that exercise on the Roman chair affects the lumbar extensor muscles in a fashion similar to exercise on the dynamometer.

Kearns et al. (87) also evaluated lumbar extension muscle activation during isolated (stabilized) and nonisolated (unstabilized) lumbar extension exercises. Twelve male subjects completed two dynamic repetitions at 50% and 90% of their 1-RM on a lumbar dynamometer with its pelvic restraint mechanisms intact, a Roman chair, and straight-leg dead lifts. Surface EMG activity was recorded from the gluteal, hamstring, and erector spinae musculature during exercise. At 50% of the 1-RM, erector spinae muscle activation was significantly higher during Roman chair exercise than during dynamometer and dead lift exercises. At 90% of the 1-RM, erector spinae activation was significantly higher during exercises on the Roman chair and dynamometer than during dead lifts, with no significant difference between the Roman chair and

dynamometer. Gluteal and hamstring activation at 50% and 90% of the 1-RM was greater during the Roman chair exercise than during the dynamometer and dead lift exercises. The investigators concluded that the differences in lumbar extensor muscle activation between exercises on the Roman chair and dynamometer may be due to loading differences attributed to the counterweight on the dynamometer designed to offset torso mass.

The 1-RM for the Roman chair and dead lift exercises in the study by Kearns et al. (87) was determined by placing hand-held metal plates against the chest and gripping a barbell, respectively, and performing a dynamic repetition. Fifty percent and 90% of the weight of the hand-held metal plates and barbell, respectively, were used for the EMG analyses. The load attributed to upper body mass was not taken into consideration for Roman chair and dead lift exercises. Therefore, the actual loads for these two exercises probably exceeded 50% and 90% of the true 1-RM, and EMG comparisons with exercise on the dynamometer were likely not valid. However, this study still provided useful information by noting that similar muscles groups, namely the lumbar extensors, were active during trunk extension exercise on both the Roman chair and dynamometer.

Efficacy of the Variable Angle Roman Chair (Fig. 11-3)

A back extension machine has recently been developed to allow for the performance of progressive resistance exercise in a relatively inexpensive and portable manner. This lumbar extension machine (BackStrong International, Rego Park, NY) is a variable angle Roman chair (VARC) that can be adjusted from 75 degrees relative to horizontal to 0 degrees relative to horizontal in 15-degree increments. As the angle from horizontal decreases on the VARC, the load applied to the low back extensor muscles increases (64). Specifically, the surface EMG activity of the lumbar paraspinal muscles during exercise increases progressively and consecutively between all six angles, from 75 to 0 degrees. Furthermore, lumbar paraspinal EMG activity

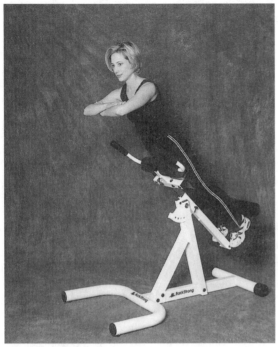
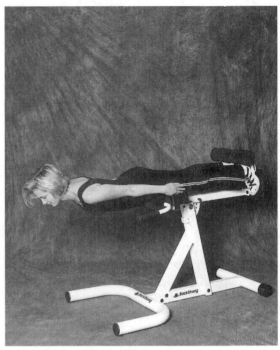

A   **B**

Fig. 11-3 The variable angle Roman chair. Although this piece of equipment can replicate a standard Roman chair **(A)**, the muscular requirements are changed if it is positioned as shown in **(B)**. (Trunk is close to vertical in starting position; ending position is depicted in both **A** and **B**). (*Courtesy of Backstrong International*, Rego Park, NY).

increases progressively during VARC exercise by positioning the subject's hands and arms farther away from the axis of rotation in the lower lumbar spine. Because there is a strong positive linear relationship between the magnitude of EMG activity observed and the amount of muscle mass recruited during exercise (70,88), the VARC is capable of providing a mechanism for progressive resistance lumbar extension exercise (64).

Although the VARC appears to allow for variable loading, the device lacks the sophistication to quantify load in a classic sense. Furthermore, it is not known whether progressive resistance exercise training on the VARC can accommodate the increases in training load necessary for strength gains. Therefore, there is a need for mechanisms to accurately quantify load during back extension exercise on the VARC and other Roman chair devices and during exercise training on these devices.

RECOMMENDATIONS FOR THE PRESCRIPTION OF RESISTANCE EXERCISES

The American College of Sports Medicine (ACSM) has established guidelines for the prescription of resistance exercises for the development and maintenance of muscular strength and muscular endurance (89). These guidelines recommend a minimum of one set of 8 to 12 repetitions to volitional fatigue, at least two times per week. These guidelines are appropriate for resistance training of the lumbar musculature. It is important to recognize that certain exercises are contraindicated in many pathologic conditions. Individuals with LBP should consult their physician before beginning an exercise program. In general, the guidelines established by ACSM (89) are appropriate for people with LBP with the following considerations:

1. Initial level of fitness in patients with LBP is often low. Appropriate resistance should be selected to allow a minimum of 8 to 12 repetitions.

2. Although rehabilitation programs will often target the weak lumbar musculature, a well-rounded exercise program that incorporates exercises for the development of muscular strength and muscular endurance of all the major muscle groups is recommended.

3. Because the lumbar extensor muscles are not significantly recruited during many trunk extension activities, careful attention should be given to incorporating appropriate exercises specifically for the low back. Lumbar extension dynamometers and Roman chair exercise machines have both been shown to actively recruit the lumbar extensors during trunk extension exercise. Stabilization of the pelvis may be required to maximize improvement in functional capacity. More research is needed to document the efficacy of alternative exercise devices.

Muscular strength and endurance represent just two components of physical fitness. Exercises for the development of aerobic capacity, flexibility, and a healthy body composition should be included.

SUMMARY

Low back pain is one of the most common and costly medical problems in our society. Although the specific role of exercise in the prevention and rehabilitation of LBP is uncertain, many causes of LBP have been attributed to poor physical conditioning. Muscular strength and muscular endurance of the lumbar extensor muscles can be improved with properly prescribed progressive resistance exercise using lumbar dynamometers or Roman chair devices. Because the lumbar extensor muscles work in conjunction with gluteal and hamstrings when performing the normal activities of daily living, the lumbar muscles rarely encounter an overload stimulus sufficient to develop good functional capacity. Some attention to stabilization during lumbar extension exercise may be required

for the most effective improvements. In addition to the development of lumbar muscle strength and endurance to overcome structural weakness, a well-rounded exercise program that involves resistance training exercises for all of the major muscle groups and aerobic exercise for the development of cardiovascular conditioning and activities that promote flexibility are important.

REFERENCES

1. Pollock, M., et al. Muscle, in *Rehabilitation of the Spine: Science and Practice*, S. Hochschuler, et al., editors. 1993, St. Louis: Mosby. p. 263–284.

2. Bogduk, N., and L. Twomey. *Clinical Anatomy of the Lumbar Spine*. 1990, New York: Churchill Livingstone.

3. Bogduk, N. A reappraisal of the anatomy of the human lumbar erector spinae. *J Anat* 1980, 131(3): p. 525–540.

4. MacIntosh, J., and N. Bogduk. The morphology of the lumbar erector spinae. *Spine* 1987, 12(7): p. 658–668.

5. MacIntosh, J., and N. Bogduk. The attachments of the lumbar erector spinae. *Spine* 1991, 16(7): p. 783–792.

6. Kirkaldy-Willis, W., editor. *Managing Low Back Pain*, 2nd ed. 1988, New York: Churchill Livingstone.

7. Kalimo, H., et al. Lumbar muscles: stucture and function. *Ann Med* 1989, 21: p. 353–359.

8. Panjabi, M., et al. Spinal stability and intersegmental muscle forces: a biomechanical model. *Spine* 1989, 14: p. 194–200.

9. Mattila, M., et al. The multifidus muscle in patients with lumbar disc herniation. *Spine* 1986, 11(7): p. 732–738.

10. Zhu, X., et al. Histochemistry and morphology of the erector spinae muscle in lumbar disc herniation. *Spine* 1989, 14(4): p. 391–397.

11. Rantanen, J., et al. The lumbar multifidus muscle five years after surgery for a lumbar intervertebral disc herniation. *Spine* 1993, 18(5): 568–574.

12. Rantanen, J., et al. Lumbar muscle fiber size and type distribution in normal subjects. *Eur Spine J* 1994, 3(6): p. 331–335.

13. Ng, J., et al. Relationship between muscle fiber composition and functional capacity of back muscles in healthy subjects and patients with low back pain. *J Orthop Sports Phys Ther* 1998, 27(7): p. 389–402.

14. Thorstensson, A., and H. Carlson. Fiber types in human lumbar back muscles. *Acta Physiol Scand* 1987, 131: p. 195–202.

15. Mannion, A., et al. Muscle fiber size and type distribution in thoracic and lumbar regions of erector spinae in healthy subjects without low back pain. *J Anat* 1997, 190: p. 505–513.

16. Mannion, A., et al. Fiber type characteristics of the lumbar paraspinal muscles in normal healthy subjects and patients with low back pain. *J Orthop Res* 1997, 15: p. 881–887.

17. Haggmark, L., et al. Muscle fiber type changes in human skeletal muscle after injuries and immobilization. *Orthopedics* 1986, 9: p. 181–185.

18. Graves, J., et al. Health and fitness assessment: muscular strength and endurance, in *American College of Sports Medicine Resource Manual for Guidelines for Exercise Testing and Prescription.* 1998, Baltimore: Williams & Wilkins. p. 448–455.

19. Gibbons, L., et al. The association of trunk muscle cross-sectional area and magnetic resonance imaging parameters with isokinetic and psychosocial lifting strength and static back muscle endurance in men. *J Spinal Disord* 1997, 10(5): p. 398–403.

20. Jorgensen, K. Human trunk extensor muscles: physiology and ergonomics. *Acta Physiol Scand* 1997, 160(S637): p. 1–58.

21. Reid, J., and P. Costigan. Trunk muscle balance and muscular force. Spine 1987, 12(8): p. 783–786.

22. McArdle, W., et al. *Exercise Physiology: Energy, Nutrition, and Human Performance.* 1991, Philadelphia: Lea and Febiger.

23. Cassisi, J., et al. Trunk strength and lumbar paraspinal muscle activity during isometric exercise in chronic low back pain patients and controls. *Spine* 1993, 18(2): p. 245–251.

24. Mayer, T., et al. Quantification of lumbar function. Part 2: sagittal plane trunk strength in chronic low-back pain patients. *Spine* 1985, 10(8): p. 765–772.

25. McNeill, T., et al. Trunk strengths in attempted flexion, extension, and lateral bending in healthy subjects and patients with low back disorders. *Spine* 1980, 5: p. 529–538.

26. Mooney, V., and G. Andersson. Controversies: trunk strength testing in patient evaluation and treatment. *Spine* 1994, 19(21): p. 2483–2485.

27. Mooney, V., et al. Relationships between myoelectric activity, strength, and MRI of the lumbar extensor muscles in back pain patients and normal subjects. *J Spinal Disord* 1997, 10(4): p. 348–356.

28. Risch, S., et al. Lumbar strengthening in chronic low back pain patients: physiological and psychosocial benefits. *Spine* 1993, 18: p. 232–238.

29. Battie, M., et al. Isometric lifting strength as a predictor of industrial back pain reports. *Spine* 1989, 14(8): p. 851–856.

30. Mannion, A. The influence of muscle fiber size and type distribution on electromyographic measures of back muscle fatigability. *Spine* 1998, 23(5): p. 576–584.

31. Biering-Sorensen, F. Physical measurements as risk indicators for low back trouble over a one year period. *Spine* 1984, 9: p. 106–119.

32. Kankaapaa, M., et al. Age, sex, and body mass index as determinants of back and hip extensor fatigue in the isometric Sorensen back endurance test. *Arch Phys Med Rehabil* 1998, 79: p. 1069–1075.

33. Luoto, S., et al. Static back endurance and the risk of low back pain. *Clin Biomech* 1995, 10(6): p. 323–324.

34. Hultman, G., et al. Body composition, endurance, strength, cross-sectional area, and density of mm erector spinae in men with and without low back pain. *J Spinal Disord* 1993, 6(2): p. 114–123.

35. Morris, J., et al. Role of the trunk in stability of the spine. *J Bone Joint Surg* 1961, 43A: p. 327–333.

36. Hemborg, B., et al. Intra-abdominal pressure and trunk muscle activity during lifting IV. The causal factors of intra-abdominal pressure rise. *Rehabil Med* 1985, 17: p. 25–38.

37. Davis, J., et al. The value of exercises in the treatment of low back pain. *Rheumatol Rehabil* 1979, 18: p. 243–247.

38. Linton, S. The relationship between activity and chronic back pain. *Pain* 1985, 21: p. 289–294.

39. Mannion, A., and P. Dolan. Electromyographic median frequency changes during isometric

contration of the back extensors to fatigue. *Spine* 1994, 19(11): p. 1223–1229 1994.

40. Kumar, S., et al. Human trunk strength profile in flexion and extension. *Spine* 1995, 20(2): p. 160–168.

41. Shirado, O., et al. Concentric and eccentric strength of trunk muscles: influence of test postures on strength and characteristics of patients with chronic low-back pain. *Arch Phys Med Rehabil* 1995, 76: p. 604–611.

42. Hides, J., et al. Evidence of multifidus wasting ipsilateral to symptoms in patients with acute/subacute low back pain. *Spine* 1994, 19(2): p. 165–172.

43. Hides, J., et al. Multifidus recovery is not automatic after resolution of acute, first episode low back pain. *Spine* 1996, 21(23): p. 2763–2769.

44. Rissanen, A., et al. Effect of intensive training on the isokinetic strength and structure of lumbar muscles in patients with chronic low back pain. *Spine* 1995, 30(3): p. 333–340.

45. Leggett, S., et al. Restorative exercise for clinical low back pain: a prospective two-center study with 1-year follow-up. *Spine* 1999, 24(9): p. 889–898.

46. Nelson, B., et al. The clinical effects of intensive, specific exercise on chronic low back pain: a controlled study of 895 consecutive patients with 1-year follow up. *Orthopedics* 1995, 18(10): p. 971–981.

47. Mooney, V., et al. The effect of workplace based strengthening on low back injury rates: a case study in the strip mining industry. *J Occupat Rehabil* 1995, 5: p. 157–167.

48. Sandefur, R. Use of problem-based learning methods in the chiropractic college classroom. *J Chiropract Educ* 1990, 4: p. 81–83.

49. Manniche, C., et al. Intensive, dynamic back exercises for chronic low back pain. *Pain* 1991, 47: p. 53–63.

50. Manniche, C., et al. Clinical trial of intensive muscle training for chronic low back pain. *Lancet* 1988, 24: p. 1473–1476.

51. Nelson, B., et al. Can spine surgery be prevented by aggressive strengthening exercises? A prospective study of cervical and lumbar patients. *Arch Phys Med Rehabil* 1999, 80: p. 20–25.

52. US Department of Health and Human Services. *Clinical Practice Guideline #14: Acute Low Back Problems in Adults*. 1994, Rockville, MD: Public Health Service.

53. Pollock, M., et al. Effect of resistance training on lumbar extension strength. *Am J Sports Med* 1989, 17(5): p. 624–629.

54. Graves, J., et al. Effect of training frequency and specificity on isometric lumbar extension strength. *Spine* 1990, 15(6): p. 504–509.

55. Tucci, J., et al. Effect of reduced frequency of training and detraining on lumbar extension strength. *Spine* 1992, 17(12): p. 1497–1501.

56. Li, Y., et al. Neuromuscular adaptations to back extension strength gains. *Med Sci Sports Exerc* 1998, 30(5): p. S207.

57. Foster, D., et al. Adaptations in strength and cross-sectional area of the lumbar extensor muscles following resistance training (abstract). *Med Sci Sport Exerc* 1993, 25(5): p. 547.

58. Fleck, S., and W. Kraemer. *Designing Resistance Training Programs*. 1987, Champaign, IL: Human Kinetics.

59. Graves, J., et al. Pelvic stabilization during resistance training: its effect on the development of lumbar extension strength. *Arch Phys Med Rehabil* 1994, 75(2): p. 210–215.

60. Mayer, J., et al. Specificity of training and isolated lumbar extension strength. *Med Sci Sports Exerc* 1998, 30(5): p. S206.

61. Parkkola, R., et al. Response of the trunk muscles to training assessed by magnetic resonance imaging and muscle strength. *Eur J Appl Physiol* 1992, 65: p. 383–387.

62. Lee, S., et al. Comparative analysis of two lumbar strength training apparatuses on low back strength, in *Comprehensive Spine and Joint Care-From Exercise to Outcomes*. Department of Orthopedics and OrthoMed Centers. 1996, La Jolla: University of California at San Diego. p. 213–214.

63. Fujita, S., et al. Effect of non-isolated lumbar extension resistance training on isolated lumbar extension strength. *Med Sci Sports Exerc* 1997, 29(5): p. S166.

64. Mayer, J., et al. Electromyographic activity of the lumbar extensor muscles: the effect of angle and hand position during Roman chair exercise. *Arch Phys Med Rehabil* 1999, 80(7): p. 751–755.

65. Alaranta, H., et al. Non-dynamometric trunk performance tests: reliability and normative data. *Scand J Rehabil Med* 1994, 26: p. 211–215.

66. Ito, T., et al. Lumbar trunk muscle endurance testing: an inexpensive alternative to a machine for evaluation. *Arch Phys Med Rehabil* 1996, 77: p. 75–79.

67. Rissanen, A., et al. Isokinetic and non-dynamometric tests in low back pain patients related to pain and disability index. *Spine* 1994, 19(17): p. 1963–1967.

68. Schoene, M. *Back Machines: A Waste of Money?*, in *The Back Letter.* Philadelphia: Lippincott Williams & Wilkins. 5(7): 8.

69. Nachemson, A. Disc pressure measurements. *Spine* 1981, 6: p. 93–97.

70. Moritani, T., and H. De Vries. Re-examination of the relationship between the surface integrated electromyogram (iEMG) and force of isometric contraction. *Am J Phys Med* 1978, 57(6): p. 263–277.

71. Dolan, P., and M. Adams. The relationship between EMG activity and extensor moment generation in the erector spinae muscles during bending and lifting activities. *J Biomech* 1993, 26(4): p. 513–522.

72. Soderberg, G., and J. Barr. Muscular function in chronic low back dysfunction. *Spine* 1983, 8: p. 79–85.

73. Holmes, J., et al. Erector spinae activation and movement dynamics about the lumbar spine in lordotic and kyphotic squat lifting. *Spine* 1992, 17(3): p. 327–333.

74. Shirado, O., et al. Flexion-relaxation phenomenon in the back muscles. A comparative study between healthy subjects and patients with chronic low back pain. *Am J Phys Med Rehabil* 1995, 74(2): p. 139–144.

75. Toussaint, H., et al. Flexion relaxation during lifting: implications for torque production by muscle activity and tissue strain at the lumbosacral joint. *J Biomech* 1995, 28(2): p. 199–210.

76. Triano, J., and A. Schultz. Correlation of objective measures of trunk motion and muscle function with low back disability ratings. *Spine* 1987, 12: 561–565.

77. Flicker, P., et al. Lumbar muscle usage in chronic low back pain. *Spine* 1993, 18(5): p. 582–586.

78. Alexiev, A.R. Some differences of the electromyographic erector spinae activity between normal subjects and low back pain patients during the generation of isometric trunk torque. *Electromyogr Clin Neurophysiol* 1994, 34: p. 495–499.

79. Veiersted, K. The reproducibility of test contractions for calibration of electromyographic measurements. *Eur J Appl Physiol* 1991, 62: p. 91–98.

80. Thelan, D., et al. Lumbar muscle activities in rapid three-dimensional pulling tasks. *Spine* 1996, 21(5): p. 605–613.

81. Zedka, M., et al. Comparison of surface EMG signals between elctrode types, interelectrode distances, electrode orientations in isometric exercise of the erector spinae. *Electromyogr Clin Neurophysiol* 1997, 37: p. 439–447.

82. Sihvonen, T., et al. Averaged (rms) surface EMG in testing back function. *Electromyogr Clin Neurophysiol* 1988, 28: p. 335–339.

83. Thelan, D., et al. Cocontraction of the lumbar muscles during the development of time-varying triaxial moments. *J Orthop Res* 1995, 13: p. 390–398.

84. Tan, J., et al. Isometric maximal and submaximal trunk extension at different flexed positions in standing. *Spine* 1993, 18(16): p. 2480–2490.

85. Graves, J., et al. Quantitative assessment of full range-of-motion isometric lumbar extension strength. *Spine* 1990, 15(4): p. 289–294.

86. Udermann, B., et al. Effect of pelvic restraint on hamstring, gluteal, and lumbar muscle emg activation. *Arch Phys Med Rehabil* 1999, 80(4): p. 1176–1179.

87. Kearns, C., et al. Muscle activation during isolated and non-isolated lumbar extension exercises. *Med Sci Sports Exerc* 1997, 29(5): p. S165.

88. Moritani, T., and H. De Vries. Neural factors versus hypertrophy in the time course of muscle strength gain. *Am J Phys Med* 1979, 58(3): p. 115–130.

89. American College of Sports Medicine. ACSM position stand on the recommended quantity and quality of exercise for developing and maintaining cardiorespiratory and muscular fitness, and flexibility in adults. *Med Sci Sports Exerc* 1998, 30(6): p. 975–991.

CHAPTER 12

EFFICACY OF THERAPEUTIC EXERCISE IN LOW BACK REHABILITATION

Wendell Liemohn

Laura Horvath Gagnon

BIOMECHANICAL CONSIDERATIONS IN EXERCISE PRESCRIPTION

SUMMARY

INTRODUCTION

It has been estimated that 90% of all patients with nonspecific low back pain (LBP) will recover within 6 weeks regardless of treatment (1). Following such a procedure with an athlete anxious to return to competition would not be appropriate; moreover, it should not be appropriate for anyone, whether the individual is a blue-collar laborer or an account executive. The primary goal of exercise in the amelioration of back pain is to prevent and reduce pain and to gain flexibility and strength (2). For the athlete, the goal is to be able to return to competition.

EXERCISE INTERVENTION RESEARCH

In this chapter, the efficacy of different exercise interventions reported in the literature dealing with LBP is examined. Many factors can limit reviews such as this:

- The quality of the randomized controlled trials (RCTs) is not always good; moreover, in some research, no attempt is made to conduct RCTs.
- Patients' clinical categories of LBP are not typically delineated, which could prejudice the findings with respect to any specific treatment regimen. For example, if an individual had damaged facet joints and used an extension bias exercise program, improvement would not be likely.
- Even in studies with a good RCT design, the clinician's skill level could affect the results. For example, clinicians who use McKenzie's protocols may have completed anywhere from zero to four McKenzie courses. Thus, they would not be expected to administer precisely identical treatments.

Even though rest can bring about recovery, the arguments for exercise are strong. As tissue heals, it needs to form flexible, strong connections in line with the direction in which stress to the tissue is usually applied. Graded exercise can introduce these forces, whereas rest does not. Moreover, joint surfaces need motion to ensure proper nutrition through imbibition; conversely, bed rest decreases nutrition to the area that needs it the most. Lastly, exercise can elevate mood, facilitate endorphin release, and counter the low feelings associated with dealing with an injury (3).

Several major reviews of studies in which exercise intervention has been a treatment for LBP have been published in the past 15 years; we summarize two of the major reviews. One of these was conducted by the 1987 Quebec Task Force on Spinal Disorders (QTFSD) (4); this exceptionally comprehensive review examined 469 studies that had been published by December 1985. Subsequently, several prodigious reviews were published including studies by Faas (5), Campello et al. (1), and van Tulder et al. (6). However, because these reviews overlap in time and examine many of the same studies, we have chosen to present only the review done by van Tulder et al. (6). Next to the QTFSD study, this may be the most comprehensive review conducted on the efficacy of exercise for LBP.

1987 Quebec Task Force on Spinal Disorders (4)

In 1987 the QTFSD published a monograph for clinicians on the management of activity-related spinal disorders. Because RCTs are considered the gold standard in intervention research, they were of particular interest in this project. Of the 469 studies that the QTF reviewed that were published through 1985 (most of these studies were published between 1976 and 1985), only 18% were RCTs. In their monograph the QTF reported that no single therapeutic intervention was found to be effective in the treatment of chronic LBP (i.e., none met the QTF's RCT criteria for efficacy). With reference to the 18% of the studies that were

RCTs, the QTF indicated that only 56% of these were considered to have acceptable methodologic quality. The state of the art of RCTs in this period was less than ideal.

van Tulder et al. (6)

These researchers conducted a systematic review of RCTs published between 1966 and 1995 on treating acute and chronic LBP. Acute LBP was defined as pain persisting 6 weeks or less, and chronic LBP was defined as pain persisting 12 weeks or more. With these criteria, they rated the studies on (a) methodologic quality, (b) relevance of outcome measures, and (c) levels of evidence. Based on the data collected in these three areas, they then categorized the studies as being either high- or low-quality RCTs. One hundred fifty research studies met their inclusion criteria; of these 68 evaluated treatments of acute LBP, and 81 evaluated treatments of chronic LBP (one study evaluated both). Although this research examined all types of interventions (e.g., bed rest and manipulation), only those studies that specifically addressed exercise interventions are discussed in this section.

For acute LBP, 10 studies addressed exercise intervention. van Tulder et al. found that only two of these 10 met the "high-quality" criteria that they had established for RCTs. The remaining eight RCTs were classified as being of low quality. Because the two studies that were rated high quality reported negative results for exercise, van Tulder et al. concluded that exercise therapy is no more effective than other conservative treatments for treating acute LBP. It should be pointed out that this does not necessarily mean that there are no exercise approaches that are effective in treating acute LBP; rather, it means that no studies were found that met the criteria that the researchers had established for inclusion in their research. For example, if the McKenzie's diagnostic system was used for preselecting patients to participate in the use of McKenzie exercises for acute LBP, RCT inclusion criteria would not be met and hence high quality would not be obtainable.

For chronic LBP, 16 studies addressed exercise intervention. van Tulder et al. determined that three of these were high-quality RCTs and that the remaining 13 were low-quality RCTs. Because the three high-quality RCTs all reported positive results, they concluded that there was strong evidence for the effectiveness of exercise in treating chronic LBP. These three studies are discussed in the next section. High-quality RCTs have numerous traits that are not always seen in low-quality RCTs; these traits can range from obvious qualities, such as having a good subject number, to less understood factors, such as ensuring that the procedure used to randomize subjects to treatment groups will stand up to the strictest scrutiny.

High-Quality RCTs for Chronic LBP

These three studies are presented chronologically. Because some of these research studies have very lengthy titles, each is listed under the descriptive title that we chose.

Transcutaneous Electrical Nerve Stimulation (TENS) and Exercise for Chronic LBP (7)   Criteria for participation in this research included having LBP for at least 3 months, ability to keep twice weekly appointments, a physical examination by the investigative team, and no prior use of TENS. Of the 543 telephone responses to recruitment, 145 subjects were eventually enrolled in the program. The dependent variables included a comprehensive health status questionnaire, a self-assessment of level of activity, one analog scale on pain and one on improvement, an ordinal scale of pain frequency, and three physical measures (straight-leg raise, spine and hip flexion, and the Schober test). Patients were then assigned to the four treatment groups as follows: (a) 36 to TENS alone, (b) 37 to TENS plus exercise, (c) 36 to no exercise and sham TENS, and (d) 36 to sham TENS and exercise. The two exercise groups spent approximately 25 min performing three relaxation exercises followed by nine flexibility and stretching exercises. All groups met twice a week for 4 weeks;

the period with investigators was approximately the same regardless of treatment group. Those in the two exercise groups also exercised at home, which added an average of 16 exercise periods to the eight performed under supervision. The sham-TENS and TENS units were used approximately 25 days by both groups; however, the sham-TENS patients used their equipment approximately 28 min more each day. Heating pads were made available to all subjects, and they often used the heating pad before their stretching exercises. In addition to keeping journals, the investigators questioned patients about compliance and checked to see whether they were blinded to the sham-TENS use. The systematic checks showed excellent compliance; moreover, 84% of the sham-TENS users guessed that they had functioning units. (After the investigation was completed, 68% of the sham-TENS patients and 68% of the TENS patients wished to continue using the equipment.) The following findings were reported:

- There was no significant treatment effect for TENS users in relation to measures of pain, function, and back flexion.
- Exercise resulted in significant improvement in self-rated pain scores, pain frequency reduction, and greater levels of activity when compared with patients who did not exercise.
- No statistically significant or clinically important differences resulted in any measure between subjects receiving sham TENS and true TENS.
- For chronic LBP, TENS may only offer a placebo effect.

Intensive Exercise Protocols   This includes an excerpted report by Manniche et al. (8) and a more complete report by the same group (9); both were cited in the review by van Tulder et al. (6) but were treated as one. The second intensive exercise protocol designated as high-quality research was that done by Hansen et al. (10). Ironically, the intensive exercises Hansen et al. used were the same as those used by Manniche et al. (8,9), but the length of training and the contrast training regimens were different.

Manniche et al. (8,9).   These investigators studied 105 chronic LBP patients who met exacting criteria for inclusion in this research, aspects of which were reported in the two journals cited. The dependent variables included the Low Back Pain Rating Scale that had previously been developed by Manniche to address three separate dimensions of LBP, namely pain, disability, and physical impairment. The measures used to evaluate physical impairment included a back extensor endurance test, a modified Schober test, and a functional mobility test. A single observer blinded to group placement of the patients collected all data; the patients were then randomly assigned to one of three groups. Group A received thermotherapy, massage, and isometric exercises for the lumbar spine and was, in essence, a control group. Groups B and C performed the same three progressive resistance exercises, with group B performing only 20 repetitions, or one-fifth of group C's regimen; each training period lasted 45 min (Figs. 12-1 to 12-3). The exercises were (a) pull to neck, (b) trunk lifting, and (c) leg lifting. Group C followed a very intensive training regimen in which they did 10 repetitions of each exercise, took a 1-min break, and then did 10 more repetitions, following the same routine until each exercise had been done 50 times. There was then a 15-min rest in which hot packs were applied. The entire routine was repeated until 100 repetitions were done of each exercise; each training period lasted 90 min. (In the first 2 weeks of this training the program was graduated, and the 100 repetitions of each exercise were reached in the third week of training.) Thirty sessions of this training were given over a 3-month period: three times a week for the first month and two times a week for the second and third months. At 3 months, a statistically significant difference was found between group C and the other two groups. The scores for group A stayed qualitatively the same. Although 42% of group B improved, the researchers contended that this could have been a placebo effect. By the end of the third month, 74% of the intensive exercise group (group C) improved in all disease variables measured; however, at 1 year, only the patients who continued the

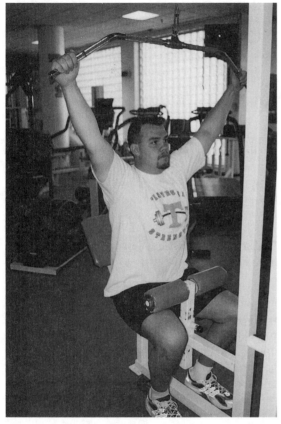 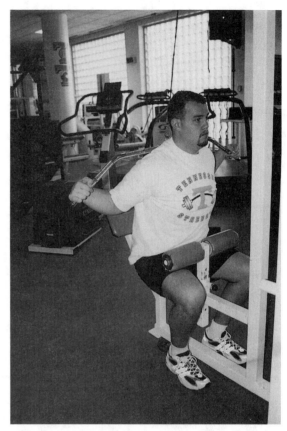

Fig. 12-1 This pull-to-neck exercise is comparable to the one reported by Manniche et al. (8,9).

exercise program at least once a week were significantly better. There were other select findings from this study:

- Intensive exercises can be most appropriate for some patients.
- It may take up to 3 months before some patients will benefit from these intensive exercises.
- To remain symptom free, patients should continue on the program with a minimum of one workout each week.
- Because of the compounding of intensive strengthening exercises with hyperextension training, it is uncertain whether either aspect of the training could alone produce the positive results, or whether a synergism exists between the two.

- The success of this program may be due in part to the stringent protocol that was followed. For example, patients were carefully monitored during their training, and there was a maximum of two to three patients with each physical therapist in the initial workouts.
- If others wish to employ this intensive exercise protocol, Manniche et al. (9) recommend that this type of training be preceded by both a clinical and a radiologic examination by a physician.

Hansen et al. (10). Patients were employees of the Scandinavian Airline System who had subchronic or chronic LBP. Subchronic LBP was defined as a current spell lasting 4 weeks or more or with at least two pain episodes per month during the previous year.

Chronic LBP was defined as a current spell lasting 3 months or longer. Patients were interviewed using a questionnaire and indicated their pain level with a visual interval scale. They were given a physical examination and a radiographic examination; the physical examination included a measurement of lumbar angle by inclinometry, trunk flexion and extension strength were measured with a dynamometer, and sagittal range of movement was measured with a flexicurve. A group of 180 patients met

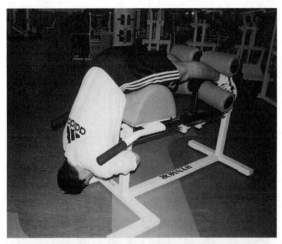

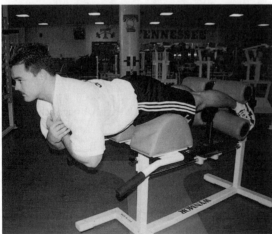

Fig. 12-2 This trunk lifting exercise is comparable to the one reported by Manniche et al. (8,9). However, their subjects were told to lift the trunk to the greatest possible extension of their hips and spine.

inclusion criteria, and they were randomized into two treatment groups and one placebo control group. They were assigned to (a) intensive dynamic back muscle training (essentially the same exercises as those shown in Figures 12-1 to 12-3, with 300 repetitions), (b) standardized physical therapy (included traction, flexibility, ergonomic counseling, and isometric exercises for the back and abdominal muscles), and (c) placebo control (hot packs and traction). It was concluded that intensive therapy seemed most effective for those with light jobs and those with hard physical occupations tended to benefit from physiotherapy.

Recent Randomized Controlled Trials and Postsurgical Studies

The more recent studies have not been examined in comprehensive reviews such as the one done by van Tulder et al. (6). Moreover, the inclusion criteria set forth in the prior reviews precluded including the examination of the efficacy of exercise with postsurgical patients. We present a brief summary of those studies meeting those criteria. To make it easy for the reader to make comparisons between studies, we have chosen to summarize each study by using the evaluative categories suggested by Koes et al. (11) as a template. Although we used their categories, we did not use their guidelines to determine a numeric score for the studies that we reviewed. Nevertheless, the information presented should enable readers either to make their own summary judgments or to decide which studies they would like to peruse in their entirety. The RCT studies subsequent to 1995 are presented chronologically; these are followed by the RCT studies in which postsurgical patients formed at least part of the study population. The evaluative categories delineated by Koes et al. (11) are used as a format for this presentation.

Kuukkanen and Malkia (12)

Study Population. The study included 90 patients (mean age = 39.9 years) with nonspecific subacute LBP.

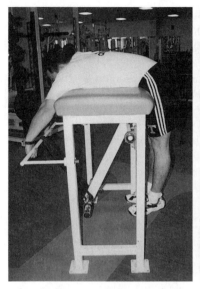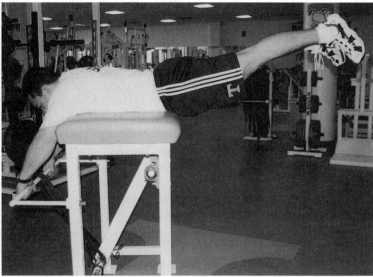

Fig. 12-3 This leg lifting exercise is comparable to the one reported by Manniche et al. (8,9). However, their subjects were told to lift the legs to the greatest possible extension of their hips and spine.

Interventions. Patients were randomized into an intensive training group, a home exercise group, and a control group. Exercises for the intensive group included strength and endurance training twice a week at the clinic, and patients were encouraged to exercise at home; this group exercised an average of 3.1 times per week. The home exercise group followed the same principles as the intensive group and exercised an average of 3.5 times per week. The control group was free to choose any treatment protocol they wished.

Measurement of Effect. Patients were evaluated at the end of the 3 months of training and 3 and 6 months after the completion of training. Performance on isometric and dynamic strength tests, the Oswestry, and a second questionnaire designed to determine pain and daily energy expenditure levels were the dependent variables.

Results. Back pain intensity and functional disability decreased significantly in the two groups that exercised. Both groups showed increased muscular performance at every test session, whereas the control group showed no significant change in muscular performance.

Conclusion. It is possible to increase muscular strength and endurance significantly in LBP patients and to decrease back pain intensity in 3 months with progressive resistive exercises. Moreover, the researchers noted that these positive results appeared to be more permanent in the home exercise group. However, these researchers did not specifically delineate the types of exercises done by the different training groups.

Kankaanpaa et al. (13)

Study Population. Subjects were 59 middle-aged patients with nonspecific chronic LBP for more than 3 months. Exclusion criteria included patients with nerve root compression, disc prolapse, previous back surgery, and radicular symptoms below the knee.

Interventions. The subjects were randomized into either an active or a passive rehabilitation group. The active group participated in 12 weeks (two times a week for 1.5 h) of active rehabilitation. Treatment included exercise with training units specially designed for the development of lumbar flexion, extension, rotation, and lateral flexion strength and coordination. The loads in training were gradually increased during the 12 weeks, the exercises were always performed in a painless range of motion, and the subjects trained under a physiotherapist in groups of four to five. The subjects also were instructed in home exercises. The control group received passive treatments of thermal and massage therapy once a week for 1 month and during the final 4 weeks of the active group's rehabilitation.

Measurement of Effect. The dependent variables were (a) pain intensity on a visual analog scale, (b) functional disability on a pain and disability index, and (c) muscle endurance on an isoinertial back extension testing device. Testing was done before the training, at the conclusion of training (12 weeks), and 6 and 12 months after the conclusion of training.

Results. The results showed that LBP intensity and functional disability significantly decreased after the treatment and 6 and 12 months later. Although lumbar endurance was significantly improved in the active group 12 weeks after treatment and at the 6-month follow-up, the difference was not significant at 1 year.

Conclusion. Active rehabilitation as performed in this study was effective in reducing back pain intensity and in improving functional capacity and lumbar muscle endurance in the short term. The researchers also contended that the isoinertial back endurance test is valid and that it does not have the shortcomings incumbent in typical back endurance tests (e.g., the Biering-Sorensen test) (14).

Randomized controlled trials in which patients were at least part of the subject population are covered in the next section. The reader will note that aggressive protocols by Manniche et al. were pre-

sented earlier in this chapter (8,9). In the next section, similar aggressive protocols that Manniche et al. presented to postsurgical patients are delineated.

Manniche et al. (15)

Study Population. The subjects were 96 patients between the ages of 18 and 70 years who in the preceding 4 to 5 weeks had undergone lumbar surgery for intervertebral disc protrusion.

Interventions. Program A (traditional) included mild exercises in classes of two to six patients; subjects were told to stop if pain or inconvenience occurred. It included exercises in a hot water training pool and gymnasium sessions. Program B (intensive exercises) consisted of five heavy exercises with 50 repetitions in classes of two to six patients; subjects were told that pain in the lumbar area was not a reason for stopping. The first part of the program was performed in the gymnasium and it included the extension exercises shown in Figure 12-1 plus abdominal strengthening, leg abduction and adduction, and 6 min on a training bicycle. The second part of their training was performed in a hot water training pool; subjects were told that pain was likely to occur but that it was all right if it was located in the lumbar area. Each group also received 14 h of instruction in ergonomic guidelines.

Results. Patients who participated in the high-intensity exercises had improved disability index scores; their working capacity levels at 26 weeks of follow-up were also better than those of patients in the traditional program, and these benefits were present at 52 weeks.

Conclusion. A high-intensity back exercise program that does not allow pain to be a limiting factor can provide patients with behavioral support by allowing them to attain a good "working relationship" with their new postsurgical spine and to improve functional levels. The researchers also emphasized that length of the program is critical (e.g., two times per week for 3 months).

Manniche et al. (16)

Study Population. The subjects were 62 adults who had undergone lumbar surgery for intervertebral disc protrusion no less than 14 months or more than 60 months before the start of the study. Before involvement in this research, potential subjects were asked to make a global assessment of their surgery outcome by indicating whether it was excellent, good, fair, unchanged, or poor; those indicating good, fair, or unchanged were invited to participate.

Interventions. Patients were examined by a physician and randomly assigned to two different training programs. They completed the Low Back Pain Rating Scale and a fitness test on a bicycle ergometer. Patients were randomly assigned to the hyperextension group or the extension group; the essential difference between the two is that trunk lifting (exercise 1) and leg lifting (exercise 2) were taken into hyperextension in the former group and not in the latter group. Both groups performed an abdominal strengthening exercise (exercise 3) and a lateral pull-down exercise (exercise 4). (The extension exercises and the lateral pull-down exercises shown in Figures 12-1 to 12-3 were performed but carried into hyperextension.) Patients were offered a hot pack for 20 min before exercising. Ten repetitions of exercises 1 through 3 were done with a 1-min rest between exercises; 50 repetitions of exercise 4 were done without rest. The program was repeated after a 5- to 10-min rest; there were two treatments per week (lasting 60 to 90 min) and 24 training sessions over a 3-month period.

Measurement of Effect. Measurements used to register physical impairment included (a) a modified Biering-Sorensen back endurance test, (b) a modified Schober test, and (c) a functional mobility test.

Results. Although both groups improved, the differences between groups at the end of training were negligible and not of practical significance. Only the hyperextension group increased significantly on the modified Schober test; however, approximately one-third of this group had transient (1 to 14 days) LBP that was attributed to the hyperextension exercises.

Conclusions. As Manniche and his colleagues indicated in previous research (8,9), training should be performed two to three times each week for at least 3 months; in this research they also suggested the inclusion of cardiovascular training.

Bendix et al. (17)

Study Population. The subjects were 123 patients between the ages of 18 and 59 years with disabling chronic LBP; the two most frequent diagnoses were nonspecific lumbago with or without sciatica and previous disc surgery.

Interventions. Patients were randomly assigned to three different treatment programs; the physician performing the pre- and posttreatment examinations was blinded to the assignment. Program 1 ran for 39 h per week for 3 weeks; follow-up was 1 day per week (6 h) for 3 weeks. Training was in groups and included aerobics, progressive resistance training with machines, stretching, and work hardening. Program 2 ran for 2 h twice a week for 6 weeks; treatments included 45 min of aerobics (plus coordination and stretching activities) and 45 min of progressive resistance training on machines. Program 3 followed the same schedule as program 2, but each session included 15 min of warm-up exercises (but not aerobics), 45 min of progressive resistance training on machines, and 75 min of pain management training.

Measurement of Effect. All patients were evaluated 13 months after completing their training program; this evaluation included the completion of a questionnaire on work, sick leave, pain and disability levels, medication, and participation in physical activity. The physical testing for all three groups included muscle strength and endurance evaluations; groups 1 and 2 were also measured for cardiovascular fitness. Other data collected included health care contacts, days of sick leave, and pain and disability levels.

Results. Group 1 had significantly better scores on all variables, including higher work-ready rates, fewer contacts with the health care system, and lower pain scores. Subjective reports of disability showed that group 1 was doing better at 1 year than at the start of the research and that the other groups showed no difference. Physical activity participation was significantly higher in group 1 than the other groups. There were no differences between groups 2 and 3 in most parameters.

Conclusion. The functional restoration program used by group 1 was superior to the less intense programs from the patients' point of view and from a total economic perspective (e.g., return to the work force and less medical care). The researchers also stated that, although this intensive program may be effective in a Scandinavian country, it may not be as effective in less socialized countries such as the United States.

BIOMECHANICAL CONSIDERATIONS IN EXERCISE PRESCRIPTION (18)

In the last section of this chapter, we have chosen to tap into the prodigious research of McGill (18). Although this research is not an RCT, it is based on some of the extensive research that he has conducted on biomechanical evidence for prescribing exercises for specific LBP patients. He stated that the clinician who chooses the optimal exercise for a patient with LBP draws on both science and clinical experience. After concluding that science alone presently provides insufficient guidance to identify the ideal exercise for each situation, he suggested that exercises can be chosen from a biomechanical perspective after taking into account

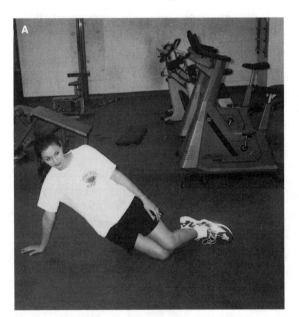 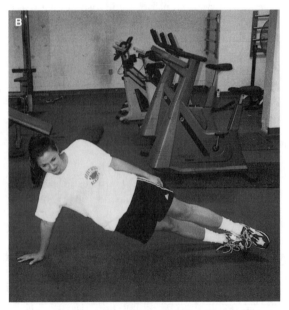

Fig. 12-4 Two levels of an isometric horizontal side support exercise are shown. In **(A)**, the hand and lower legs are in contact with the floor; in **(B)**, the hand and only one foot are in contact with the floor. In McGill's (18) depiction of this exercise, the arm is bent at the elbow, and the forearm rather than just the hand supports the weight of the body. This exercise is discussed in Chap. 8 (see Fig. 8-10).

the objectives for the patient. He added the following suggestions:

- Low back exercises may be more beneficial if performed daily.
- The "no pain, no gain" axiom may not always apply.
- General exercise programs that include cardiovascular components are often effective.
- It is unwise to perform full range bending after rising in the morning because of fluid imbibition in the disc.
- The horizontal side support exercise challenges the lateral obliques and the quadratus lumborum; this seldom used exercise appears to have merit (Fig. 12-4).
- Muscular endurance exercises may have a greater protective value than strength exercises.
- Some persons may not experience reduction in pain or increase in function in less than 3 months.
- By preselecting or categorizing patients, knowledge of resultant tissue loads can reduce injury risk.

SUMMARY

In this chapter we have endeavored to summarize efficacy studies on RCT on exercise intervention for LBP. Even though RCT research has improved markedly in the past 15 years, many questions remain unanswered. The reader may have noted that a disproportionate number of the good RCT studies were conducted in Northern European countries, providing evidence that socialized medicine presents opportunities for research that can contribute to the conundrum.

REFERENCES

1. Campello, M., Nordin, M., Weiser, S. Physical exercise and low back pain. *Scand J Med Sci Sports* 1996, 6(2): p. 63–72.

2. Malkia, E., and B. Kannus. Editorial: low back pain-to exercise or not to exercise? *Scand J Med Sci Sports* 1996, 6(2): p. 61–62.

3. Nutter, P. Aerobic exercise in the treatment and prevention of low back pain. *Occup Med* 1988, 3: p. 137–145.

4. Spitzer, W.O., LeBlanc, F.E., Dupuis, M., et al. Scientific approach to the assessment and management of activity-related spinal disorders. A monograph for clinicians, Report of the Quebec Task Force on Spinal Disorders. *Spine* 1987, 12(7S): p. S9–S59.

5. Faas, A. Exercises: which ones are worth trying, for which patients and when? *Spine* 1996, 21(24): p. 2874–2879.

6. van Tulder, M.W., Koes, B.W., Bouter, L.M. Conservative treatment of acute and chronic nonspecific low back pain. A systematic review of randomized controlled trials of the most common interventions. *Spine* 1997, 22(18): p. 2128–2156.

7. Deyo, R.A., Walsh, N.E., Martin, D.C., et al. A controlled trial of transcutaneous electrical nerve stimulation (TENS) and exercise for chronic low back pain. *N Engl J Med* 1990, 322: p. 1627–1634.

8. Manniche, C., Hesselsoe, G., Bentzen, L., et al. Clinical trials of intensive muscle training for chronic low back pain. *Lancet* 1988, 2: p. 1473–1476.

9. Manniche, C., Lundberg, E., Christensen, I., et al. Intensive dynamic back exercises for chronic low back pain: a clinical trial. *Pain* 1991, 47(1): p. 53–63.

10. Hansen, F.R., Bendix, T., Skov, P., et al. Intensive, dynamic back-muscle exercises, conventional physiotherapy, or placebo-control treatment of low-back pain-a randomized, observer-blind trial. *Spine* 1993, 18(1): p. 98–108.

11. Koes, B.W., Bouter, L.M., van der Heijden, G. Methodological quality of randomized clinical trials on treatment efficacy in low back pain. *Spine* 1995, 20(2): p. 228–235.

12. Kuukkanen, T., and E. Malkia. Muscular performance after a 3 month progressive physical exercise program and 9 month follow-up in subjects with low back pain. A controlled study. *Scand J Med Sci Sports* 1996, 6(2): p. 112–121.

13. Kankaanpaa, M., Taimela, S., Airaksinen, O., et al. The efficacy of active rehabilitation in

chronic low back pain: effect on pain intensity, self-experienced disability, and lumbar fatigability. *Spine* 1999, 24(10): p. 1034–1042.

14. Biering-Sorensen, F. Physical measurements as risk indicators for low-back trouble over a one-year period. *Spine* 1984, 9(2): p. 106–119.

15. Manniche, C., Skall, H.F., Braendholt, L., et al. Clinical trial of postoperative dynamic back exercises after first lumbar discectomy. *Spine* 1993, 18(1): p. 92–97.

16. Manniche, C., Asmussen, K., Lauritsen, B., et al. Intensive dynamic back exercises with or without hyperextension in chronic back pain after surgery for lumbar disc protrusion—a clinical trial. *Spine* 1993, 18(5): p. 560–567.

17. Bendix, A.F., Bendix, T., Lund, C., et al. Comparison of three intensive programs for chronic low back pain patients: a prospective, randomized, observer-blinded study with 1-year follow-up. *Scand J Rehabil Med* 1997, 29(2): p. 81–89.

18. McGill, S.M. Low back exercises: evidence for improving exercise regimens. *Phys Ther* 1998, 78(7): p. 754–765.

INDEX

Note: Page numbers followed by letters *f* and *t* refer to figures and tables, respectively.

A

Abdominal bracing, 32
  sample exercises, 32*f*, 174*f*, 175*f*, 177*f*, 178*f*
Abdominal hollowing maneuver, 172–174, 173*f*
  with bridging movement, 173, 174*f*
  in dynamic stabilization training, 177
  goal of, 174
  with leg movements, 173, 173*f*
  in quadruped position, 174*f*, 174–175
  substitution patterns in, 173
Abdominal muscles, 16–20, 18*f*
  and erector spinae, 20, 21*f*
  flexion exercises and challenge to, 17*t*
  in football players, 108
  importance of, 17
  methods used to develop, 16–17, 19*f*, 174–178*f*
  strength assessment of, 81*f*, 81–82
  in trunk stabilization, 30
Abdominal strengthening exercises
  comparison of, 17*t*
  considerations in prescribing, 13–16
Achilles tendon, tightness in, effect on spine, 41
Active assisted exercise, aquatic, 208
Active exercise, aquatic, 208
Active isolated stretching (AIS), 59–60, 60*f*
Active knee extension (AKE) test, 50*f*, 50–51
  nonballistic, 59
Acute stage, 168
  of arthritis, aquatic therapy for, 206–207
  of low back pain, exercise programs for,
      168–171
Acuteness, 168
Adaptive shortening, 146–147
Aerobic activity
  aquatic, 209
  for arthritis patients, 205

and cardiovascular health, 90
and disc nutrition, 92–93
and low back pain prevention, 93
and low back pain rehabilitation, 93–94
and mental health, 95–96
and spine health, 90–94
Age
  and arthritis, 204
  and low back pain, 100
  and lumbosacral range of motion, 41–42
  and passive extensor moment, 30
  and stenosis, 69
  and stroke volume, 190
AIS. *See* Active isolated stretching
Alexander, Frederick Matthias, 163
Alexander technique, 163–166
  application to low back pain, 165–166
  principles of, 163–164
  research on, 165
American Arthritis Foundation, 210
Ankle(s)
  in sit-and-reach test, 52, 53*f*
  tightness in, effect on spine, 41
Annulus fibrosis, 8, 9*f*
Anterior element injury, 102
  in basketball, 106
  in football, 107–108
  in golf, 111
  in gymnastics, 113
  in racquet sports, 116
  in rowing, 117
  in running, 122
  in swimming, 125
  in weight training, 129
Anterior longitudinal ligament, 12, 12*f*, 13*f*
Anterior sacroiliac ligament, 13*f*

NOTES

NOTES

NOTES

NOTES

NOTES

NOTES

NOTES

NOTES

NOTES

NOTES

NOTES

NOTES

NOTES

NOTES